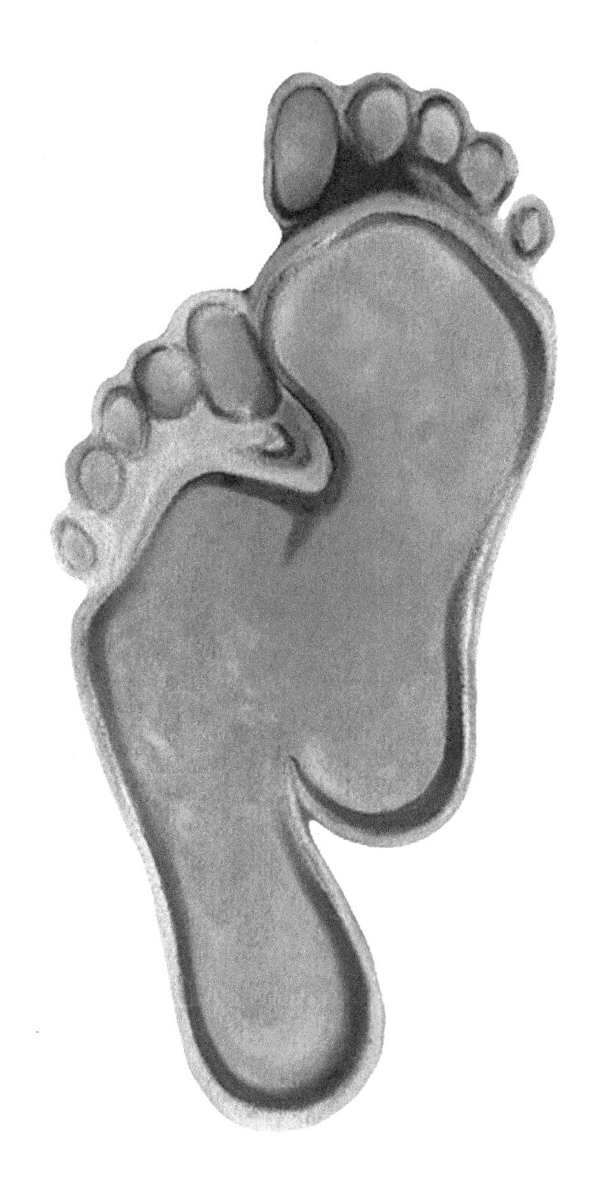

Integrative Reflexology®

Theory and Practice

Integrative Reflexology® is a form of bodywork that includes massage techniques and energy work.

Any information in this book is not intended to replace or give medical advice.

You should always consult your physician about any health concerns.

This book is intended to offer supplemental support to help the body balance.

Integrative Reflexology®

Theory and Practice

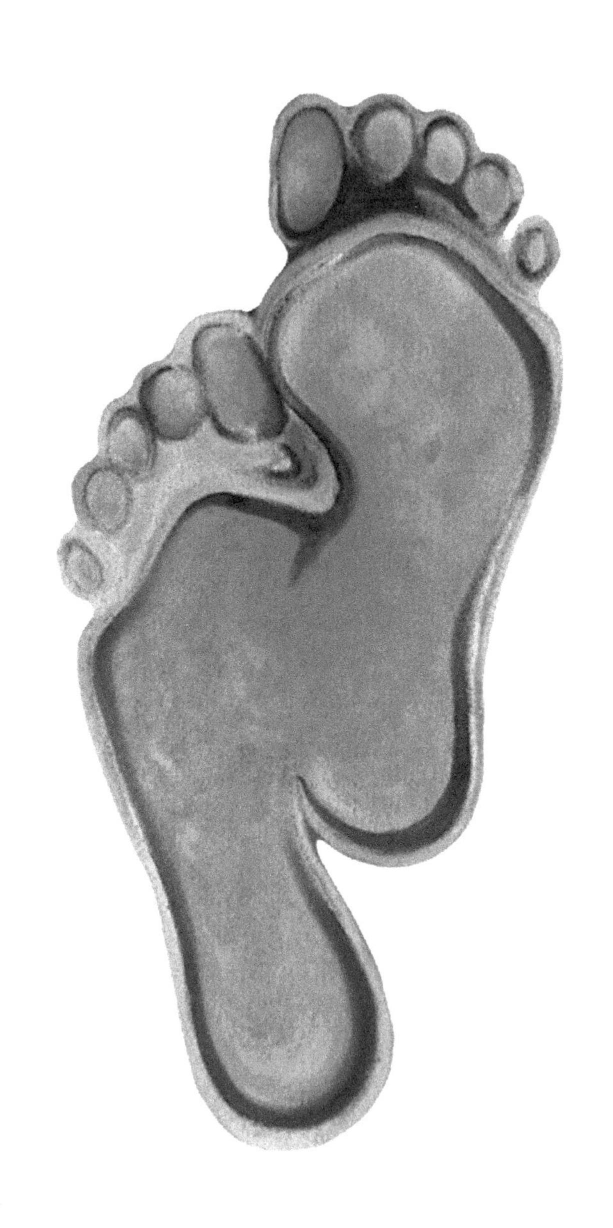

Integrative Reflexology®

For more information, please contact:
Claire Marie Miller Seminars
877.319.5772
info@clairemariemiller.com
www.clairemariemiller.com

Integrative Reflexology®
Nurturing the Mother®, Pregnancy & Postpartum Massage
Nurturing the Mother®, Fertility Massage

Manufactured in the United States of America

Paperback ISBN: 978-0-9818491-7-1
LCCN: 2016000000
HEA014000 HEALTH & FITNESS / Massage & Reflexotherapy

Special Thanks to Many Who Have Helped this Book Evolve

Writing Assistance—Courtney Rosser

Editing—Sun Butler, Lucie Pollard Branham

Design and Layout—Hill Goodwin

Art: Jeff Hackney, Hill Goodwin, Meghan Lubker, Victor Crutchfield, Taj Vaccarella

Photographs—Briana Brough, Hill Goodwin

Foot Models—Melina Piluras, Nico Sidell Morrison, Gini Bell

To all my students who believe in the healing energy, knowledge, and practice of Integrative Reflexology®. My students have taught me well.

It "takes a village" to produce a book, and many years to grow the information.

This book has been in production since 1993.

Table of Contents

Hand and Meridian Chart

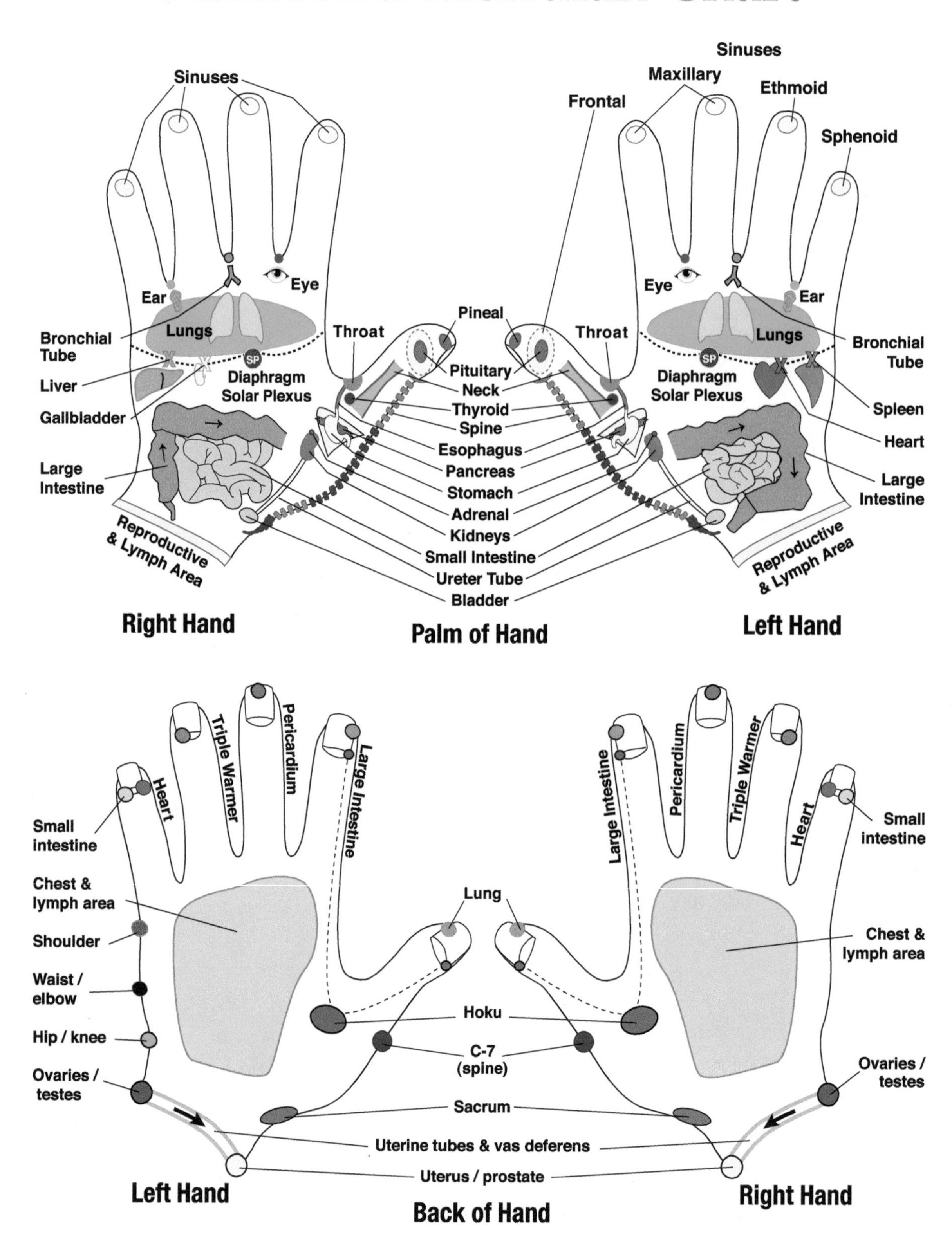

Foot Chart

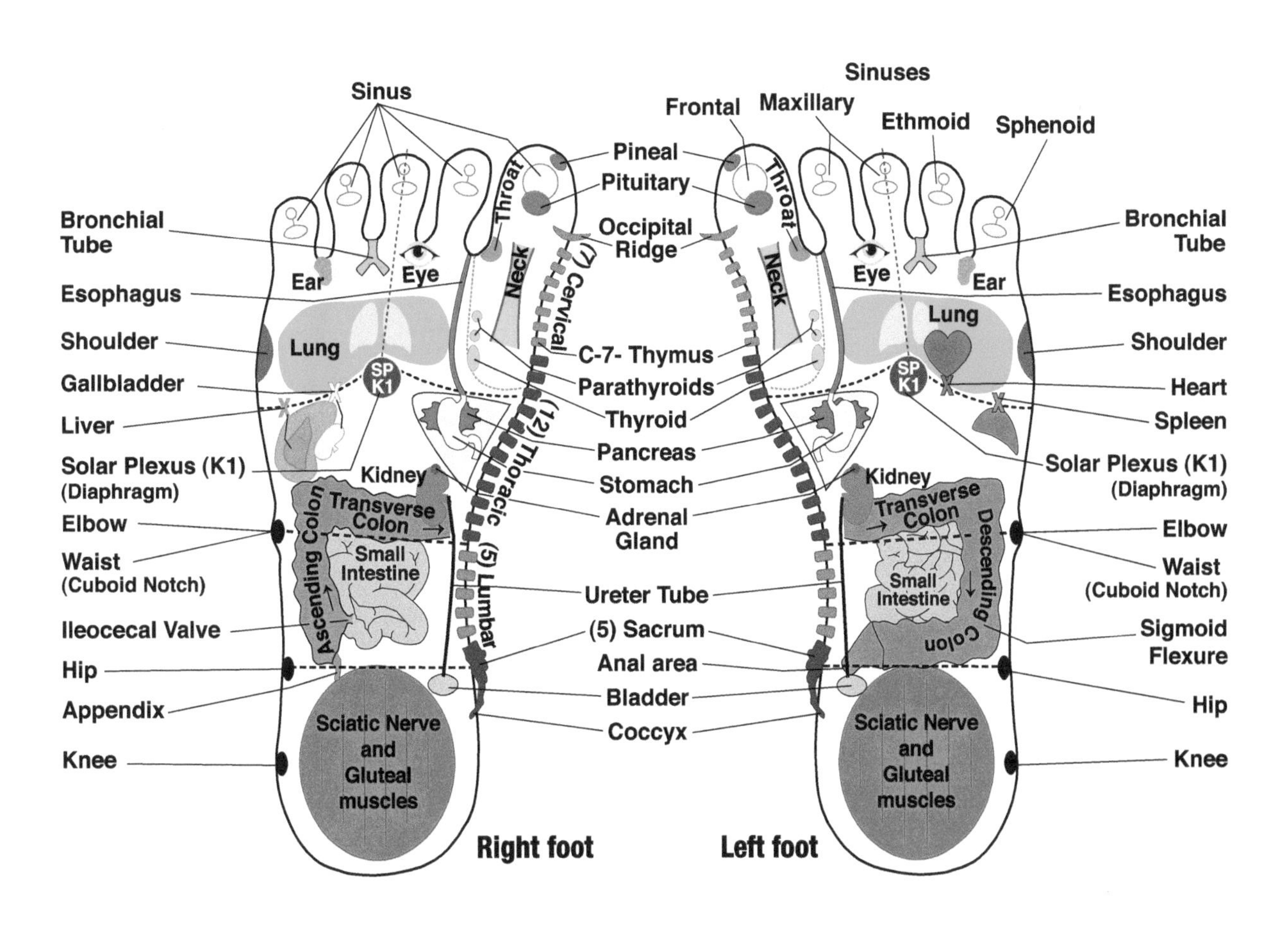

Sinus
Sinuses
Frontal
Maxillary
Ethmoid
Sphenoid
Pineal
Pituitary
Throat
Bronchial Tube
Occipital Ridge
Eye
Ear
Neck
(7) Cervical
Esophagus
Shoulder
Lung
C-7- Thymus
Parathyroids
Gallbladder
SP K1
Heart
Liver
Thyroid
Spleen
Pancreas
(12) Thoracic
Solar Plexus (K1) (Diaphragm)
Kidney
Stomach
Transverse Colon
Adrenal Gland
Elbow
Waist (Cuboid Notch)
Ascending Colon
Small Intestine
Descending Colon
(5) Lumbar
Ureter Tube
Ileocecal Valve
(5) Sacrum
Sigmoid Flexure
Anal area
Hip
Appendix
Bladder
Coccyx
Knee
Sciatic Nerve and Gluteal muscles
Right foot
Left foot

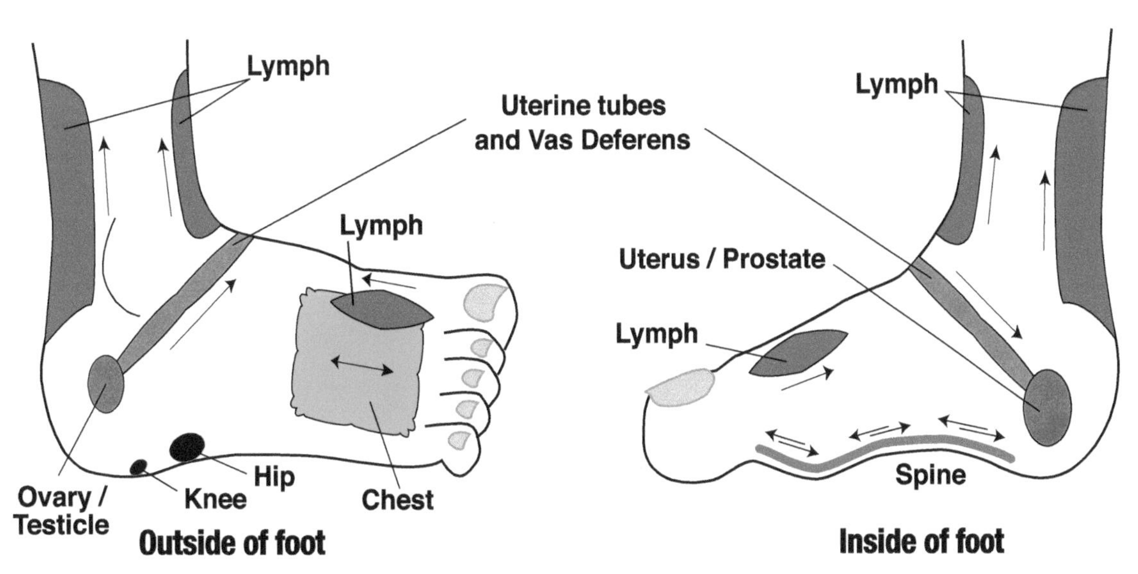

Lymph
Uterine tubes and Vas Deferens
Uterus / Prostate
Chest
Hip
Knee
Ovary / Testicle
Spine
Outside of foot
Inside of foot

in · te · grate

v.

: 1630s, to render (something) whole

: 1802, to put together parts or elements and combine them into a whole

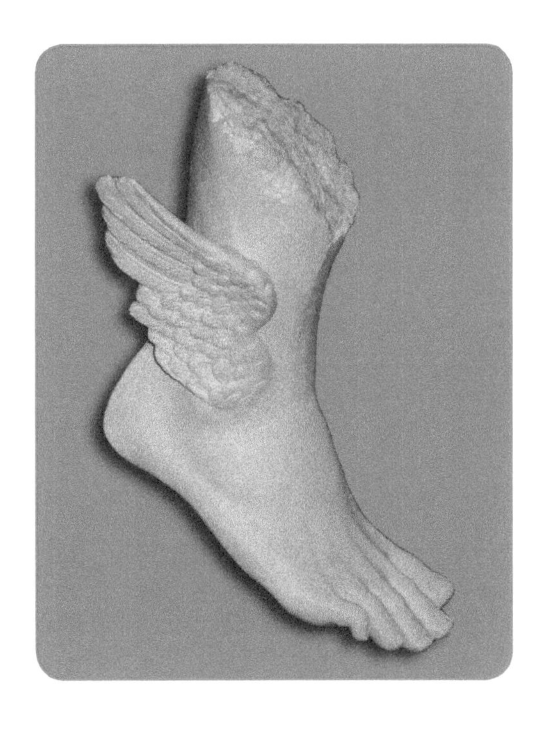

1
History of Integrative Reflexology®

Feel your feet and the 100,000 nerve endings in each foot that are ready for stimulation. Your continued health relies on that stimulation. If you are not going barefoot, then you need reflexology.

> *"Integrative Reflexology® works primarily on the feet. It can tap into and open up the systems and organs to allow your body to transport important information about the source and nature of any neurological and metabolic imbalances within the body."*
> *—Claire Marie Miller*

A Personal Journey

My journey with reflexology began in 1979, during my second semester at the Boulder School of Massage Therapy. As part of my training, I attended an introduction course in reflexology where I received my first reflexology session and saw my first reflexology foot chart. As a result of the work I received on my feet during that workshop, I had a powerful emotional release and was surprised by its intensity; it touched me at the core of my being. To this day, I still have a vivid memory of that first reflexology session and how deeply relaxed I became. The deep state of relaxation I experienced allowed me to access feelings I was holding deep inside, of which I was unaware. This was still early enough in my bodywork career that I had not yet learned about somatic release—the therapeutic release of stored emotions. I could not believe that all of that experience came from work on the feet. My deep curiosity would then guide me through many years of study and practice on the path of understanding how reflexology works.

My fascination with the human condition, illness and health care began at the tender age of 16, while volunteering at a local hospital where I spent most of my time in the radiology department. Looking at x-rays, literally looking into the body, was amazing to me. A year later, immediately after graduating high school, I made the choice to attend radiologic technology training. I loved seeing live anatomy in the form of x-rays. My career as an x-ray tech cemented my lifelong intrigue with the body.

Another experience in my youth that was influential in my choice to pursue alternative health and healing was the development of a thyroid goiter. After a year of medication (Synthroid) to treat the goiter, there was still a benign cyst or tumor on the thyroid gland. Surgery to completely remove the gland was the next step. Preferring to avoid surgery at all cost, I explored alternative methods of treatment. In my search I was introduced to Hatha yoga poses and in particular the shoulder stand. Upon reading further about the shoulder stand—that it balances the thyroid gland—I worked on spending five minutes in the position for thirty days straight. I had no teacher, only a book to guide me. After the thirty days, I was retested and the radioisotope scan showed that the tumor or cysts had completely disappeared. This was an "aha" moment for me—proof that there was another way to get well other than conventional medicine and in my case, surgery. My passion for Hatha yoga had taken root.

Soon after my healing experience with yoga, on July 7, 1977, I quit my job as an x-ray specialist in the Heart Catheterization Lab at Johns Hopkins Hospital and embarked on a journey across the country to California. My pioneering spirit was awakened.

Due to my extensive skills in a variety of x-ray work, I got a job immediately upon my arrival in Ventura, California. Little did I know that my world and my perception of the world were about to be radically altered. In Ventura, I was introduced to a teacher who was pivotal in my life—Isha Chandi taught Hatha Yoga and was also a full-blooded Native American healer in the Chumash tribe. Isha put me on the fast track of studying and eventually teaching yoga. Isha also gave me my first experience receiving bodywork, in the form of massage. In trying to describe these experiences, all I can say is "other-worldly."

The next teacher to enter my path was Dolores, an astrologer and Isha's dearest friend. My love of algebra and geometry in high school made sense of the planetary circles, angles, and degrees of signs. The stars gave me a powerful gift. For the first time in my life, I really liked myself for exactly who I am.

The third teacher to enter this powerful incubation period was Rosalyn Bruyere. At that time, Rosalyn was the first laboratory-proven psychic and healer. Her friend and colleague, Dr. Valarie Hunt, had set up many experiments to challenge Rosalyn's skills and gift. The scientific proof of her abilities was documented in a physics lab at UCLA. By the time I met Rosalyn, she had already published her internationally acclaimed book *Wheels of Light*. Energy healing, and chakra balancing were the essences of her excellent instruction. She also played a pivotal role in affirming my choice to study massage in Boulder, CO.

Over the summer of 1978, I embarked on a period of intense study with these three teachers. By October of 1978, my decision to move to Boulder, CO was made. I packed up my red VW bug with all my belongings and headed off to Boulder via San Francisco and Lake Tahoe. The journey was met with some challenges—being robbed of many of my belongings in San Francisco, falling in love with my future husband in Lake Tahoe and arriving in Boulder with no clue how any of this was going to work. With 200 applicants and only 40 available spots, I felt fortunate to secure one of the coveted places to begin my training at the Boulder School of Massage Therapy (BSMT).

The program at BSMT was a 1000-hour training in massage therapy certification. The school had three core courses—Swedish massage, Asian medicine, and Reichen massage (a model that combined structural and emotional releases). My training in all of these subjects became the basis for what has become my lifelong work and practice.

Swedish massage focuses on circulation of the blood along with lymphatic flow. It is a classic model of massage that uses long strokes toward the heart to clear the proximal (toward the torso) aspect of the limb before moving down the limb to the most distal portion. I was drawn to the lymphatic connection in Swedish massage. The importance of addressing the lymph system in the body was established as a theme for me in all of my forms of bodywork. It helped that I had also performed lymph angiograms as an x- ray technician and had a strong visual image of this system.

The second semester core subject was Asian Medicine. Over the 12 weeks of that semester we learned a complete shiatsu massage addressing all the Chinese meridians. Another class within that semester was devoted to understanding the five-elements model of Asian medicine. I found this model fascinating with its incorporation of the seasons, emotions, foods and so much more. Understanding the roles that the toes and fingers play in the energetic pathways of the meridians was a valuable background for my future work with reflexology. The book, *Staying Healthy with the Seasons*, was included in this part of the curriculum and today, 37 years later, it is still my go-to source for understanding the meridians.

The final semester of the program was focused on Reichian massage, which included body reading and massage techniques for releasing the energetic blocks that prevent the free-flowing movement of the recipient's energy. Reichian massage was based on Wilhelm Reich and Alexander Lowen's powerful somatic work related to the body's structure. Their work was naturally connected to the newly evolving therapy of the times called Rolfing, which focused deeply on the structural experience of our body and the connections within that structure. The Rolf Institute was also located in Boulder, CO and many of the instructors at BSMT were either Rolfers or in training to become Rolfers. This way of viewing the structure of the body struck a cord with me and deeply influenced the way I saw the feet and their impact on the body. When I learned that Ida Rolf, the founder of Rolfing, called the feet the "tattletalers" of the body, I thought to myself, "this is why foot reflexology gives us so much valuable information." This semester of somatic learning informed the experience I had had during the reflexology workshop.

Looking back, I can see how my training at the Boulder School of Massage Therapy laid the foundation for the four-theory approach to reflexology—structure, zones, meridians and psychoneuroimmunology. It is now clear that during that time in Boulder I was in the early days of a lifelong mission to understand and create this unique model of working with and observing the body through the feet.

Upon graduation from BSMT, I moved to Lake Tahoe, California on my 25th birthday. I married two weeks later, began a family and established my practice as a massage therapist. In Tahoe, I made a friend who owned her own health supplement store, "Pepper's," which was named after her sweet dog. It was at her store that I found *The Foot Book*, by Devaki Berkson. This book presented a multifaceted approach to reflexology. It included a variety of techniques, interesting herbal additions to the foot soaks, dietary recommendations, yoga poses to support related areas of the body, positive affirmations and visualizations. Holistic health care was the model for this style of reflexology and I embraced it and practiced what I learned from this book on all of my clients. As much as I loved this book and all of its great information, what I did not like was the reflexology chart in the book. I found it to be confusing. So, I began drawing my own foot reflexology charts based on my knowledge of the human body through x-rays as well as my work with clients and the results they experienced. The charts that I began drawing then have evolved, over decades, into the Integrative Reflexology® charts in use today. My students continually affirm that these charts are clear, easy to use for foot and hand reflexology and that the drawings offer a logical and intuitive sense of the anatomy of the body as it applies to the feet. When creating the charts. I simply drew on what made sense to me based on my knowledge of human anatomy and my experience as a massage therapist and with foot reflexology.

Lake Tahoe, a skiing and hiking vacation destination, proved to be a great place to build my clientele and promote natural health. Reflexology was one of my most requested bodywork therapies. I am sure that I worked on at least 1000 feet during the years of building a thriving massage practice in Lake Tahoe. All of my massage clients received detailed reflexology within their bodywork session. I began to observe in each session how the feet guided me in the massage, showing me where in the body to focus and apply deeper techniques. What I assessed in the feet—the tender, swollen or misaligned areas—was exactly aligned with what I felt in the body.

While teaching foot reflexology classes at Lake Tahoe Community College, I began to develop the systematic approach and method that would eventually form Integrative Reflexology®. The format of working the foot from head-to-toe and the rhythm of back and forth stimulation from foot to foot came naturally as I shared my passion with my students and taught reflexology from the background of my training as a massage therapist.

Reflexology permeated all that I did during that time in my life, from general massage to pregnancy massage, labor massage, fertility massage and infant massage. This may be a result of my own development and experience with reflexology and massage—I have always seen reflexology as a part of massage and not separate to massage. Many years after my time in Lake Tahoe, at the North Carolina Massage Board, I was asked if reflexology is energy work or bodywork? My answer is: it is both bodywork and energy work, it is not separate.

In 1988, equipped with all of this experience, knowledge and a full family, my husband and I moved our family to the east coast and settled in Chapel Hill, NC. Before we had even settled into our decision to make Chapel Hill our home, I had written to Rick Rosen who had a massage school in the area.

Soon after arriving, I began teaching reflexology and pregnancy massage courses for Rick at his school. This was the perfect opportunity for me to continue to develop these modalities and the protocols that I continue to teach today. The classroom I taught in began as a yurt and later blossomed into the beautiful campus and the Body Therapy Institute at South Wind Farm in Siler City, NC. My connection with BTI was to be one of the most pivotal in my career as a teacher and innovator in the field of massage therapy.

Then, in 1990, I taught the first Nurturing the Mother® workshop and certification course in pregnancy and postpartum massage at Camp New Hope in Chapel Hill, NC. Reflexology was utilized in much of the pregnancy massage to relieve discomforts, bring on labor and to support postpartum healing. To leave the feet out of the protocol was not an option, despite having heard, in later years, that one should not work on a pregnant woman's feet. Rather, I have used the beneficial results I have seen with my clients and myself as evidence to dispel this myth.

In 1993, I wrote the first of my reflexology manuals, called *Bring the Feet to Life*. The name and the manual came to me in a dream and initiated the development of a new certification program—"Bring the Feet to Life with Integrative Reflexology." Within a few years I chose to reverse the name, and eventually dropped the "Bring the Feet to Life" subtitle, to settle on Integrative Reflexology®, a registered trademark name.

The Integrative Reflexology® method naturally evolved with a massage therapy approach. I often thought about how I could use massage in one area as a way to stimulate the body as a whole. The feet were the answer to that inquiry.

When the Integrative Reflexology® method became a certification as a specific therapy in 1993, it was with the intention to teach primarily to massage therapists who wanted to integrate reflexology into their massage therapy session and/or use it as a stand-alone therapeutic session. Over the years, I have found that Integrative Reflexology® has drawn the interest of estheticians, energy workers, caregivers and others who are not certified in massage but who want to learn this powerful form of healing. While learning Integrative Reflexology® students repeatedly tell me, "it just makes sense." This method was created organically, through the experience of what made sense to me and my body, so to hear others reflect that it makes sense to them serves as affirmation that I have succeeded.

To date, thousands have been trained in Integrative Reflexology®, and are now performing the method successfully worldwide. It is a very unique approach to an ancient healing art.

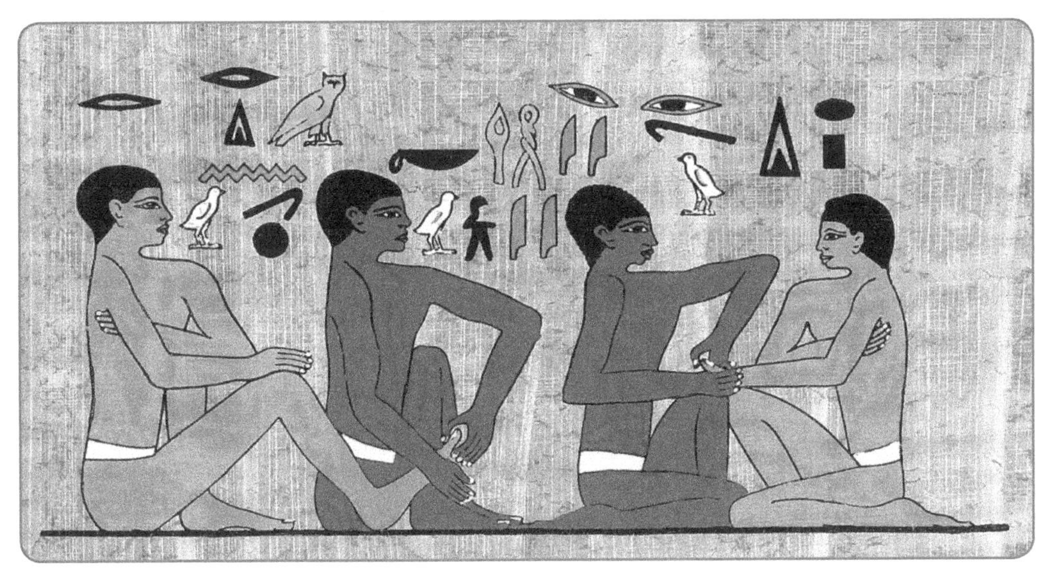

Fig 1.1
Egyptian pictographs from the tomb of the ancient Egyptian physician Ankhmahor (2330 B.C.)

The Ancient Healing Art of Reflexology

"Your feet walk upon the earth and through this your spirit is connected to the universe."

—Jenny Wallace, Cherokee healer

Reflexology is as old as walking barefoot—our bare feet are pumiced by rocks, roots and leaves, stimulated by the texture of the Earth, and serve as a connection between the magnetic energy flowing through the Earth and our own nervous system. In a workshop I teach at the North Carolina beach, my students take therapeutic walks on the sand, totally barefoot, with a foot soak in the salts of the ocean. That is reflexology Nature's way.

Stimulating the feet for healing purposes is known to have been part of the ancient health care modalities used by our ancestors all over the world. Christine Issel, in her book, *Reflexology: Art, Science & History*, states that "[n]o one culture can claim to have 'discovered' reflexology, because different forms of working on the feet to effect health have been used by people all over the world since the beginning of time." Many ancient cultures directly connected the health of the body to the health of the feet.

Egyptian pictographs are the oldest documentation that can be interpreted as depicting reflexology. The tomb of the ancient Egyptian physician,

Ankhmahor (2330 B.C.), contains six wall carvings that honor his skills as a physician. Among those six is a scene depicting reflexology.

We also see the importance of the feet reflected in the rituals of many cultures. Anointing of the feet is a ritual in ancient Christianity which entails washing the feet as a symbol of the spiritual connection made by humbling oneself in honor of another spiritual being. In many Native American cultures, the feet are the spiritual connection to the vital force of Mother Earth. The 'Blessingway' is a Navajo ceremony for birthing mothers in which the prayers of the community are symbolically ground into cornmeal and the birthing mother receives those prayers as the cornmeal is massaged into the soles of her feet. I have both performed this ancient ritual for a mother to be, and received the blessings for my daughter and myself a few weeks before her birth. The peacefulness that follows the ritual is palpable, and it is intended for the mother to carry that feeling of peace and calm into the birth. After my Blessingway, my daughter, Danielle, had a very peaceful, gentle, underwater home birth. I can personally speak to the power of prayers I received through cornmeal massaged into my feet.

Further evidence is seen throughout history of the use of the feet as a form of healing and as access to working with other parts of the body. In Europe in the 1500s, the terms 'reflex' and 'zones' began to be used in reference to health and the body. During this time, people were using pressure therapy and noticing correlations between working certain areas of the body to achieve effects in other areas of the body. However, it is not until the late 1800s and early 1900s that we begin to see a large influx of publications about studies, practices and theories related to foot reflexology.

In 1893, Sir Henry Head published work related to the effects of zones of the body. He found that "[t]he bladder can be excited to action by stimulating the sole of the foot, and movements of the toes can be evoked by filling the bladder with fluid." (Issel. 1990). Head charted zones of the body according to the spinal segments to which they belonged. "Head's zones," as they became known, were later refined into the dermatomes that are known and used today (Issel, 1990).

Following Head's work, in 1917 Drs. Edwin F. Bowers and William Fitzgerald published a manual called *Zone Therapy*. The manual maps out 10 longitudinal zones of the body. In Dr. Fitzgerald's studies and experiments, elastic bands were used to compress the fingertips, which allowed him to perform minor surgery without any anesthetic. While this work was not well received by the Western medical establishment of the time, it was noticed and pursued by Dr. Joe Shelby Riley. Riley studied zone therapy with Dr. Fitzgerald and then became one of the most untiring developers of zone therapy. With his first book, *Zone Therapy Simplified*, published in 1919, he made the first detailed diagrams of the reflex points on the feet (Issel, 1990).

Dr. Riley's research assistant, Eunice Ingham, continued the studies laid out in his book and developed an even more comprehensive approach to zone therapy. She separated work on the reflexes of the feet from the more general field of zone therapy. Ingham has since become known as the 'Grandmother of Reflexology'. Her work expanded zone therapy, and she created a detailed map of the reflex points on the feet. Her two books, *Stories the Feet Can Tell* (1938) and *Stories the Feet Have Told* (1963), are reflexology classics. Her system of reflexology continues to be used today by her nephew, Dwight Byers, and the International Institute of Reflexology in St. Petersburg, Florida (Issel, 1990).

Reflexology Today

Today the world of reflexology continues to grow and expand into new arenas. One trend that began to take root in the 1990s was the standardization and accreditation of the profession of reflexology. The American Reflexology Certification Board (ARCB) was founded in 1991 specifically for this purpose. They act as an accrediting board to test professional reflexologists and ensure public safety. They require 300 training hours in foot and hand reflexology in order to qualify to take the exam and become certified in the practice of reflexology.

The Reflexology Association of America (RAA) is a non-profit organization that was formed in 1995 and has as its mission to "elevate and standardize the quality of reflexology services available to the public." The RAA, along with the ARCB, exists in order to strengthen the integrity of the professional field of reflexology.

The many forms of reflexology that exist today are as varied as the practitioners who offer this service. As with any healing practice, the fundamentals and history of reflexology are the same, but the lens through which one applies their knowledge is colored by one's own life experience. This is true for Integrative Reflexology®. Integrative Reflexology® was originally created as a certification course for massage therapists and others who already have a license to touch, which includes a basic foundation in anatomy, physiology, pathology, contraindications, ethics and business practices. Integrative Reflexology® is not intended to be a comprehensive course in the above topics. If you, the reader, have a desire to practice reflexology as a profession, and you do not have a background in the healing arts, you are encouraged to further your training before you begin a professional practice. The Reflexology Association of America and any affiliated training programs are an excellent source for such a venture.

Reflexology is an ever-evolving form of healing. While some want to standardize the practice of reflexology in order to validate it within the scientific community, it is necessary to honor the reality that Christine Issel points out:

"Reflexology is not only a science but also an art. It is a science, because it is based on physiological and neurological study. Reflexology is an art, because much depends on how skillfully the practitioner applies his knowledge and the dynamics which occur between the practitioner and the client."

Part 1

Theory of Integrative Reflexology®

Integrative Reflexology® is a four-theory approach to reflexology. Each of the four theories serves as a different lens for understanding how reflexology works and how we can view the body in a holistic way. By considering four different theories we, as practitioners, are honoring the complexity of the human body and the complexity of what our client is experiencing. This approach creates space for the body's innate wisdom to provide the healing offered through an Integrative Reflexology® session.

The first theory of Integrative Reflexology® is ***Structural Alignment Theory***. This theory explains the physical component of reflexology—how physical manipulation of the feet can translate to physical changes in the rest of the body.

The second theory of Integrative Reflexology®, ***Zone Theory***, shows how the body can be mapped out into different zones and those zones provide a tool for locating reflex points on the feet.

The third theory of Integrative Reflexology® is ***Meridian Theory***. This theory shows how the meridian pathways begin and end on the feet and hands and how, by noticing the correlation between reflex points and meridians, we can gain insight into our client's condition. These insights offer clues as to how we might support the client's body in returning to a state of balance.

Lastly, the fourth theory of Integrative Reflexology® is ***Psychoneuroimmunology Theory***. This theory is based on the connection between the nervous system, the immune system and the emotions. It shows us how we can simultaneously improve brain chemistry, activate a calming effect in the nervous system and stimulate the lymph system to clear toxins out of our body, all through an Integrative Reflexology® session.

As you explore each theory of Integrative Reflexology®, reflect on how the information provided applies to your own body and your own experience of life. Integrative Reflexology® is an experiential approach. As you read, you will find that "it just makes sense."

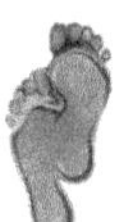

Keep an eye out for "Foot" Notes in each chapter. They will offer practical applications of the information provided. The yin/yang will mark the "Foot" Notes in Chapter 4, Meridian Theory.

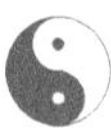

2

Structural Alignment Theory

Structural Alignment Theory of Integrative Reflexology® serves to explain the physical component of reflexology and how physical manipulation in the feet can create physical changes in the rest of the body.

Structure of the Foot

When you begin to talk about structural alignment of the feet, you must begin with the three arches that create the fundamental structure of the foot—the medial arch, the lateral arch and the transverse arch. These three arches work together to create the stable base that our entire body stands on. They create the width that supports our balance from side to side, the length that propels us forward and backward, and the stability that gives us strength. They also create the springiness that allows our body to adjust to fluctuations we encounter in walking and standing. Anatomically, the structure of the three arches is crucial to proper alignment, posture and gait. As a holistic approach to foot reflexology, Integrative Reflexology® looks beyond the basic anatomy of the arches and associates each of the three arches to either the body, mind or spirit (Fig 2.1).

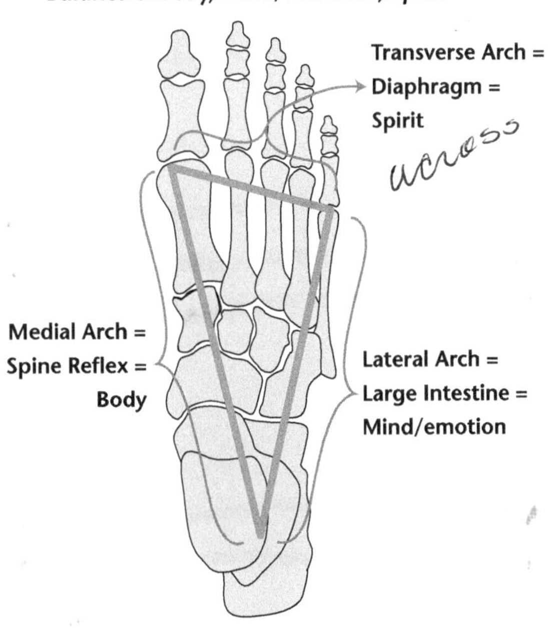

Fig 2.1
Anatomical arches of the feet

In reflexology, the inner or medial arch correlates to the spine. In Integrative Reflexology®, it is also related to the body—the physical foundation of our being. Without the spine, there is no structural framework to the body. Flat or pronated feet (where the arch is rolled inward) compress the spinal reflex and affect the foot's ability to adjust to shifts in weight. This quality in the feet could potentially affect one's sense of strength and physical presence in the world and one's ability to respond in a flexible way to the fluctuations in life. High arches often present as curvature of the spine, which is also a misalignment. A structurally aligned medial arch supports a healthy foot and a healthy spine. It creates strength and stability through flexibility.

The lateral arch correlates to the large intestine in reflexology and is also related to the mind in our holistic model. The large intestine is a place where water re-absorption and storage takes place, and the belly center is the energetic home to our emotions. Standing on the outside of the feet compresses the lateral arch and the reflexes of the ascending or descending colon. This stance can represent holding back or holding onto something emotionally and energetically. Over time, this posture can lead to elimination problems, including irregular bowel movements or constipation.

The transverse arch correlates to the diaphragm muscle in traditional reflexology and is related to the spirit in our holistic model. The diaphragm is the major muscle involved in our ability to breathe. In Latin origins, 'Spiritus' means breath, the soul, vigor—that which animates life. Thus, the diaphragm muscle is what gives life to the body. When our transverse arch is constricted, our breath and our spirit are also constricted. It is not uncommon to see a person kick off a pair of too-tight shoes and then breathe a sigh of relief.

In the context of Integrative Reflexology®, noticing the structure of the arches can help to inform us about what might be happening in the bigger picture of the client's whole body. We may also consider how the structure translates to the client's state of body, mind and spirit.

Fascia

This theory has its roots in the fascia. Fascia is the connective tissue web that is constant from the big toe to the top of the head, wrapping around every muscle, bone and organ, creating our body's physical pattern of alignment. Tom Myers, in his book, *Anatomy Trains,* writes about fascia: "It binds every cell in the body to its neighbors and even connects...the inner network of each cell to the mechanical state of the entire body." Due to the fact that fascia exists as a continuous web throughout the body, when fascia in one area is bound up with tension, that tension is reflected throughout the whole system and affects the posture and alignment of the whole body. Thus, by unbinding the fascia in one area of the body, tension can be released throughout the system. In this way, fascia can be a key in understanding how reflexology works on a physical level.

As Tom Myers expresses, "[f]ascia is, in fact, our system of Biomechanical Regulation—just as our circulatory system is a chemical regulator and the nervous system is a timing regulator—and needs to be studied and treated as a system, not only as a series of parts" (Fascia, 2016).

The feet are the meeting place of all of these systems—fascial, circulatory, nervous, lymph and meridian.

Ida Rolf played a significant role in the world of bodywork as it relates to fascia. She developed Rolfing—a method of bodywork that focuses on manipulating and releasing the fascial tissue. In her book *Rolfing*, Rolf calls the feet the 'great tattletalers.' She says, "to achieve correct body alignment, one must begin with the feet." When you look at someone's feet, you can gain insight into the state of their body's alignment and potential well-being.

Fascial Effects in Reflexology

There was a student in one of my courses with a heel spur on his right heel. The spur was easy to palpate—hard and gritty in the center of the heel. I asked him if I could palpate his gluteal muscles, since the area of the spur was reflective of his right gluteal muscles. As I reached under him, I found his wallet exactly where his heel spur was reflected. This represents a fascial connection—the wallet was pulling and

Balanced alignment of the foot in standing is the first step to proper alignment of the rest of the body. Balanced alignment of the foot occurs when the center of the heel, the ball of the little toe, and the ball of the great toe form a balanced triangle. In Hatha yoga, a balanced stance is created by standing with both feet parallel, the great toes touching, the heels slightly apart, the toes spread and lengthened, the arch lifted and knees soft. This stance assists in proper placement of the sacrum in the pelvis, which then assists in proper alignment of the rest of the spine. In proper body alignment, bone is over bone, so there is less stress on the muscles and more ease in the organs and nerve flow throughout the body. The standing postures in yoga re-educate the student and the student's body to what it feels like to be in proper standing alignment. Achieving more proper alignment then decreases the stress on the entire structure.

...lar self-care discipline ...oper foot alignment and ... Tai Chi, one moves slowly and ...rom foot to foot in a synchronized ...e arches are stimulated with each shift ...e body weight. By stimulating the arches ...nd rocking on the feet, we wake the feet up and allow them to more accurately transmit important sensory information about balance to the rest of our body (Howell, 2010). Studies have shown that when senior citizens practice Tai Chi on a daily basis they experience fewer falls and break fewer bones (Watson, 2012).

Physical self-care disciplines, such as Hatha Yoga and Tai Chi, can help us achieve more proper alignment through a balanced stance. I recommend trying the sample exercises included at the end of this chapter and noticing how they bring awareness to your stance. Over time, you may notice that they cause you to shift your stance. Once you have experienced them yourself, you can consider sharing them with your clients to help them achieve a healthier standing posture.

Assessing Structural Alignment

Lets look at a common stance that many people adopt for an extended period of time. Notice in the image, the figure with hand on hip, weight on one leg with the same hip thrown out and knee locked. This posture is what I call the "teenage stance." In assessing this stance, you will notice that it throws the pelvis and knee completely out of alignment. You will observe that if their weight is on the outside of their right foot, the lateral arch, along with the reflex areas of the ascending colon, liver and right kidney are compressed. This pattern of compression can also be observed by inspecting the soles of their shoes for patterns of wear and tear. When the places on the bottoms of the feet that correlate with these points are palpated, they may be found to be tight due to the increased weight and pressure the area receives, as well as the fascial twisting throughout the body due to the mis-alignments. Nerve flow throughout their body may also be impaired. The practitioner of reflexology can stimulate the tight areas in the feet in order to increase the nerve flow, break up congestion, free the fascia and restore energy to the impaired region.

If the client returns to the habit of standing in this misaligned way, they will present with the same tightness in future sessions. By bringing your client's attention to their posture, the wear in their shoes, and the resulting tightness in their feet, you have an opportunity to both treat and educate your client.

Toe alignment is also to be considered when working with structural alignment. The fascial web extends all the way out into the toes. The first and second toe work together to align the direction of our gait as we move forward. The outer toes then assist in maintaining balance and stability for the foot, which is transferred into the body. One can feel this happening in a balancing pose in yoga—the three outer toes work to hold the posture. This function is also seen in barefoot cultures where individuals have very wide feet.

Toe imbalances manifest as bunions, hammertoes, Morton's toes and ingrown toenails, all of which demonstrate the foot coming out of alignment. When the foot is out of alignment, the client will modify their gait and posture in order to alleviate the pain or discomfort and to maintain balance. Over time, this can establish patterns in the body that can be difficult to undo through bodywork alone. This may also lead to the need for specially designed shoes and sometimes even surgery. Toe spacers such as Correct Toes® are a non-invasive way to help restore toe alignment (Fig 2.3). When using them, one may notice how the shift in the toes and feet translates to shifts throughout the body.

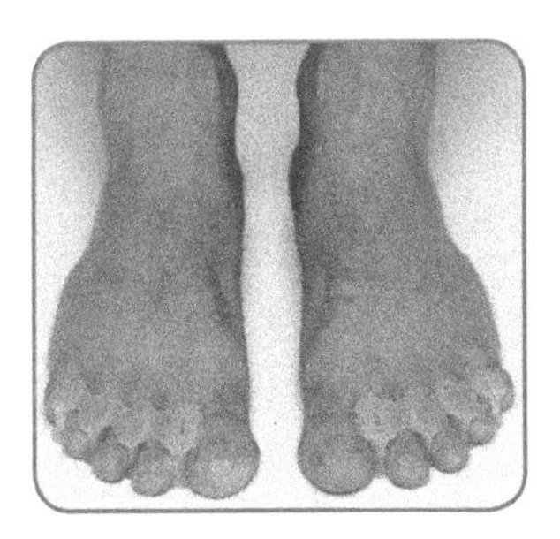

Fig 2.3
Correct Toes® toe spacers

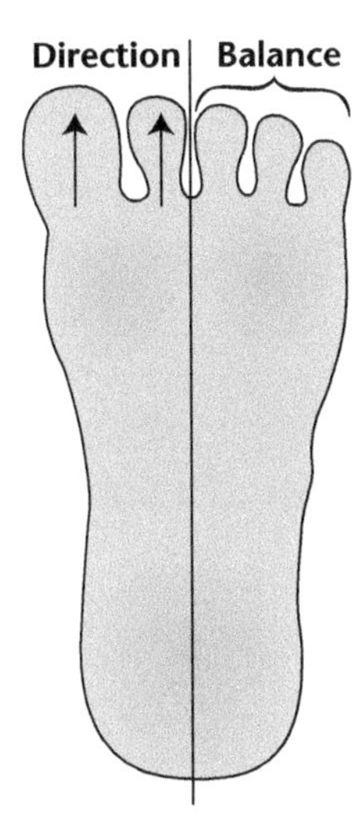

Fig 2.2
Functions of properly aligned toes

As a reflexologist, if you observe misalignment of the toes, understand that the source of that misalignment may be mechanical—from structural misalignment in the body, or energetic—from blocked energy that is connected to that particular toe. As we continue to move through the four theories of Integrative Reflexology®, the toes and their alignment will continue to be of importance.

Cultural Stances - How Culture Effects Your Posture

There are a variety of cultural practices that are considered normal today, or have been considered normal in the past, which compromise structural alignment. One dramatic example of an ancient cultural practice that results in severe structural compromise of the feet is Chinese foot binding, which was done in the name of beauty from 950-1912 A.D. Girls and women endured this painful process for the status that it brought, but then had to be carried from place to place because the binding left them with essentially no foot structure of their own by which to be supported. This is an example of how a cultural practice was used to constrict women's freedom by constricting their bodies and ultimately constricting their ability to thrive in life. One could say similar things, to a lesser degree, about pointed-toe, high heel shoes today.

Ballet is another example of a culturally accepted and celebrated practice that compromises a person's structural alignment. Ballet dancers do a lot of work en pointe (on the tips of the toes) (Fig 2.4), which creates a great deal of compression on the great toe and along the medial arch of the foot, which is related to the entire spine in reflexology. This consistent and intense pressure and compression may account for the high incidences of back and leg injuries in ballet dancers as they age. The great toe is also where the reflex areas for the pineal and pituitary glands are located. The pituitary gland is the master gland that secretes 16 different hormones. From a reflexology perspective, the compression of the great toe due to dancers being en pointe could be a cause for the hormonal imbalances that ballet dancers are known to experience.

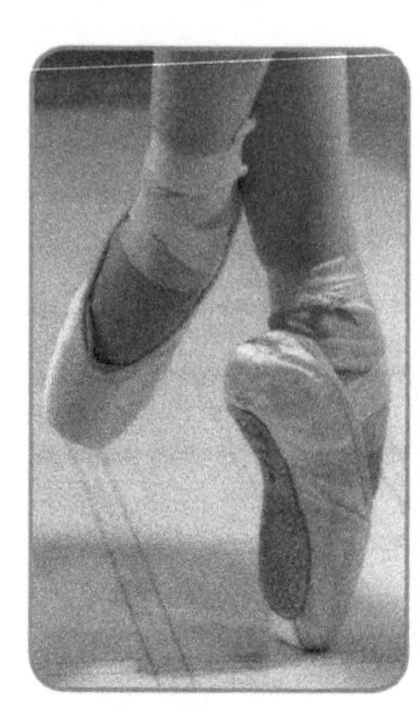

Fig 2.4
En pointe in ballet

Shoes are another negative contributor to proper structural alignment across cultures. Shoes are not now, nor have they ever been, a friend to our feet. Shoes, socks, nylons and other foot coverings all compress the feet. Some shoes compress across the ball of the foot, the reflexology area that corresponds to the diaphragm muscle. When the foot is consistently compressed in this way, constricted breathing may become a habitual pattern in the body. Unfortunately, the shoe industry is often focused on appearances rather than comfort. Throughout the world and throughout time, beauty, power, and fashion have influenced footwear. Our western culture adopted shoes

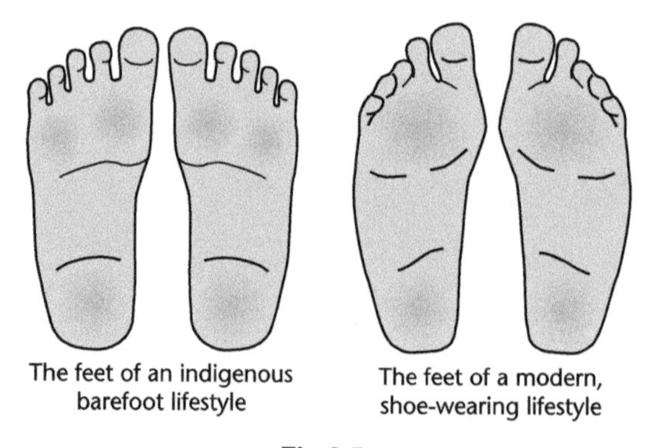

Fig 2.5
The shape of barefoot vs. shod feet

with narrow, high heels and pointed toes as a symbol of a woman's beauty, power and sexual appeal. In fact, these shoes create a degree of physical frailty in those who wear them because postures are thrown out of balance and the body becomes less grounded and therefore unstable. In order to stand upright, a person in high heel shoes must exaggerate the curvature of their spine, as seen in Figure 2.6. When one habitually wears high heel shoes, this unnatural spinal alignment becomes their everyday posture. High heel shoes can also cause ankle injuries and broken bones due to their instability. Considering the effects that high heel shoes can have on our body, it's a potentially high price to pay for looking sexy.

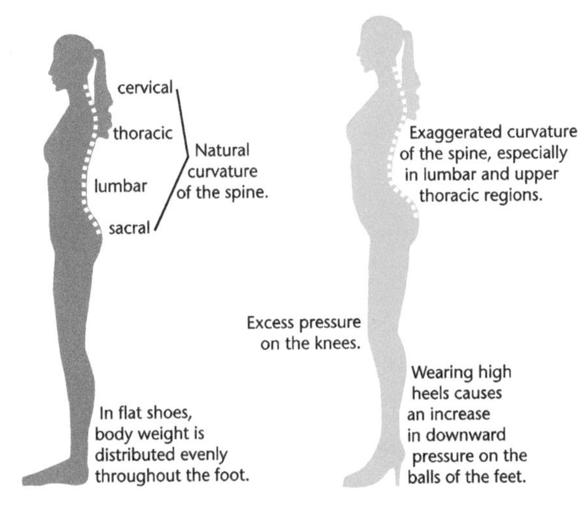

Fig 2.6
How high heels change our postural alignment.

The cultural effects of footwear are not limited to women. Many cowboy boots are extremely pointed and were designed to be used when riding horseback and putting your foot into the stirrup. A reflexology student in Bozeman, Montana shared that after relocating to the area and adopting the western attire, including cowboy boots, he grew a fine bunion in only six months. He no longer wears the boots, but the bunion remains.

Once we begin to take a holistic approach to reflexology, it is difficult to ignore the effects of some of the cultural practices we have always taken for granted. I encourage people to begin to notice for themselves how their shoes affect their whole body.

It is no surprise that there is a movement afoot, to go barefoot! Daniel Howell's book, *The Barefoot Book*, gives many excellent reasons why the human was designed to be barefoot. He states, "the key to good foot health is barefoot locomotion—moving along the ground on your bare feet." Dr. Howell points out that there is nothing natural about shoes. In fact, being barefoot is natural—the human foot is designed to do everything we need it to do without shoes. Shoes actually hinder the foot's ability to fully communicate and inform the rest of the body. As Dr. Howell points out, "the skin on the sole of the foot contains an unusually high concentration of receptors and nerves. These nerves allow the foot sole to provide the brain with sensory feedback information regarding the terrain upon which you're treading . . . being able to feel the ground is crucial to proper walking and running." This feedback helps protect the joints in our body, which have relatively few pain receptors, from undue impact when walking and running. Wearing shoes diminishes the feedback from these receptors in the feet, causing us to change our gait without all of the information our body needs for optimal functioning.

What is Proper Footwear? How To Guide Our Clients

I firmly believe that it is necessary to inform clients of the importance of caring for their feet. Care of the feet includes one's choice of footwear. During the initial intake, you might want to assess your client's shoes and discuss how they effect their structural alignment. Suggestions on footwear need to take into account the client's age, weight, job requirements, and current foot and structural challenges. A shoe that works for one person may not give another person what they need.

Today there is an explosion in the corrective shoe industry. From Birkenstocks in the 1970s, to the minimal shoes from Merrell or Nike, the Earth shoe with its negative heel, and the Vibram five-finger toe shoes, it is hard to know what to choose.

I suggest to clients that they begin the process of choosing shoes by considering the surface upon which they will be walking on a daily basis. Many jobs entail walking, standing and working on a very hard and unforgiving floor. In this environment, the sole of the shoe needs to have adequate cushion to compensate for the hard floor. Some clients may consider adding an insert to further offset the hard surface. It is also necessary to consider arch support when choosing a shoe. Some clients will need strong arch support, especially as they grow older and their arches drop. The barefoot shoes may prove to be too flat for these individuals. Others already have strong arches and prefer to have less support and more freedom of movement within their shoes. The size of the toe box of the shoe needs to be wide enough to allow the ball of the foot and the toes to spread out in a natural way. I believe a wide toe box is a must for shoes, in order to promote healthy toe alignment. There should be flexibility in the sole of the shoe so it can bend across the toe and metatarsal joint line as the client pushes off in walking.

If your clientele includes families with small children, please encourage them to keep children barefoot or in moccasins (soft-soled shoes) for as long as possible. This allows the children to develop strong yet supple arches, which will help develop a strong and supple spine.

Structural Alignment Exercises

These exercises are a great tool for expanding our awareness of our posture as well as for improving our balance and foot strength. I recommend practicing these exercises for yourself in order to have a felt experience of each exercise. In this way, you will know what you are recommending to your clients and will be better able to guide them in their practice.

Postural Awareness

Observe your own stance and ask yourself these questions:

- Are your feet parallel or is one foot turned in or out?
- Is more of your weight on one foot or the other?
- Do you feel weight more in your heels or your toes?
- Are you able to feel your inner or outer arches on either foot making contact with the ground?
- Are your knees soft and open in the back of the knee or are they locked?
- Are your hips centered over your feet?
- Are your pelvis and sacrum hanging in neutral position?
- Are your shoulders open, with arms dropped at your sides?
- Is your chin gently tucked in with your neck soft on the shoulders?
- Does your body feel balanced over your feet?

Make your observations, think about them, remember how you feel, and then write them down. Try to do this for yourself daily for a week, with the intention of bringing awareness to your postural patterns. Awareness is the first step to changing a habit that does not serve your health. This habit may be how you stand, the placement of your feet, or the shoes you choose to wear.

The information gained from this exercise can be valuable to the client who is experiencing chronic back pain from a learned habit of standing, sitting or walking. With new awareness, that client can choose to change their habit by changing their posture or shoes.

Tai Chi Stance

Stand with your feet hip-width apart. Relax the backs of your knees (knees slightly bent). Allow your pelvis to drop and tuck slightly under. Your weight should be evenly distributed on both your feet. Arms are relaxed at your side, shoulders dropped and head and neck gently lifted. Begin your movement by placing weight on your right heel, moving the weight to the ball of your little toe, then to the ball of your great toe. Then shift the weight to the heel of the left foot, to the ball of the little toe, and around to the ball of the great toe. Shift your weight back to the heel of the right foot and repeat the exercise as many times as necessary until you feel the flow and the figure 8 pattern in your feet. Then you can reverse the direction. Your shoulders and hips should move in unison with the feet. While doing this exercise, shift your awareness fully into the soles of your feet. Try it before you walk or run and see if you notice a difference in your stride.

Tiger's Mouth

This yoga exercise promotes the development of a healthy medial arch. The exercise requires someone to help you by placing his or her hand as pictured above. Then you will lift the arch of your foot by contracting it into the hand holding the top of the foot, which is the "tiger's mouth" (Fig 2.7). Your heel and toes stay on the ground while you lift your arch. This exercise will help you feel the muscles used in developing a healthy arch. Picking up items with your toes also strengthens the medial arch of the foot. If you are able to do that, keep doing it.

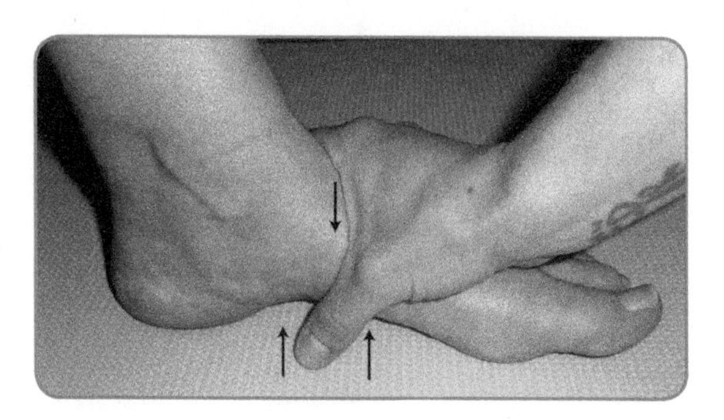

Fig 2.7
Tiger's Mouth exercise

Conclusion

By incorporating physical disciplines that promote proper alignment into our daily activities, we create more balance in our lives. Remember the triangular structure of the foot, with the body, mind and spirit connection to the arches.

When feet are wide and connected to the ground, and the triangle of the arches is fully engaged in standing, we are balanced on our own two feet. Standing on your own two feet becomes the metaphor for the way we live our life—stable and strong in body, mind and spirit. When the foot is in proper structural alignment, that balance can be translated to the rest of the body.

Integrative Reflexology® is one way that we can offer our clients support in achieving more structural balance in their lives.

3

Zone Theory

Zone Theory of Integrative Reflexology® is based on zone therapy, or reflex zone therapy, which is the dominant theory that forms the foundation of modern reflexology. The idea behind zone therapy is that the body can be mapped out into different zones, and therapeutic effects can be achieved in one area by working on another area of the same zone. When applied strictly to the feet, the zones become a location tool for finding reflex points that correspond to the body.

While the fundamentals of this theory are agreed upon across all schools of reflexology, the exact placement of the reflex zones on the feet varies widely. Since the location of the zones on the feet is the foundation for the layout of the reflex points, this variability in placement of the zones results in variability between reflexology charts. This variability often leads to confusion amongst reflexology students. It is at this point that the art of reflexology comes into play.

Inevitably, beginning practitioners of reflexology will use the reflexology chart from their training. Then, through practice, they may develop their own sense of exactly where the points are, which may differ from the placement of the points on the chart. This is where the practitioner learns to follow their sense and trust the feedback and results they experience with their clients. Zone Theory of Integrative Reflexology® and the chart included in this book are a result of this exact process. The chart has evolved over decades of practical work and it continues to be fine-tuned. While the chart itself is an evolving work of art, the theory behind the zones is a more substantiated and universal piece of the reflexology puzzle.

Zone Therapy Past and Present

We visited the early history of zone therapy in the introduction. It took us through the work of Drs. Fitzgerald and Bowers who authored *Zone Therapy* and established the 10 longitudinal zones in the body (Fig 3.1). Their successor, Dr. Riley, wrote *Zone Therapy Simplified*, diagrammed reflexes on the feet and added eight horizontal zones to the 10 longitudinal zones of his predecessors. This was in 1919; since that time, the reflexology zones have evolved to what practitioners of reflexology use today (Issel, 1990).

It is generally agreed that there are four horizontal zones on each foot, along with the 10 longitudinal zones. Each major contributor to the field of reflexology uses the zones slightly differently. Zone Theory of Integrative Reflexology® uses four horizontal zones that correspond to the four anatomical cavities of the body—cranial, thoracic, abdominal and pelvic.

The general layout of the horizontal zones is in alignment with the joint lines of the foot bones. In this alignment, the metatarsophalangeal joint at the base of the toes delineates the first zone. The second zone line is located at the phalange-metatarsal joint line, where the ball of the foot meets the arch. The third most commonly used zone line is located at the metatarsal-tarsal joint

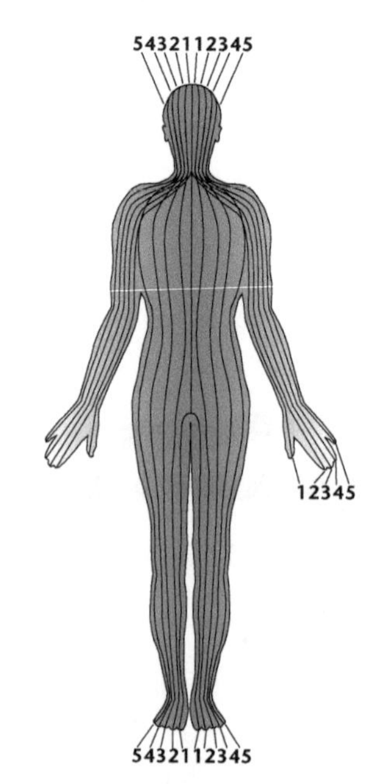

Fig 3.1
Fitzgerald's 10 longitudinal zones

line, at about the mid-point of the arch of the foot. This is also one of the most commonly found variations in interpretation of the horizontal zones. While all charts agree that this line is an accurate delineation of the waistline, some use it only as a landmark dividing the upper and lower abdomen within one zone, while others use it to define a zone. The final zone line is located where the arch of the foot meets the heel.

Constructing a New Reflexology Chart

As previously explained in the introduction, the Integrative Reflexology® chart has been created based on anatomical knowledge from my experience as an x-ray tech and decades

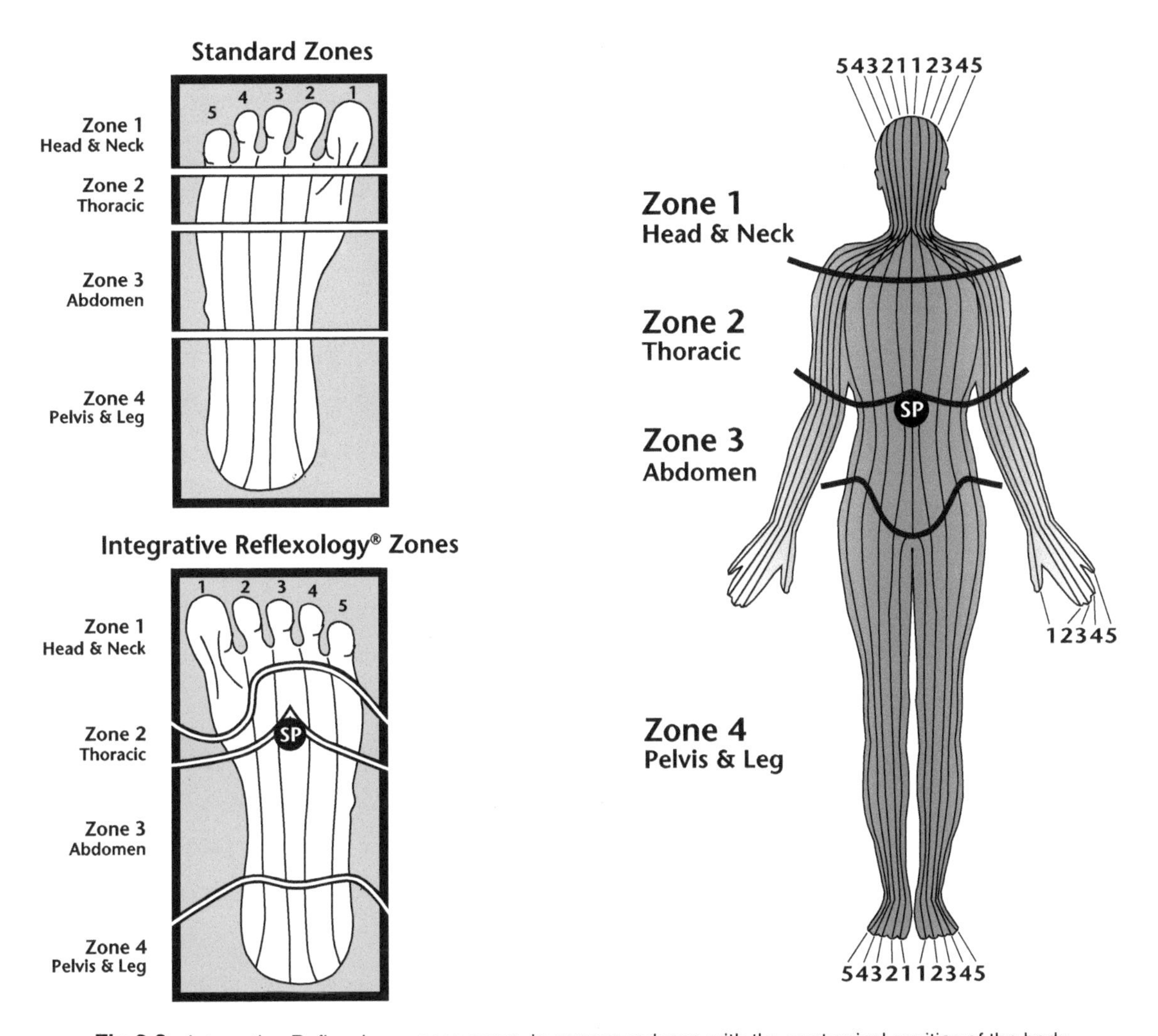

Fig 3.2 - Integrative Reflexology zones curve, in correspondence with the anatomical cavities of the body

of hands-on application. The Integrative Reflexology® zones curve with the curves of the body. The dividing lines that create the 4 horizontal zones align with the membranes that separate the four cavities of the body (cranial, thoracic, abdominal, pelvic).

The first zone corresponds to the cranial cavity and includes reflex areas for the brain, pineal gland, pituitary gland, hypothalamus, thyroid, parathyroids, sinuses and the neck. Traditional reflexology uses the neck of the great toe as the neck reflex. I have experienced the neck reflex area as extending further down the great toe, across the metatarsophalangeal joint. Anatomically, the neck includes the seventh cervical vertebra and the thyroid. Based on this anatomical fact, these reflex points are included in the neck reflex area of Integrative Reflexology®. In practical application, clients

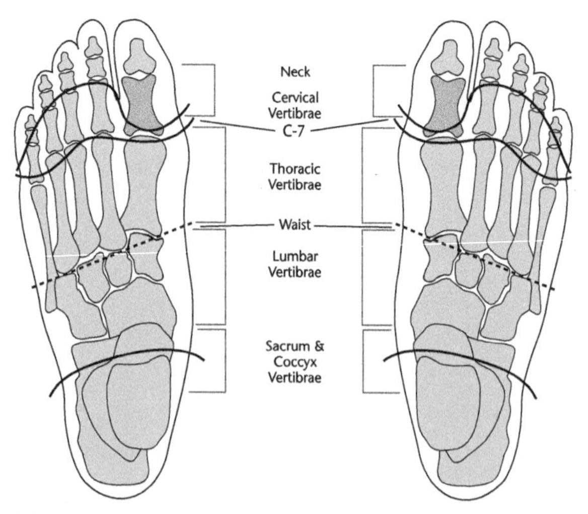

Fig 3.3 - Spine reflex areas based on the horizontal zones

have experienced elongation and relief in their neck when the neck reflex is stimulated through traction of the great toe.

The second zone corresponds to the thoracic cavity and includes the reflexology areas of the lungs, bronchi, heart and esophagus. The line of demarcation between the second and third zone corresponds to the diaphragm muscle and mimics its curve in the body.

The third zone corresponds to the abdominal cavity and includes reflex areas for all of the digestive organs and glands—the stomach, pancreas, spleen, liver, gallbladder, large and small intestines, kidneys and adrenal glands. In Integrative Reflexology®, the waistline is used as a landmark for locating specific reflexology points, not as a zone line. Anatomically, the waistline is not a dividing membrane between cavities of the body. Rather, it is a landmark that divides the upper abdomen, which includes the stomach, pancreas, liver, gallbladder, spleen, transverse colon and the kidneys, from the lower abdomen, which holds most of the large intestine and the small intestine. In this way, the third zone includes reflex areas for the entire abdominal cavity.

The fourth zone corresponds to the pelvic cavity and includes reflex points for the lower part of the large intestine, the sigmoid colon, the anus, the reproductive organs and the bladder.

Zone Theory of Integrative Reflexology® also differs from some other schools of reflexology in the location of the solar plexus point. Integrative Reflexology® considers the Chinese meridian system when placing the solar plexus point on the foot and chart. In the Chinese meridian system, the solar plexus is located at the exact same point as Kidney 1 (Fig 3.4)—in the middle of the sole of the foot. In that system, each foot is treated as the whole body rather than only half the body, as seen in traditional reflexology. In traditional reflexology, if the zones are viewed as a grid in continuation with the rest of the body,

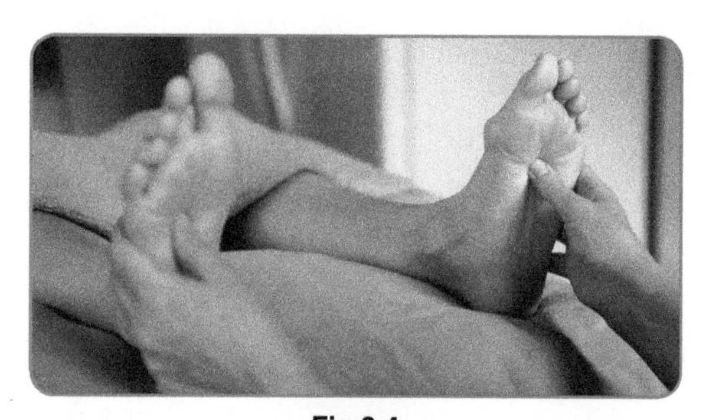

Fig 3.4
Solar plexus reflex point and Kidney 1 meridian point

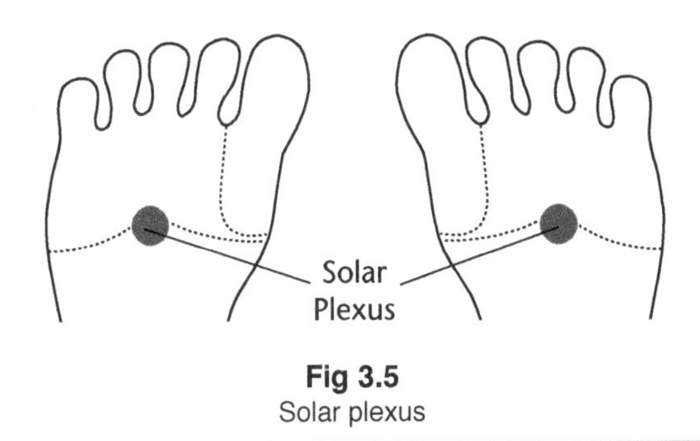

Fig 3.5
Solar plexus

then the left foot corresponds to the left side of the body and the right foot corresponds to the right side of the body. While this perspective is suitable for locating some of the reflexology points, limiting ourselves to this perspective does not allow for accurate placement of the solar plexus point. Anatomically, the solar plexus is located in the center of the torso, inferior to the diaphragm muscle. In order to accurately translate this to the foot, each foot must also be perceived as the whole body, which then allows the solar plexus point to lie in the center of the foot, just below the reflex area for the diaphragm. In the meridian system, this is Kidney 1.

The energetic effects of the solar plexus reflex area (also Kidney 1) are calming and soothing to clients. The overlapping of these two points is one of the most obvious demonstrations for the need to consider multiple systems in your practice of reflexology. There are many ways in which different systems of reflexology overlap and integrate with each other. For this reason, it is advisable to consider Zone Theory as a basic and general location system, not as an exact and absolute map of the foot and reflex areas.

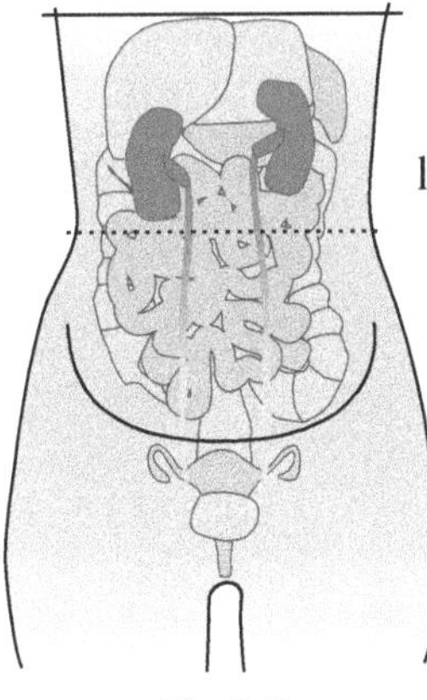

Fig 3.6
Anatomical position of the kidneys

The kidneys are example of an organ whose location varies significantly across reflexology charts. The anatomical location of the kidneys is such that the base of each kidney aligns with the waistline and the last posterior rib, just lateral to the spine (Fig 3.6). Based on this anatomical placement, the zones, as defined by Integrative Reflexology®, support the location of the kidney reflex point above the waistline on the foot. Other reflexology charts have the waistline passing through the middle of the kidney reflex, or even have the kidney below the waistline. This placement simply does not correlate with the anatomy of the body.

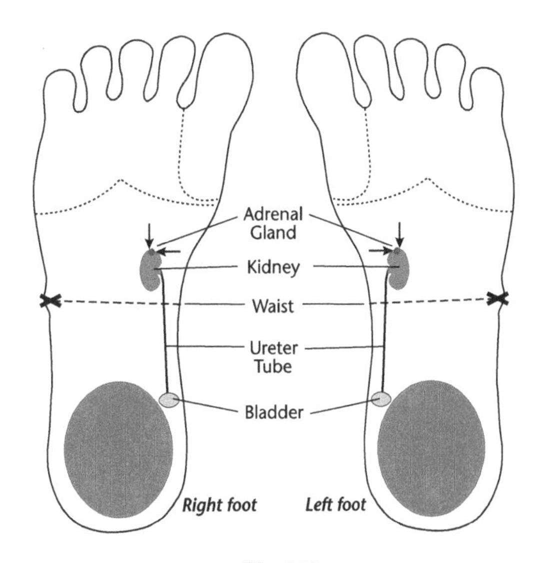

Fig 3.7
Reflexology of the kidney system

ther common disparity nd between reflexology arts is the location of the transverse colon of the large intestine. A number of charts place the entire large intestine below the waistline, while, anatomically, the transverse colon of the large intestine sits above the waistline (Fig 3.8). The splenic flexure, which is the transition point between the transverse colon and the descending colon, actually sits below the left anterior ribs.

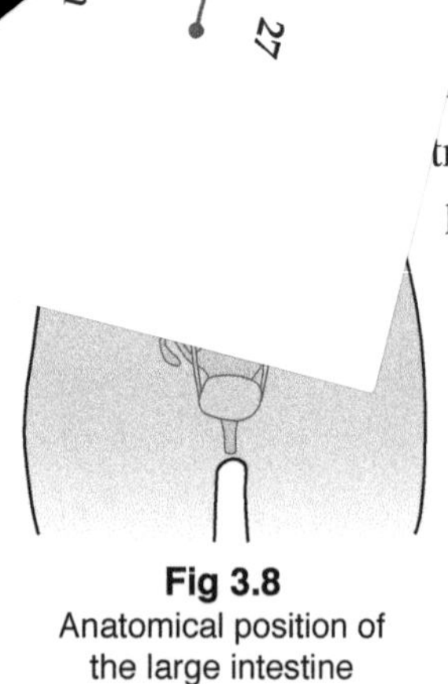

Fig 3.8
Anatomical position of the large intestine

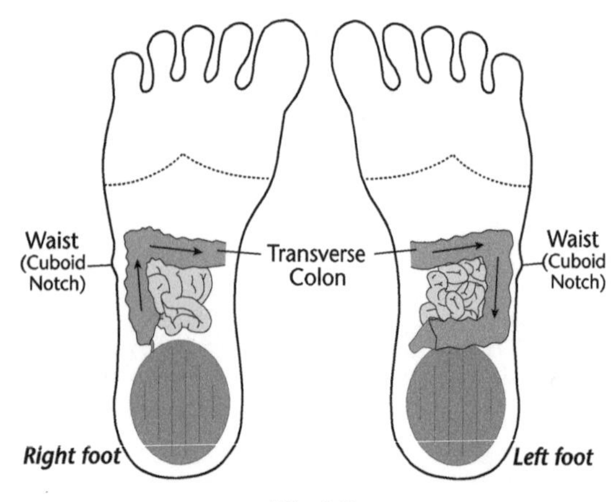

Fig 3.9
Reflexology area for the large intestine

The liver and gallbladder reflex points also vary across the many reflexology charts. Based on the location of the solar plexus reflex in the center of the foot, below the diaphragm line, the liver reflex in Integrative Reflexology® is lateral to the solar plexus, below the right fifth metatarsaophalangeal joint line. The gallbladder point lies next to the liver point medially, at the base of the fourth metatarsaophalangeal joint on the right foot. This placement of the gallbladder point on the right foot is in alignment with the gallbladder meridian along the fourth metatarsal on both feet. The heart and spleen reflex points are located in these positions on the left foot—on the fourth metatarsal for the heart and the fifth metatarsal for the spleen.

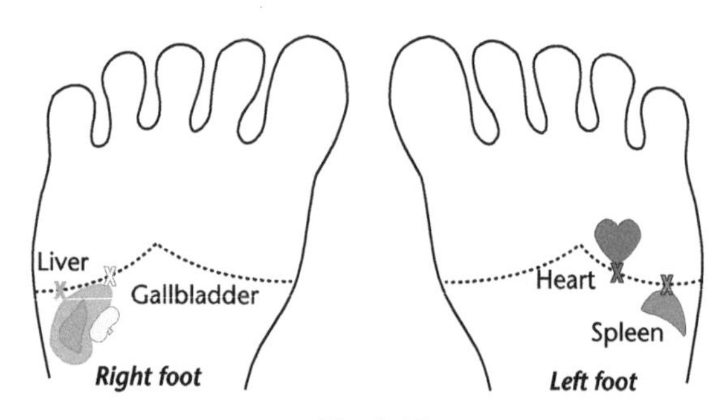

Fig 3.10
Reflexology points for the liver, gallbladder, heart and spleen

Conclusion

Zone Theory of Integrative Reflexology® is derived greatly from the underlying theory that informs all of reflexology. Zone Theory has refined those traditional ideas into a map of the foot that makes sense anatomically, has proven itself therapeutically, and has been positively received by students for decades; students of Integrative Reflexology® consistently report that this chart "simply makes sense." Like all reflexology students, you will use this chart as a guide to start with and you will inevitably deviate from it as you work with clients and refine your skills.

4

Meridian Theory

An Eastern approach to reflexology

Meridian Theory of Integrative Reflexology® is where the Eastern influence meets the Western practice of reflexology. Reflexology has its roots in the Chinese meridian pathways. Of the 14 main meridians, 12 begin or end on the fingers and toes. The meridian pathways also tend to exist in alignment with the vertical zones of reflexology. When you consider these similarities, it is clear to see how these two practices overlap. Chinese medicine and the meridians provide a vast well of information for the healing arts. In order to narrow your focus for the use of meridians in Integrative Reflexology®, it is advisable that you read through this chapter on meridians with an inquisitive mind. Your main focus will be to learn where the meridian begins or ends—on which finger or toe, and learn to apply that in a reflexology session. Later, you will learn to assess and integrate the connection between the muscles and each meridian. Finally, you will learn to incorporate information from the client's health history to inform your work with the meridians and reflexology points.

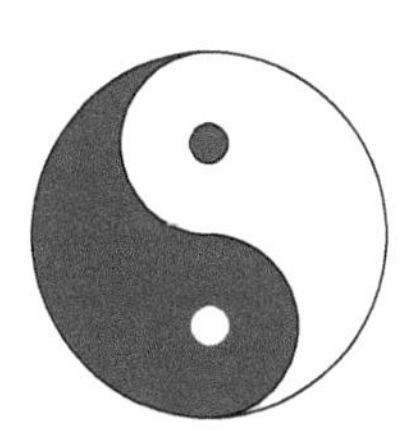

Chinese Medicine

When using an Eastern approach to reflexology, you must gain some understanding of the historical and theoretical basis for Chinese medicine. This ancient system of health care dates back at least 5000 years and is based on the belief that balance is the key to good health. The famous yin-yang circle is a symbol of balance. The symbol conveys the idea that within the light (yang) there is darkness (yin), and within the darkness (yin) there is light (yang). Balance is not a static experience, but a state of continual change and movement within a larger system (Dougans, 1992).

The ancient Chinese understood, at a fundamental level, that this balance exists in the macrocosm of the universe as well as in the microcosm of our bodies. They understood that the natural changes that take place in the world around us also take place within us. Based on this observation, they established five elements that refer to conditions or states of being, rather than material elements. These elements are Earth, Wood, Fire, Water and Metal. Each of these elements is, in turn, associated with a variety of factors—season, climate, body organ, sense, personality, emotion, and sound to name a few (Dougans, 1992).

The five elements, and the various factors associated with them, are the basis for a detailed system of observing a patient that is the foundation of Chinese medicine. By taking note of observable qualities such as strong food affinities or dislikes, seasonal preferences, and personality tendencies, a Chinese medicine practitioner can learn about a client's temperament and determine where their system (their body) is out of balance. They can then connect the imbalance to one of the five elements, which can also be related to the seasons of the year and times of the day. Each of these categories of information, including the element, is also specific to a meridian in the body. The meridians are what bring the elements and their qualities into the physical body. They are the access point through which a practitioner can work to re-balance the system.

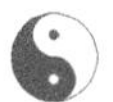

Reflexology and the meridians

When working with clients, I always use a combination of meridian information and reflexology assessment to create a treatment plan for the current therapeutic session. A pregnant client presented with pain in her lower back, hips and iliotibial band along the outer thigh. Based on this, I worked the reflexology points for the hip, knee, and lower back. The client had also expressed that she was grieving the loss of her father, had just recovered from pneumonia, and was constipated. With this information, I chose to do muscle release techniques along the quadratus lumborum, which is the muscle associated with the lung and large intestine meridians and the emotions of grief and letting go. The reflexology gave immediate relief for the hip, knee and lower back. When the client returned for the next session, she reported that the constipation was gone and she felt emotionally lighter.

The Meridians

A meridian is an invisible channel through which Chi (life force energy) flows in a specific pattern or pathway through our body. If the meridian is clear and balanced, then energy can flow through it unencumbered, contributing to a healthy system. If a meridian is congested, then the energy cannot flow as easily and this will cause congestion in the system, resulting in deficiency or excess in the meridian.

Over time, if untreated, this congestion can present as a physical symptom in the body. In a balanced system, all of the meridians are clear and open, without excess or deficiency, and they easily adjust to an ever-changing system. While this is an ideal state of balance for the body, the reality of our everyday lives makes it difficult to attain this state. As an Integrative Reflexology® practitioner, understanding and utilizing both the reflexology points and the meridians will deepen your ability to support a client achieving an optimal state of balance.

Another example of balance in this system is that all of the meridians exist in a paired relationship, one being the yin meridian and one being the yang meridian (Fig 4.1). The yin meridians carry the gentle, dark, feminine, soft and yielding energies. The yang meridians rule the strong, light, masculine, hard and assertive energies. As a practitioner, always address the yin or yang partner meridian when you notice and treat one meridian or organ that is not functioning optimally.

YIN	YANG
Lungs	Large Intestine
Kidney	Bladder
Liver	Gallbladder
Heart	Small Intestine
Pericardium	Triple Warmer
Spleen	Stomach

Fig 4.1
The paired yin and yang meridians

In the Integrative Reflexology® method, we focus on twelve of the fourteen main meridians that are directly related to fingers and toes of hand and foot reflexology. These 12 meridians exist in the six, paired yin/yang relationships listed in the chart above. Each pair of meridians is also associated with one of the five elements of Chinese medicine. The 12 meridians will be expanded on later in the chapter, along with their corresponding element, season and observable qualities. The two meridians not addressed in the Integrative Reflexology® method include the governing vessel (yin) and the conception vessel (yang). The governing vessel travels up the center of the spinal column, along the head, to the front of the face. The conception vessel runs up the front of the body and meets the governing vessel between the nose and upper lip. These two core meridians do not exist in the feet or hands, thus are not addressed by a reflexology session.

The flow of energy through each of the meridians has a peak time of day. Those peak times correspond to the natural rhythms of the human body over a twenty-four hour period. Fatigue at certain periods of the day can be an indication of an imbalance in the meridian associated with that time of day. An imbalance can also be reflected by a surge of energy at a certain time of day. Relating a person's daily rhythm and energy levels to the meridians can tell a story about potential imbalances in their system.

Table of Meridians

SEASON	Autumn	Winter	Spring	Summer	Late Summer
ELEMENT	Metal	Water	Wood	Fire	Earth
CLIMATE	Dry	Cold	Wind	Heat	Humid/Damp
EMOTION	Grief	Fear	Anger	Love	Worry/Empathy
SOUND	Crying	Groaning	Shouting	Laughing	Singing
TASTE	Pungent	Salty	Sour	Bitter	Sweet
COLOR	White	Black/Blue	Green	Red	Yellow/Brown
SENSE	Smell	Hearing	Sight	Taste	Touch
PERSONALITY	Artist	Philosopher	Commander	Lover	Peacemaker
YIN ORGAN & TIME OF DAY	Lungs 3–5 AM	Kidney 5–7 PM	Liver 1–3 AM	Heart 11 AM –1 PM Pericardium 7–9 PM	Spleen 9–11 AM
MUSCLES	Coracobrachialis, Deltoids, Diaphragm, Serratus anterior	Iliacus, Psoas, Upper trapezius	Pectoralis major, Rhomboids	(Heart) Subscapularis (Pericardium) Adductors, Gluteus maximus, Piriformis	Extensor pollicis longus, Latissimus dorsi, Trapezius, Triceps
YANG ORGAN & TIME OF DAY	Large Intestine 5–7 AM	Bladder 3–5 PM	Gallbladder 11 PM–1 AM	Small Intestine 1–3 PM Triple Warmer 9–11 PM	Stomach 7–9 AM
MUSCLES	Hamstrings, Quadratus lumborum, Tensor fascia latae	Fibularis muscles, Sacrospinalis (erector spinae), Tibialis anterior, Tibialis posterior	Anterior deltoid, Popliteus	(Small Intestine) Internal oblique, Quadriceps femoris, Rectus abdominis, Transverse abdominis (Triple Warmer) Gastrocnemius, Gracilis Sartorius Soleus Teres minor	Brachioradialis, Levator scapula, Neck muscles, Pectoralis major

Fig 4.2

The daily rhythm can also be expanded to a yearly rhythm, incorporating how a person feels during the seasons of the year and thus adding to the story about where energy may be excessive or deficient.

As you read through the meridian chart in Figure 4.2 and the detailed information for each season and meridian, keep an open, inquiring mind. First, see what fits for you in your health and then expand your awareness to consider the clients with whom you work. Do not use each piece of information on its own; rather, gather all the information into a holistic model that allows you to create an optimal session or treatment protocol for your individual client.

The Five Seasons of Meridian Theory

Next, we will look at each of the five seasons of Meridian Theory. Each season is associated with one of the five elements of Chinese medicine, a paired relationship of meridians, and other observable qualities (Fig 4.2). The following information is organized by season because everyone experiences the seasons of the year. If you are new to the Chinese medicine system, the seasons have a more tangible quality than the elements and meridians. We begin with autumn and the lung and large intestine meridians because Lung 1 is the beginning of the meridian flow cycle.

Autumn Season

The autumn season is a time of change. It is a time when we make the shift between the active, out-going energy of the summer into the more introverted, quiet and contemplative time of winter. We see this change taking place around us, as the leaves begin to express their true colors. At this time of the year, we slow down and open ourselves to receiving and processing new information—we enter into a course of study and go back to school. It is a time of harvest, when we reap the benefits of our hard work during the year and gather our resources in preparation for the less lucrative winter months. Autumn energies support all of these processes.

Lung Meridian (Yin)

The lung meridian begins the flow of energy through all the meridians when we are born. It begins at Lung 1, located in the soft depression just below the clavicle, and extends down the arm to the thumbnail. For nine months in the womb, our breath and nourishment are received through the umbilical cord. When we emerge at birth, the squeeze of our body through the birth canal stimulates the lung meridian, which in turn activates the lungs themselves, allowing our breath to move energy through all the meridians. A baby's cry upon being born is stimulating for the baby's lungs. The lungs and our breath are related to spirit, the non-physical part of us that brings life into our physical body.

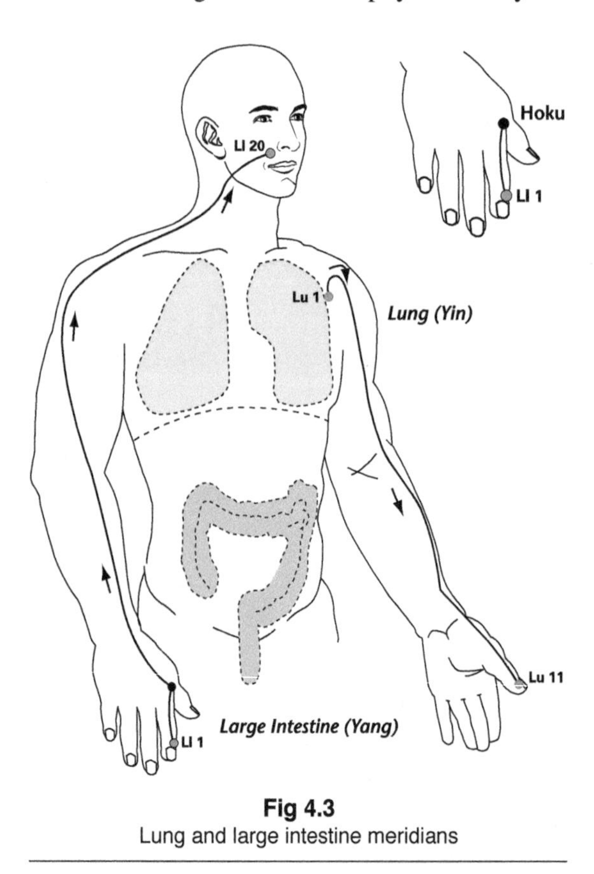

Fig 4.3
Lung and large intestine meridians

Large Intestine Meridian (Yang)

The large intestine meridian starts on the back of the index finger and extends up the outside of the arm, across the shoulder, neck and face to just beside the nose. The large intestine is an organ that is also stimulated by the squeeze through the birth canal at birth. It is critical for the baby to have the first bowel movement soon after the birth—their first elimination of waste that no longer serves them. In Chinese medicine, assessment of the bowel movements is used for diagnosis of all conditions since the large intestine is highly sensitive to stress, potentially resulting in constipation or diarrhea. Utilizing information about a client's ease of digestion may give you a focus for the therapeutic reflexology session.

Autumn Element—METAL

This is a challenging element to explain. It is about alchemical change—taking one substance and transforming it into another substance. When we breathe, oxygen goes into our body and carbon dioxide goes out. When we eat, food goes into our body and waste is excreted through a bowel movement. Our body is constantly transforming energy from one substance into another, taking in what we need and eliminating waste. This is also true of mental processes that involve taking in information and being able to process and let go of what you do not need. The metal element embodies this process of transformation.

Autumn Climate—DRY

The dampness of the late summer gives way to lower humidity and drier air in autumn. The changing climate of the autumn season correlates with the changes in our bodies. Our lungs reflect this shift. Some of us may experience breathing more easily due to the drier air, while others experience breathing difficulties due to increased allergies to the mold of decomposing leaves or other irritants in the air. Our skin and our nasal passages dry out, asking us to change how we take care of our bodies and what foods we eat.

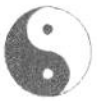 *You would give additional focus to the lung and large intestine meridian points and reflexology areas for all clients during the autumn season.*

Autumn Emotion—GRIEF and LETTING GO

Grief is a natural process in the cycle of life and change. It is necessary to grieve the end of any change in our life, before we can more fully embrace the new beginnings that blossom in its wake. By allowing ourselves to grieve, we are inviting completion and when we feel completion in a process, we can let go. Letting go is necessary to make room for the newness that wants to come into our lives.

Every autumn presents the opportunity to clean out and start fresh with a new focus. A Fall cleanse is recommended to prevent illness in the winter. It reminds our body that we are shifting into a new season and allows us to enter into the quiet of winter with clarity. Autumn is the beginning of the inward time, when emotional release in quiet contemplation benefits the mind and the body. Even the autumn trees are letting go, shedding their leaves to allow for new growth in the spring. Both organs associated with the autumn meridians let go—the lungs with exhaling and the large intestine through the bowel movement. When we recognize grief and letting go as a natural part of any cycle we are able to surrender to its energies and maintain balance.

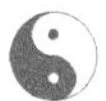 *If your client has suffered a loss of any kind, address the meridian and reflexology areas for lung and large intestine.*

Autumn Sound—CRYING

Crying is the sound we emit when we are sad and grieving. By allowing ourselves to emit cries, or to have a "good cry," we are giving ourselves permission to grieve and let go. A baby's first breath is often a cry, perhaps the beginning of letting go, of grieving the departure from the womb. By crying, we are surrendering to the process of letting go, accepting that some aspect of life is ready to leave or change. It is possible that a client will cry while receiving work on the lung meridian or the lung reflexes. This crying is a release and it is important to hold space for it to occur.

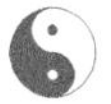 *If your client has an emotional release with crying, work the lung and large intestine meridians and reflexology areas.*

Autumn Taste—PUNGENT

The foods that are pungent would include the healing foods of garlic, onions, leeks and radishes. The therapeutic nature of these foods can de-mucous the digestive and respiratory systems. Good old-fashioned chicken soup, filled with garlic and onions, helps clear the body of excess mucous and infection. The aromas released when cutting up an onion will often clear the sinuses and tear ducts. These mechanisms of release are natural ways that our body eliminates toxins.

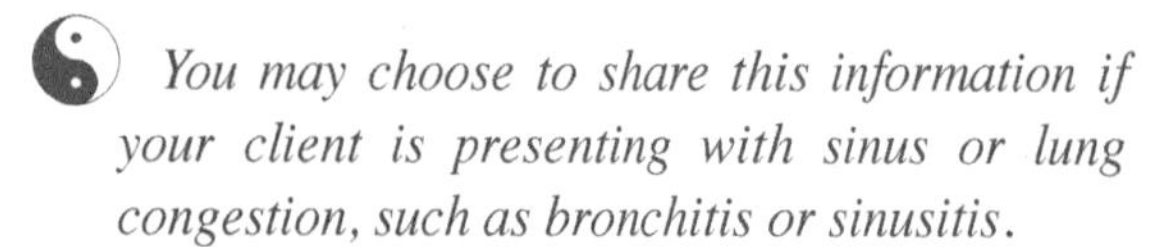

You may choose to share this information if your client is presenting with sinus or lung congestion, such as bronchitis or sinusitis.

Autumn Color—WHITE

In the Eastern part of the world, white is the color that is worn when a person is grieving. It is interesting that many of the pungent foods associated with this season—garlic, onions, leeks and radishes—are also white. White is a color associated with cleansing and purification, both processes related to letting go.

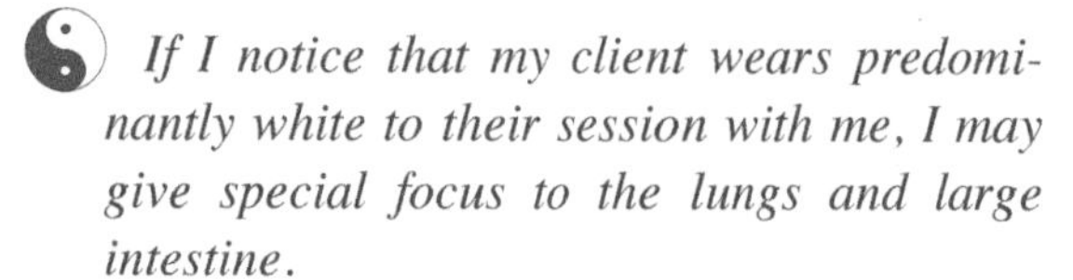

If I notice that my client wears predominantly white to their session with me, I may give special focus to the lungs and large intestine.

Autumn Sense—SMELL

The sinuses play an important role in discerning our environment. The nose protects our body by filtering out dust and debris from the air entering our respiratory system. It also warns us if the food we are about to eat is rotten. The sense of smell can educate, evoke memories and warn us of danger. Keeping your nose clear and healthy through salt washes will improve your respiratory health.

For this reason, it is important to work sinuses in conjunction with lung and large intestine issues. ***A personal example:*** *A friend, who had recently lost her mother, was plagued with a chronic and severe sinus infection on her left side (the feminine/mother side). She had not had time to grieve due to all of the work involved with being executor of the estate. She had also stated that she had not been able to cry. It may be that when this person has the time to be with her grief, the sinuses will open up and release.*

Autumn Personality—ARTIST

An artistic person who demonstrates a strong creative tendency is able to communicate and transform through art, music, and writing. They are able to change one substance or thought into something else. This is the application of the metal element and the alchemical change, which is a strong energetic component of the personality for this person. The artist is someone who expresses individuality through creativity—transforming their personal message into art.

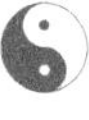 *Processing change or grief can be expressed through art therapy. Writing and creating art are valuable tools as we honor profound changes in our lives.*

Time of PEAK ENERGY for the Autumn meridians:

Lung—3-5 am

This is when the air is the freshest. It is when we rise to breathe in the new day—excellent for meditation, exercise and creating a fresh, new beginning.

 *While the lung meridian represents the beginning of the meridian flow, it can also represent the end. This time period is often referred to as "the leaving time" in hospitals, the time when it is quiet and peaceful and the patients will die.*

Large Intestine—5-7 am

This is when our bodies naturally want to eliminate the waste of our food from the day before. Noticing the qualities of our bowel movements can serve as a barometer for the quality of our diet. Many Eastern medicine practitioners inquire about the appearance of the morning's bowel movement—Is it in one piece? What color is it? Does it float or sink?—These qualities are all indicators of the health and balance of the large intestine.

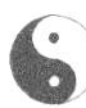 *Notice, or perhaps inquire, if the client has digestive challenges—do they comment on what time they wake up in the morning and if they have an easy morning bowel movement?*

Autumn Meridian MUSCLES

Massage therapists and body workers are advised to address these muscles during a session, along with reflexology areas and meridian points on the hand, especially the Hoku point. Chronic aches in the muscles associated with each meridian may indicate chronic imbalances in the organ of the meridian.

Lung Meridian:

CORACOBRACHIALIS
DELTOID
DIAPHRAGM
SERRATUS ANTERIOR

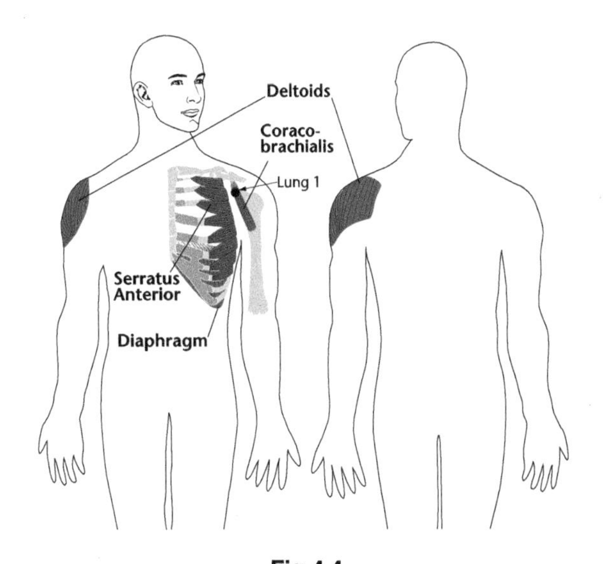

Fig 4.4
Muscles related to the lung meridian

Both the diaphragm and serratus anterior are associated with breathing. The attachment for the anterior deltoid is located in the area of Lung 1 and the coracobrachialis runs along the lung meridian.

Large Intestine Meridian:
HAMSTRINGS
QUADRATUS LUMBORUM
TENSOR FASCIA LATAE

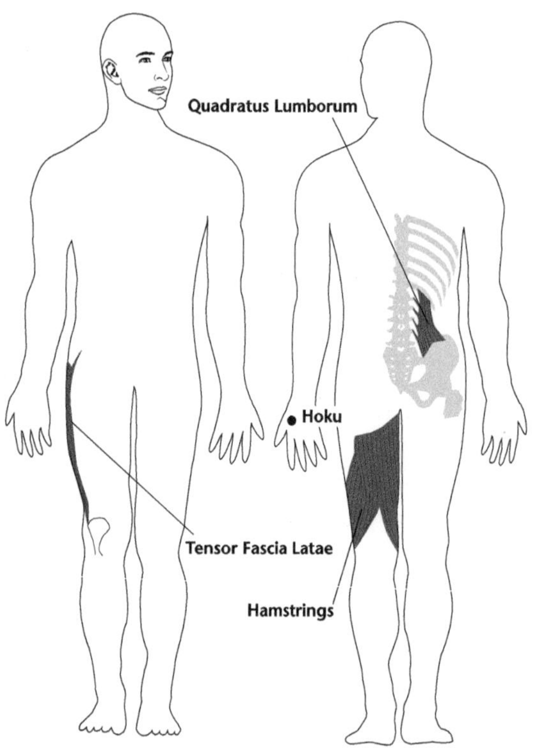

Fig 4.5
Muscles related to the large intestine meridian

The quadratus lumborum is one of the tight and tender areas that the practitioner may massage to help relieve lower back pain. Another approach may be to work the large intestine to simulate the digestive area and thereby relieve the back pain that may be caused by constipation. The combination of work on the foot reflexology areas for large intestine, the large intestine meridian points on the hand (the web between thumb and first finger called the Hoku point), as well as quadratus lumborum release techniques on the actual muscle, may have a positive effect on a client's lower back pain.

The tensor fascia latae (TFL) muscle runs along the lateral thigh from the hip to the knee. Tenderness in this area, along with hip and knee discomfort may indicate digestive challenges. The practitioner can stimulate the Hoku point to assess if the TFL tenderness is related to the large intestine, either meridian or organ. You may notice that the Hoku point on one side is more tender than on the other side. That may reflect in either the ascending colon for the right Hoku or descending colon for the left Hoku. You can then check to see if that is also reflected in the feet by working the reflexology areas that correlate to that particular section of the colon/large intestine.

The hamstring muscles are associated with the large intestine meridian as well as the bladder meridian. This correlation begs the question, could dehydration be a cause for constipation and back pain?

Winter Season

The energy of the winter season is reflected inward. It is a time for slowing down, minimizing the use of resources (both external and internal), keeping warm and quieting into stillness. Winter carries with it a calm that invites us to join its tranquility, both physically and mentally. The winter is also a time for reflecting on our life and deepening our inner philosophical being. It is an excellent season to begin a meditation practice.

Kidney Meridian (Yin)

The kidney meridian begins on the bottom of the foot at the same location as the solar plexus point in the reflexology system. It then continues up the inner leg, across the abdomen and chest, to the lower and medial portion of the clavicle. The kidneys store energy for our body and are associated with the winter, which is a time to replenish the body's reserves. The kidneys also regulate the water in our body. Fluids in our body are essential to life. They lubricate the cells, transport nutrients and gather and eliminate waste. In this way, the kidneys truly are the essential storehouse for our body, both physically and energetically. Kidney 1, the start of the kidney meridian, located on the bottom of the foot, is said to connect in with the earth and the water meridians that flow underground.

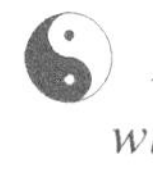

Notice that Kidney 1 overlaps with the solar plexus reflex point, both physically and energetically.

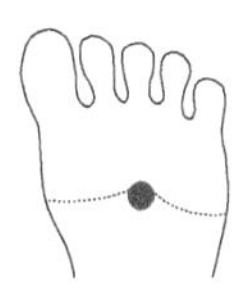

Bladder Meridian (Yang)

The bladder meridian starts at the inside corner of the eyes and bridge of the nose, follows up over the skull, down the back of the spine and the back of the legs, to the outer corner of the little toe. It is the longest meridian in the body.

The bladder holds the water in our body that is ready to be eliminated. It is also said to hold emotions until we are ready to release them.

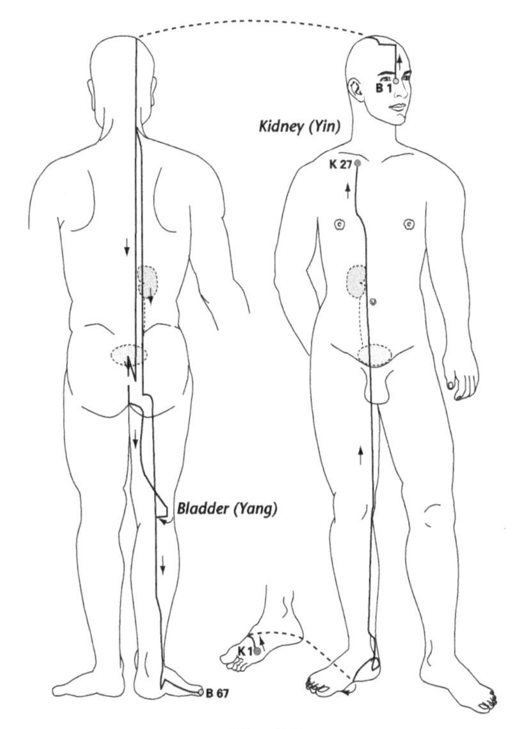

Fig 4.6
Kidney and bladder meridians

The bladder is also intimately related to our reproductive system due to its location in the pelvic cavity, in close proximity to the uterus or prostate.

Stimulation of the bladder point on the outer corner of the little toe (Bladder 67) has been shown to turn breech babies with a 40% success rate.

Winter Element—WATER

Water is the vital essence of all life on Earth, as well as in our body. The kidneys and bladder are the water organs of our body. The kidneys are responsible for filtering and balancing our fluids, while the bladder collects and releases them. Thus, the kidney and bladder meridians work to maintain fluid homeostasis in the body. The kidneys also work to balance the minerals in the body, which are essential to proper muscle function.

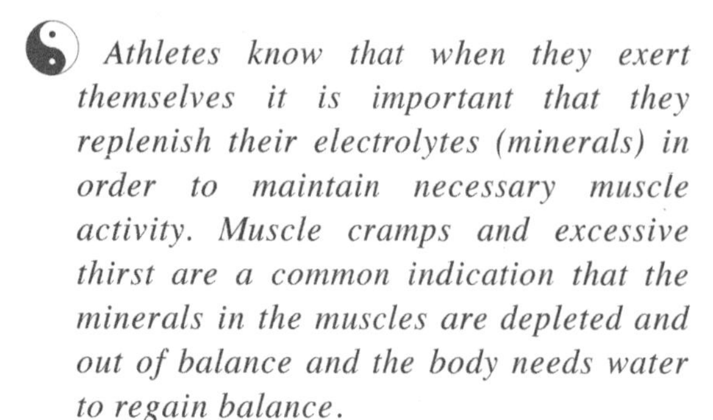
Athletes know that when they exert themselves it is important that they replenish their electrolytes (minerals) in order to maintain necessary muscle activity. Muscle cramps and excessive thirst are a common indication that the minerals in the muscles are depleted and out of balance and the body needs water to regain balance.

Winter Climate—COLD

As the temperatures drop in the winter, our body responds with its own changes. There is a desire for warmer foods, such as soups and teas that heat the body from within, in contrast to the cold outside. The cold climate gives the body and the earth a chance to rest. The cold brings quiet and a slower pace of life, which allows for introspective pursuits. Cold takes us deeper into ourselves.

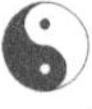
The bones are associated with the season of winter, hence the common saying "I feel it in my bones," reflecting the deep inner knowing about a situation.

Winter Emotion—FEAR

Historically, the winter months posed a real threat to survival, thus evoking the primal instinct to fear the season. Our ancestors would have feared not having enough food or heat to survive the winter. Worry and anxiety are also an aspect of fear. We become anxious and worried about the things we fear and that can stimulate the "fight or flight" response in our body. Living in this state of stress can lead to imbalances in our meridians. A balanced expression of fear would manifest as an ability to distinguish between a true and a perceived threat and then act accordingly.

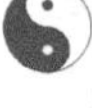
The "fight, flight or freeze" response to stress is triggered by the vagus nerve, the largest part of which runs through our solar plexus in the center of our chest. With a client who expresses fear and anxiety, consider using the solar plexus reflex point, which is also Kidney 1 in the meridian system. This point will calm and reduce anxiety. Fear can increase as we age. When

working with elderly clients, notice their emotional state. They may have a fear of falling, a fear of death, a fear of being alone. Stimulate Kidney 1 with some frequency during the session when you are working with elders.

Winter Sound—GROANING

Groaning is the natural sound we make as we settle into our quiet winter nights. It is the sound of finally being able to rest after a busy day. Bare trees groan when the cold winter winds whip through the woodland areas. We tend to groan more as we grow older.

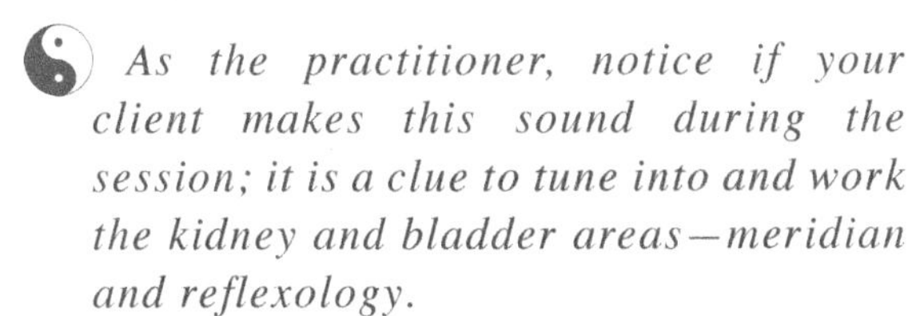

As the practitioner, notice if your client makes this sound during the session; it is a clue to tune into and work the kidney and bladder areas—meridian and reflexology.

Winter Taste—SALTY

Salt is an important component in food preservation that is necessary to sustain life through the winter. Soups are an excellent winter food, with salt being the seasoning that brings all the flavors together. The fluids in our body are extremely sensitive to and dependent on salt; too much or too little will create imbalances in the body. Salt can also be an excellent source of minerals, which are essential components to healthy cells. The kidneys are the vital organs that help to maintain the salt balance in our bodies.

Notice if your client tends to be swollen. You may ask yourself, is the swelling related to their salt intake? Swelling may also occur if the kidneys are out of balance and not processing fluid efficiently.

Winter Color—BLUE/BLACK

This is the color of the winter sky with its long, dark blue/black nights. The darkness of these colors reflects the depths of our soul, the depths of winter, and the depths of the ocean.

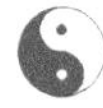

As the practitioner, you may notice what color clothing your client is currently wearing or tends to wear often. If they wear a lot of blue and/or black, focus in on the kidney reflexes and meridian points. This may seem like a silly connection to make, but this correlation can be true in both what the client wears and even the color of the foods that they are attracted to. Remember, it is a clue, not an absolute.

Winter Sense—HEARING

The organ of hearing, the ear, is thought to be the shape of a kidney. One can imagine the silence often associated with the winter—when the snow falls so quietly it is beautiful. In the silence of winter our hearing can seem more perceptive. The hearing sense often diminishes as we age into the winter of our life.

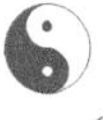

If your client presents with ear infections, earaches, ringing in the ear or diminished hearing, address the kidney reflex and meridian.

Winter Personality—PHILOSOPHER

Winter is a quiet time for retreating inward, spending time by the fire to contemplate life's mysteries. The philosopher ponders concepts and appreciates the stillness of quiet reflection. The philosopher often has a way with words, able to articulate his or her thoughts clearly. The winter is an excellent time for reading and writing since the more outward focused activities have slowed down. This personality is also reflected in the winter of our life cycle—the elder years. During this time in our lives, we slow down and look back on our life, gleaning the wisdom from what we have experienced. The elders are the ones who are able to quietly share their wisdom with the generations who follow.

My mother lived with anxiety, emotional outbursts and stress-related ulcers. She was also the first one to pick up the book I'm OK, You're OK, by Wayne Dyer. She was actually a frustrated philosopher. When I became aware of this through my study of the meridians, it completely changed how I approached my mother. I found I was able to calm her when I took a philosophical response to her outbursts. It was very healing for our relationship. She also never wore black, but always wore blue. She developed deafness and osteoporosis, both related to the winter element and the kidney and bladder meridians.

Time of PEAK ENERGY for the Winter meridians:

Bladder—3-5 pm

This tends to be a natural time for slowing down in the day. It is a good time to release fluids that have built up over the day. Workers often report feeling tired at this time of day and reaching for a caffeine drink that picks them up. One might try a cup of tea or warm liquids to transition in the flow of the day. You might feel better if you wait until this time of day to have your caffeine drink, rather than in the morning. The British may be on to something with their 4:00 teatime.

Kidney—5-7 pm

This is when we experience our last burst of energy as we enter into the evening period of the day. There is usually more activity as we transition from work to home and dinner preparations. The kidneys work with the adrenal glands where we produce the stress hormones. Kidneys are about balance, so this is an important time of day to be able to utilize personal resources in order to re-balance our system as it transitions into the evening. Many people utilize this time to manage stress through meditation or exercise.

Winter Meridian MUSCLES

Bladder Meridian:

ERECTORS

FIBULARIS (previously PERONEUS)

SACROSPINALIS

TIBIALIS ANTERIOR

TIBIALIS POSTERIOR

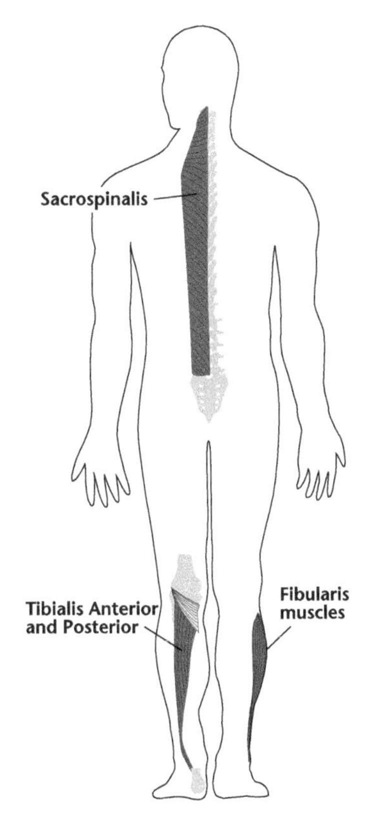

Fig 4.7
Muscles related to the bladder meridian

The bladder meridian flows along the path of these muscles. These lower leg muscles are common locations for night time muscle cramps. Sacrospinalis is closely associated with bladder problems (Dougans, 1992).

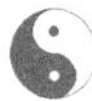 *Muscle cramps in the lower leg may be alleviated with an increase in magnesium and electrolytes.*

Kidney Meridian:

ILIACUS

PSOAS

TRAPEZIUS

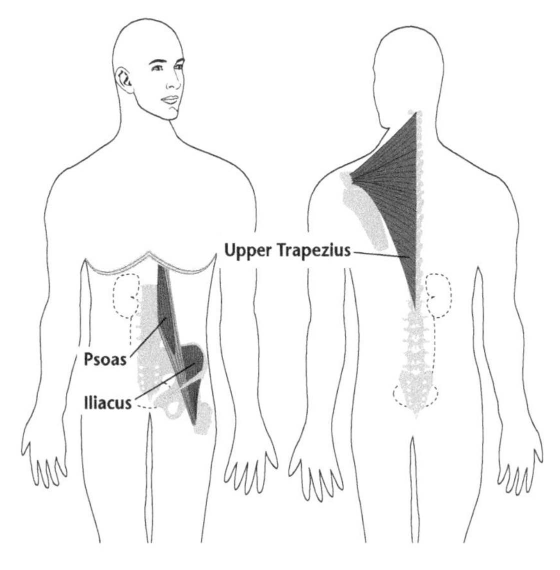

Fig 4.8
Muscles related to the kidney meridian

The iliopsoas (iliacus and psoas combined) is called the hydrating muscle and runs along the ureter, from the kidney to the bladder. It is also related to the flexor hallicus longus muscle on the foot. Plantar fasciitis can present in this muscle on the foot, implying that dehydration may play a role in the client's condition. You may recommend to your clients that they begin to notice if drinking more water/fluids during the day helps to alleviate their plantar fasciitis symptoms.

Notice that the psoas originates in the area of the solar plexus. You will learn in the next chapter that the solar plexus is also home to the vagus nerve, which plays a role in the fight, flight or freeze response in our body. Chronic stress and fear can be connected with a chronically tight psoas muscle, which can impact flow through the kidneys, both the organs and the meridian.

NOTE—The techniques for massaging along the reflex areas of the kidney, ureter and bladder are gentle in order to protect the flexor hallicus longus tendon. It is also suggested that the practitioner be gentle when doing massage in the area around the actual kidneys.

Spring Season

The season of spring is enlivening and all about new beginnings. As Mother Nature's new year, this time of year assaults all of our senses with new growth. As the weather warms, we become more active. It is the season for fertility as practiced in ancient times. We sow seeds that will become the autumn harvest. It is the time when we initiate new plans that have been developing through the cold winter months. With spring comes new awakenings and new potentials for creativity.

Liver Meridian (Yin)

The liver meridian runs from the inner great toe up the medial leg, across the groin to the ribs directly below the breast and in line with the nipple. The liver organ performs a multitude of functions—metabolizing food and hormones, cleansing blood, making and distributing bile. In this way, it is the command center for the regulation of bodily functions.

Gallbladder Meridian (Yang)

The gallbladder meridian begins at the outer corner of the eye and moves along the sides of the head, continuing in a zig-zag pattern down the lateral sides of the body to the outer corner of the fourth toe. As an organ, the gallbladder stores and

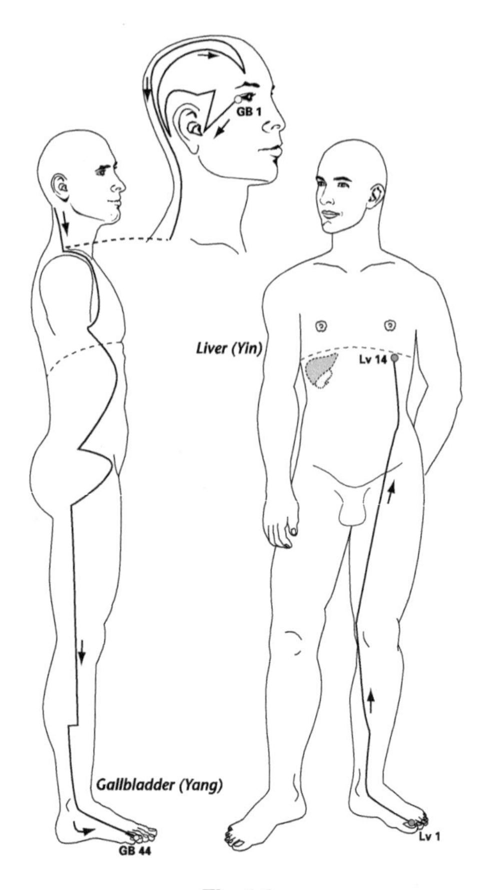

Fig 4.9
Liver and gallbladder meridians

releases bile, which is the substance that breaks down fats and aids in the digestion of fatty acids. The gallbladder meridian is said to be the one to carry out the orders of the liver commander.

According to the Nei Ching, the gallbladder rules decisions. So, angry, rash decisions may indicate an excess in the gallbladder meridian while indecision and timidity could be due to deficient energy in this meridian (Dougans, 1992).

Spring Element—WOOD

The element of wood represents new growth. The most obvious example of this new growth is the wood of the trees starting a new growth spurt in the spring. Wood also represents the strength and flexibility that trees exhibit in their constant goal of growth and expansion.

Spring Climate—WIND

The spring season comes roaring in like a lion with windy weather. It is also the tornado season. The winds of change are upon us in the spring, whether it be from our external or internal environment. Conditions of the body, such as burping frequently and being gassy, are described as having 'excess wind.' This can indicate an imbalance in the liver and/or gallbladder meridians.

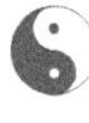

As a practitioner, the existence of excess gas would be a quality you would take note of in your assessment and then implement in your treatment plan by working with the liver and gallbladder meridians and reflex areas.

Spring Emotion—ANGER

This is an emotion that precipitates change. When we get angry, we know we are ready to grow and release what is holding us back. Spring is the season of chaos and revolutions. The windy climate may make us irritable with changes that come too quickly or violently. It is wise to take care with anger in the spring season as it may get out of control.

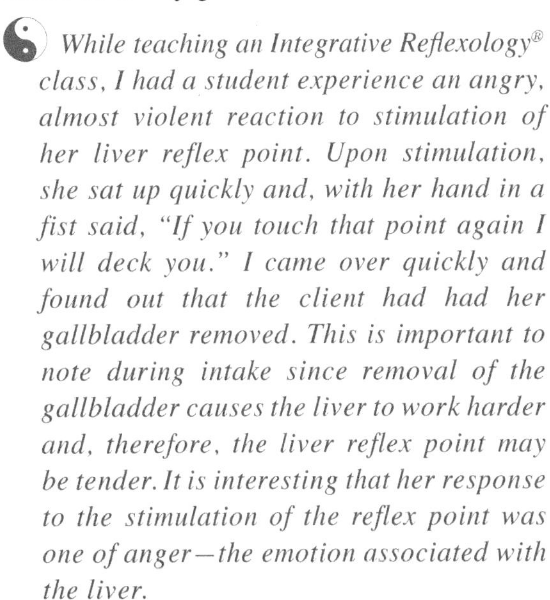

While teaching an Integrative Reflexology® class, I had a student experience an angry, almost violent reaction to stimulation of her liver reflex point. Upon stimulation, she sat up quickly and, with her hand in a fist said, "If you touch that point again I will deck you." I came over quickly and found out that the client had had her gallbladder removed. This is important to note during intake since removal of the gallbladder causes the liver to work harder and, therefore, the liver reflex point may be tender. It is interesting that her response to the stimulation of the reflex point was one of anger—the emotion associated with the liver.

Spring Sound—SHOUTING

Shouting is the obvious sound associated with anger and is a way of getting the anger out. We shout to be heard, perhaps to announce that change is happening. Shouting can allow us to express our passions. Shouting is not necessarily a negative form of expression. Sometimes we feel so alive we simply want to shout our joy to the world. In order to maintain balance in our bodies, all of our emotions need an outlet. Holding in our emotions creates tension and imbalance in our bodies.

Spring Taste—SOUR

Lemons are an excellent example of a sour food that is beneficial for cleansing in the spring. Vinegar and fermented foods that support healthy flora for our gut also have a sour taste. Doing a spring cleanse is highly recommended. A popular spring cleanse is lemon, maple syrup and cayenne. Sour foods are both alkaline and calming for the body, which can be a good balance if our anger is rising and our body is responding to that energy with more acidity.

Spring Color—GREEN

This association is evident in the beautiful green color that emerges out of winter as the grass and trees begin their new growth. Green vegetables are abundant in the spring, as the first growth in the garden. The food that grows green is the best food to clear the congestion of winter. Greens such as spinach, kale, Swiss chard and collards are also considered to be beneficial for the renewal of the liver and gallbladder organs. The color green also represents fertility. It is a happy and joyous color promising new growth for all of us.

Spring Sense—SIGHT

There are plenty of details to stimulate our sight in the spring with all the buds on the trees and flowers beginning to color the landscape. Clear vision allows us to start off on the right foot with whatever new endeavor we are pursuing. On the other hand, being blind with anger can cause a person to inaccurately assess a situation. Making willful and angry decisions is usually not a positive way to make change. In our bodies, when the liver is congested, our vision can be impaired, thus, many eye complaints can be related to the liver.

With liver cleanses, or detoxing in general, you may notice your eyesight becoming clearer. My husband is a Sun Dancer on the Pine Ridge reservation in South Dakota. Each time that he has done the full four-day fast, dance and sweat with the Sun Dance, he has noticed that his eyesight is greatly improved. For a month afterward he does not need reading glasses.

Spring Personality—COMMANDER

The commander embodies a strong, assertive personality that is capable of being heard and taking initiative. This person has the ability to shout out orders. People with this personality embody the awakening energy of springtime in that they are often highly energetic themselves, ready to take action where it is needed. The commander has a vision and can become angered if something stands in the way of manifesting that vision. At the same time, the commander has the patience to see a vision through to completion and take the action steps necessary to achieve a goal.

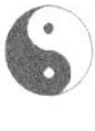

Notice the clients in your practice who tend to demand what they would like to receive in the session. It would be wise to carefully stimulate the liver and gallbladder points on these clients and see how they react.

Time of PEAK ENERGY for the Spring meridians:

Gallbladder—11 pm—1 am

This time is when the gallbladder is processing the fats we have ingested throughout the day. It is generally best to be asleep while this process is taking place. Often, those who are night owls will have a gallbladder either strong or weak in its function and perhaps an imbalance in the gallbladder meridian.

Liver—1-3 am

This is a beneficial time to be resting and allowing the liver to process and clear all that has passed through it during the day. A strong liver translates into a strong body. We cannot live without our liver. An imbalanced liver meridian can manifest as someone who prefers to be consuming alcohol during this time of the night, thereby taxing his or her liver during its peak hours, rather than allowing it to rest and rejuvenate.

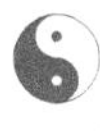

In my former career, I was an x-ray tech working the 12 midnight—8 am weekend shift in Baltimore. The 1-3 am time slot was inevitably full of alcohol-related auto accidents.

Spring Meridian MUSCLES

Liver Meridian:

PECTORALIS MAJOR

RHOMBOIDS

These are the muscles used when releasing anger in the form of boxing or punching. They are also the muscles that can convey a sense of being in charge, being a commander with your shoulders pulled back and standing in military attention.

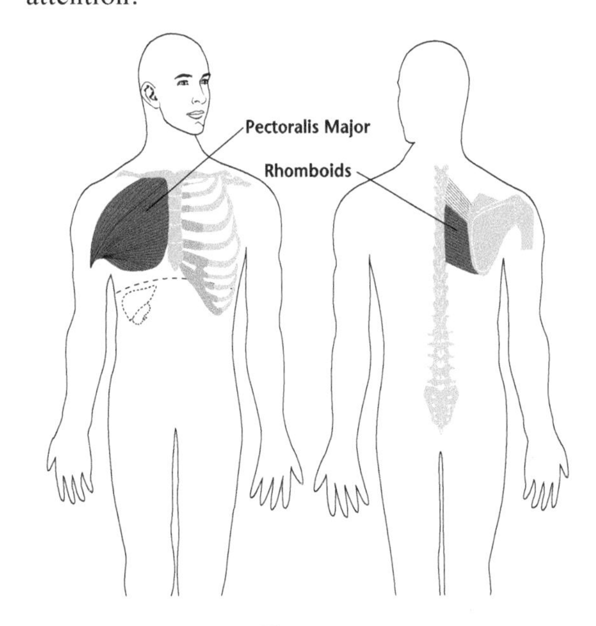

Fig 4.10
Muscles related to the liver meridian

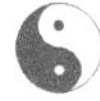

I have also found that clients who tend toward holding anger have chronic rhomboid pain between the shoulder blades. They have their backs up. This is again an indication to work the liver reflex point and the rhomboid area on the body.

Gallbladder Meridian:
ANTERIOR DELTOID
POPLITEUS

These are the muscles used when holding your ground, being unwilling to budge. It is very easy for the muscles and tendons associated with these two meridians to be inflexible. A lot of tension can be held if a person becomes willful and unable to go with the flow. There is a distinction here between strength that is flexible and strength that is rigid and unyielding. For the liver and gallbladder meridians, balance equates to strength with flexibility.

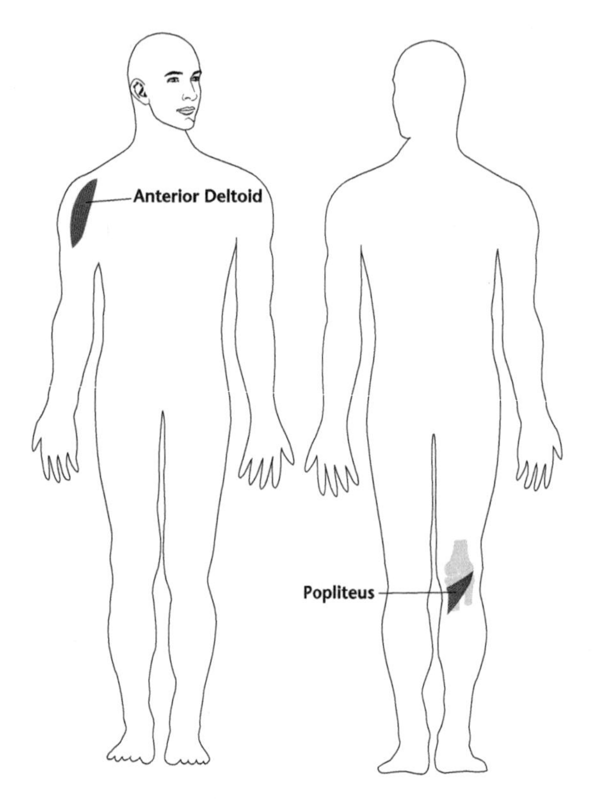

Fig 4.11
Muscles related to the gallbladder meridian

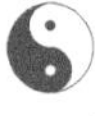

It has been interesting to notice so many of my students who have had their gallbladder removed also tend to lock their knees. This would be an observation you would want to note in your client—if they lock their knees, check to see if the gallbladder reflex point is tender.

Summer Season

Summer is a season full of energy and activity. It is a time when people are out in the community, gathering at parks and open spaces, enjoying the long days. This is the season when the sun's heat is at its peak and the sun's light is long lasting. It is a time of active growth—gardens and farmers markets overflow with an abundance of foods and flavors. The weekends are full of music festivals and street fairs. There is so much to do in the summer and the energy of the season carries our bodies through busy schedules with ease. The summer season in Chinese medicine is home to four meridians, rather than two—the heart meridian is paired with the small intestine meridian and the pericardium meridian is paired with the triple warmer meridian. The meridians for summer are all located on the hands rather than the feet. So it is necessary to include hand reflexology to stimulate these meridians for your client.

Heart Meridian (Yin)

The heart meridian begins in the axilla and continues down the inner arm, ending at the inner corner of the fifth finger, toward the ring finger. The heart organ pumps all the blood and life force energy through our bodies. The heart meridian is the energetic center that rules all we do for "love."

 *Martial Arts instructors have taught that if a person is having a heart attack, or similar event, then you should gently bite the little finger at the nail bed to stop the heart attack. I would still call emergency first!*

Small Intestine Meridian (Yang)

The small intestine meridian begins on the outside tip of the little finger and extends up the outside of the arm, around the back of the shoulder and shoulder blade, up the side of the neck, around to the cheek and outer corner of the eye, and ends at the ear. The small intestine meridian may seem like an unlikely partner to the heart meridian. But, without the powerful assimilation of nutrients that occurs in the small intestine, all other organs will slowly lose their vitality. The heart is the pump that moves all of the important nutrients absorbed in the small intestine throughout the body via the blood and plasma.

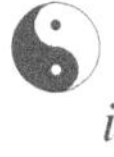 *Research into the role of the small intestine in both heart and brain function is currently expanding in health care. The small intestine is often called the "second brain." There are more neuro-receptors and increased serotonin production in this vital organ then in the actual brain. There are also immune cells in the small intestine called Peyer's patches that support our immune system based on the food we ingest.*

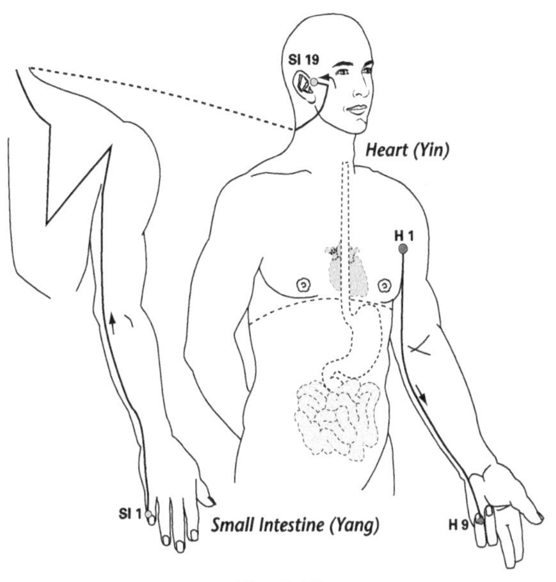

Fig 4.12
Heart and small intestine meridians

Pericardium Meridian (Yin)

This meridian is also called circulation/sex meridian. The pericardium meridian begins along the lateral side of the nipple and extends down the middle of the inner surface of the arm, to the middle finger. This meridian is associated with activity that increases circulation, especially sexual activity.

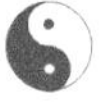 *Sex does get the heart pumping. Much of the medication used for increasing sexual ability is actually increasing general circulation.*

Triple Warmer Meridian (Yang)

The triple warmer meridian begins at the nail bed of the fourth finger, continues up the outside of the arm, over the shoulder, up the side of the neck, and around the back of the ear, to the ending point at the outer edge of the eyebrow.

The triple warmer is a unique meridian in that it is not connected to a specific organ. Rather, it refers to an energy system that regulates three physiological functions in the body. It regulates the functions of intake/respiration, digestion, and elimination so that all are working in harmony and balance for good health. Each of these functions is described as a "burner" or "cooker" for the food that is transformed into energy for the body. These "burners" are associated with one of the body's three main cavities: thorax, abdomen and pelvis. The thorax houses the function of intake/respiration. The abdomen houses the function of digestion/transformation and the pelvis houses the function of elimination.

Summer Element—FIRE

Fire represents both the heat of the day (noontime), the heat of the year (summer), and the heat of passion that fuels the summer meridians. The heat within the body is created with the circulation of blood through all the organs. The heart and the pericardium are the pumps that move the blood.

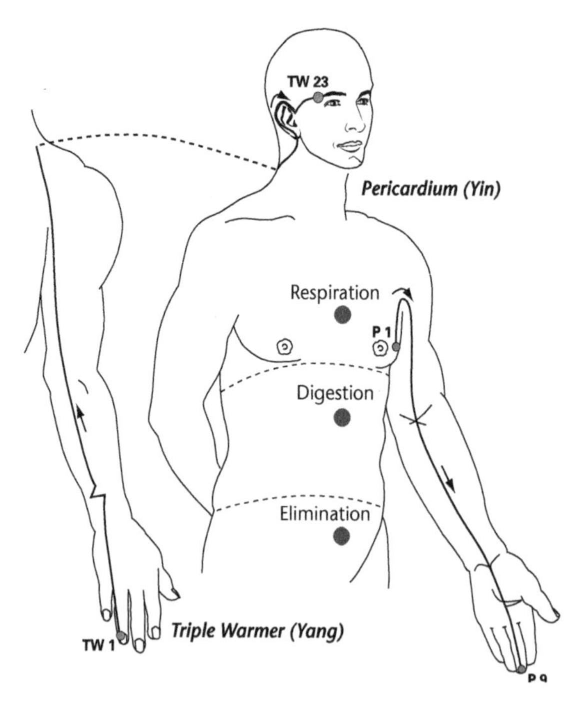

Fig 4.13
Pericardium and triple warmer meridians

Summer Climate—HEAT

The sun is at its full peak in the summer, with longs days of heat that are maintained through the night. We work hard in the summer, an appropriate amount of sweating and working in the heat can be cleansing to the body.

The four meridians for the summer season all create heat in the body. The heart pumping moves the blood (blood is heat), cooking the food in the small intestine to transport the nutrients into the blood. The pericardium assists the heart and the triple warmer is activated through physical movement that reduces stagnation in the blood.

Summer Emotion—LOVE

Love is the emotion of heat and passion, happiness and joy. It is the emotion that fuels our desire to connect with all living things. The summer is often a light-hearted, joyful time of the year when the worries of winter seem far away as we enjoy the fruits of our labor. Our love flows easily as we gather in our community. Love is an obvious fit with the heart and pericardium meridians. It is easy to be swept away with love in the warm, light summer months.

Summer Sound—LAUGHTER

Laughing is the joyous sound that accompanies the energy and activity of summer. It is also heart-healthy to laugh often. Laughing increases circulation and warmth, as well as immune responses that benefit the whole body. Laughing opens our heart and allows us to connect with others in love.

Think back to a time when you laughed so hard that your belly hurt. That form of cleansing laughter works all the way into your body, stimulating the small intestine. It can also get your bladder going!

Summer Taste—BITTER

In Chinese medicine, the bitter taste is one that can clear excessive heat from the body. Bitter greens and other bitter vegetables are good for balancing excess heat. The summer heat will cause spring greens to bolt and become bitter tasting. Bitter [illegible]
chocolate, thought [illegible]
both physically and emo[illegible]

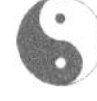

Love is the emotion of th[illegible]
often called bittersweet. Notic[illegible]
feel a sense of love so strong it fee[illegible]
sweet.

Summer Sense—TASTE

There are so many foods that grow in abundance during the summer to satisfy our taste buds. The berries of summer—strawberries, blueberries, raspberries, blackberries, cherries and more—are stimulating for both the tongue and the brain. Berries have more antioxidants than any other foods we consume and are considered to be excellent for the heart and the brain.

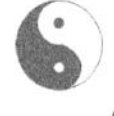

Summer is the season with the most flavorful foods. The tip of the tongue is where we get this first burst of flavor. When eating, we often have a tendency to pay less attention to the flavor of our food, and eat to fill our bellies rather than to stimulate our senses.

Summer Color—RED

The color red represents so much about summer, fire, love and the heart. Many foods of summer are red in color. The heart is full of red, oxygenated blood and strong red muscle cells. Love and passion are expressed with the color red.

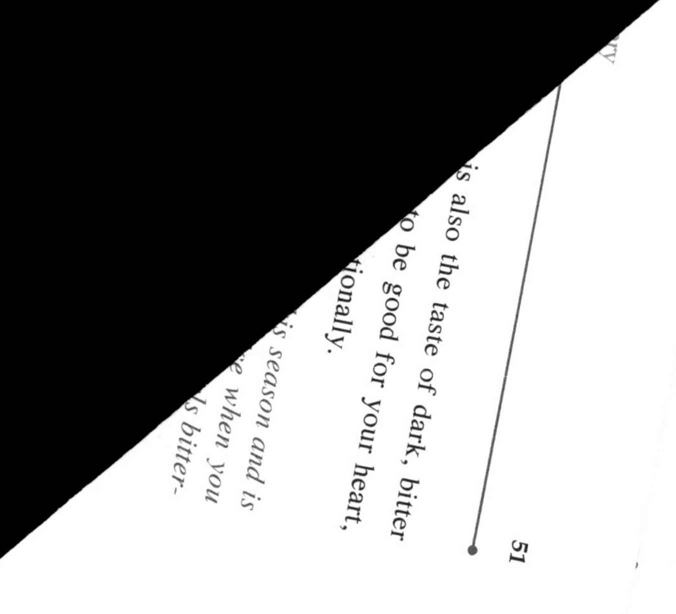

Time o...
Summer meridians:

Heart Meridian—11 am–1 pm

Historically, this was often the time that families would gather and share a big, midday meal. Sharing food releases oxytocin, the hormone that bonds us together through the energy of love. This time of day may be a great time to exercise for those with strong heart energy.

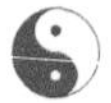 *Lunchtime exercise keeps you heart healthy!*

Small Intestine Meridian—1-3 pm

This is siesta time in many cultures, where rest and digestion of the parasympathetic system is in full swing. The small intestine is the organ for the digestion and assimilation of our food. In our modern culture, we rarely take the time for full digestion of our food. This extends into all areas of our lives, where we rush from one activity to the next, not allowing time for full digestion of the information and experiences we are encountering. This fast-paced lifestyle could be at the heart of many of our health problems.

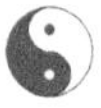 *In many countries, such as Spain, everything shuts down from 1-3 pm, after the main meal of the day. This is a natural way to digest our food and enjoy our life at a slower pace.*

Pericardium Meridian—7-9 pm

The pericardium meridian is also called the circulation and sex meridian. Before electricity was invented, it was during this time of the evening that couples often made love before retiring for the night. It is also a great time to take an evening walk, another way to exercise the heart muscle.

Triple Warmer Meridian—9-11 pm

This is when the three burners are turned on and complete the process of food digestion and elimination. This time is considered the best time to begin your night's sleep. The heavy, relaxed breathing that accompanies your sleep state supports the process of the three burners and the final process of elimination that comes in the morning with the large intestine (5:00-7:00am).

Summer Meridian MUSCLES

Heart Meridian:

SUBSCAPULARIS

The subscapularis muscle is just deep to the scapula and near the heart.

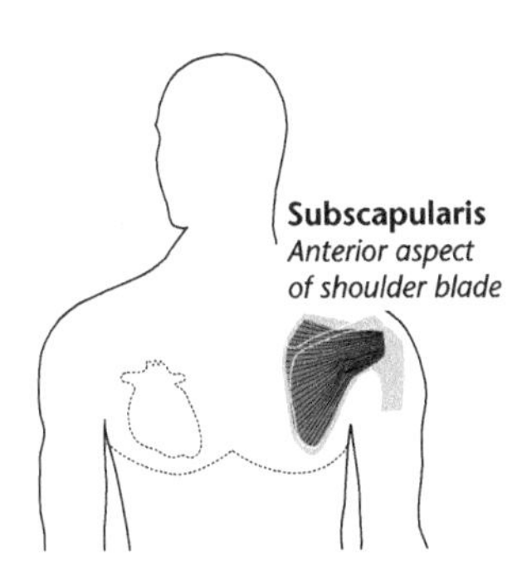

Fig 4.14
Muscles related to the heart meridian

Small Intestine Meridian:

EXTERNAL OBLIQUE

INTERNAL OBLIQUE

QUADRICEPS FEMORIS

RECTUS ABDOMINIS

TRANSVERSE ABDOMINIS

We know in modern medicine that having strong abdominals and a fit waistline often indicate a healthy heart.

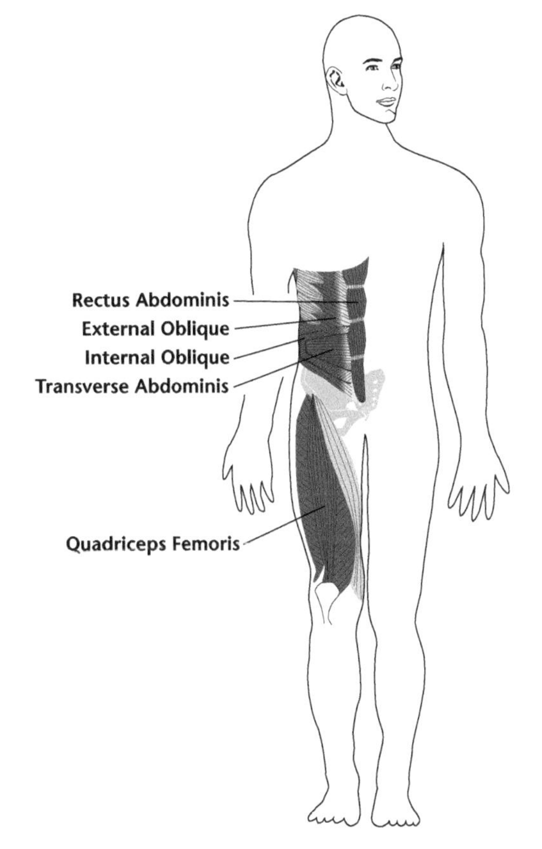

Fig 4.15
Muscles related to the small intestine meridian

Pericardium Meridian:

ADDUCTORS
GLUTEUS MAXIMUS
PIRIFORMIS

These are the muscles used for exercise, dancing and lovemaking. All three activities will strengthen the heart muscle and support the pericardium.

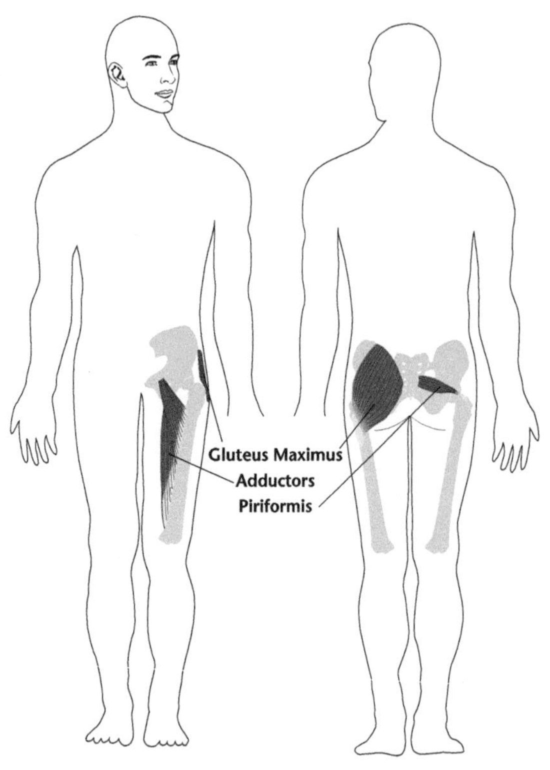

Fig 4.16
Muscles related to the pericardium meridian

Triple Warmer Meridian:

GASTROCNEMIUS
GRACILIS
SARTORIUS
SOLEUS
TERES MINOR

These are all muscles that support movement and will increase the functions of the three burners. As we move, the first burner of respiration increases oxygen uptake. The oxygen fuels the fire of digestion, the second burner. Digestion burns through the food in our body creating waste and activating peristalsis that leads to elimination, the third burner.

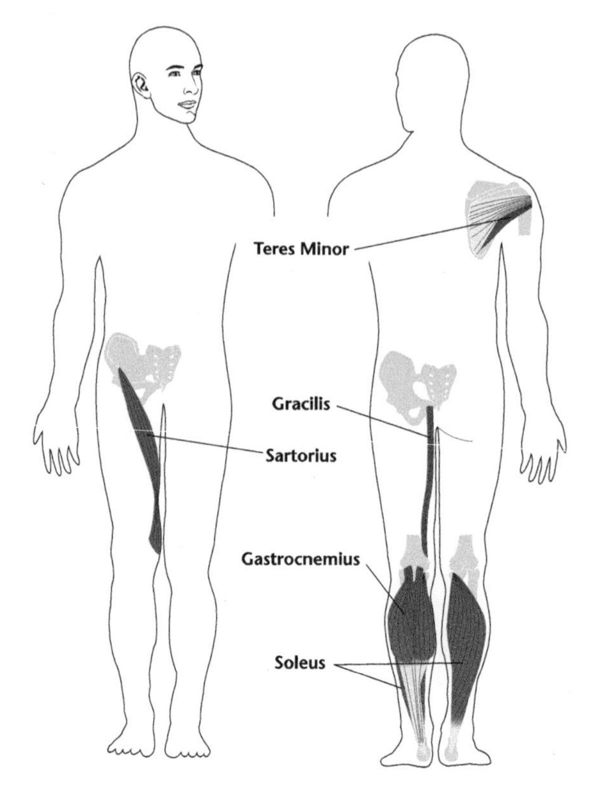

Fig 4.17
Muscles related to the triple warmer meridian

Late Summer Season

This late summer season is usually considered to be around the time summer ends and before autumn begins. This is usually a harvest time, with great abundance of pumpkins and many varieties of squash. The weather is shifting as we move into another important transition. This season can represent any important transition in a person's life journey.

Spleen/Pancreas Meridian (Yin)

The spleen meridian begins at the great toe on the inner corner of the nail bed. It continues along the inside edge of the foot, up the inner ankle and inner leg, across the inguinal area of the groin, and up the abdomen to the inner armpit area.

The spleen organ is the only organ in the lymphatic system. It supports all autoimmune functions. The spleen meridian is also connected with the pancreas and its hormonal secretions.

 *When the pancreas reflex point on the right foot is more tender, it represents the head of the pancreas and is related more to digestion. When the pancreas reflex point on the left foot is more tender, it represents the tail of the pancreas and is related more to hormones and the immune system.*

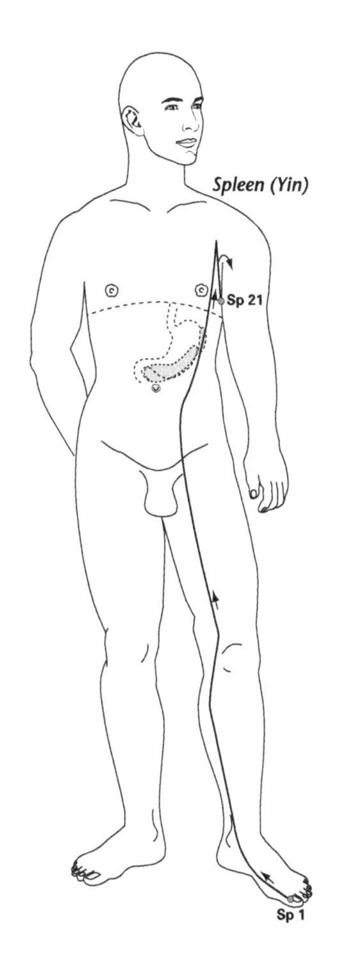

Fig 4.18
Spleen/pancreas meridian

Stomach Meridian (Yang)

The stomach meridian begins on the face just below the eye and travels down the front of the neck, across the chest and the nipple, down the abdomen, across the hip flexors, down the center of anterior thigh, along the outer edge of the knee and lateral edge of the calf muscles to end on the outer edge of the 2nd toe.

The stomach energy is activated when we see our food. Digestion begins with salivation and continues with chewing our food and mixing it with saliva before it is cooked in our stomach with the acids that breakdown the particles of food.

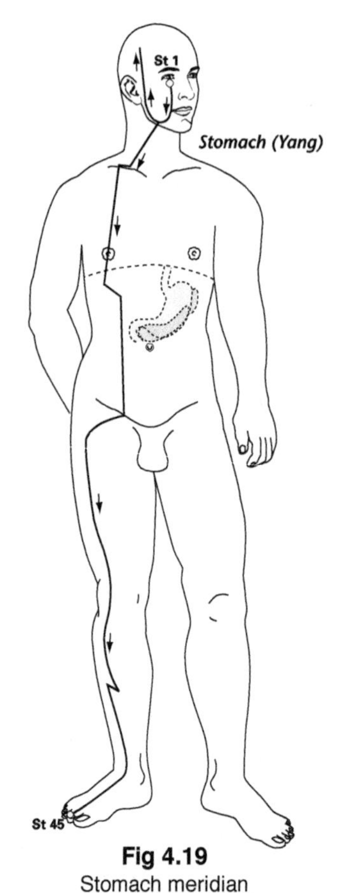

Fig 4.19
Stomach meridian

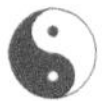 *The stomach meridian is important since food is critical to both the physical and emotional aspects of our health.*

Late Summer Element—EARTH

This is the time when the harvest is in full bloom and we reap the rewards of the earth. It is the time of giving thanks for the abundance of the earth. We also begin to preserve and store food and wood for the coming of autumn and winter. Earth is the grounded stillness that supports the space between seasons and activities. Mother Earth is a consistent resource, she is stable and solid and always available.

Late Summer Climate—HUMIDITY

This is the climate just before the dry season emerges. The tightness in the air of late summer is broken up by cooler mornings. This season is considered a transitional season, as climates move back and forth from hot to cool and wet to dry. In Chinese medicine, this season rules all seasonal transitions. Whenever weather shifts back and forth, the immune system is challenged, which is where balance in the late summer meridians can be supportive.

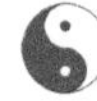 *As a practitioner, notice the weather patterns and how they effect your client's immune system. The changing weather often brings an increase in colds, sinus infections and viruses. You can stimulate spleen and lymphatic areas to strengthen the immune system.*

Late Summer Emotions—WORRY and EMPATHY

The emotion associated with the late summer season may be related to the human need to nurture and feed our family. This is most often related to the mother's energy—to take care of and protect her children. The mother's energy will also worry about her children and family—do they have enough to eat, are they safe, how can I protect them? Empathy is exhibited when we are aware of how our children are feeling. As a mother, you listen for signals in the baby's cry that it is hungry, or needing to be changed or held. This is an innate empathic skill we all have, but mothers or those who like to mother others have it in abundance. This energy can also lead to over-mothering, over-protecting and over-nurturing. Chronic worry will weaken the immune system. As with all areas of our emotional nature, balance is the key.

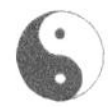 *Stress in any form is an immune suppressor.*

Late Summer Sound—SINGING

Singing boosts the immune system by activating the 200-300 lymph nodes in the neck, more than any other area of the body. Singing is also very beneficial for moving toxins out of the neck. A sore throat is often the body's first indication of illness and the need to slow down.

 *If the client presents with a sore throat, work the throat reflex and open the lymph area on the top of the foot. You can also work the spleen reflex point to support and strengthen the immune system.*

Late Summer Personality—PEACEMAKER

This is the person who tends to feed and nurture others. The peacemaker is considerate, sympathetic and thoughtful, always willing to share and help out. The peacemaker wants to provide everyone with what they need and find a fair solution for all. The imbalance to this personality is when one takes care of others too much, at the detriment to their own needs. This can take its toll on the immune system and lead to excessive worry, which creates more stress and imbalance.

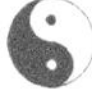 *An important meridian point is Spleen 6 on the inner leg just above the ankle. It is considered to be one of the most powerful acupressure points to stimulate the immune system for the whole body. It can also help relieve menstrual cramps.*

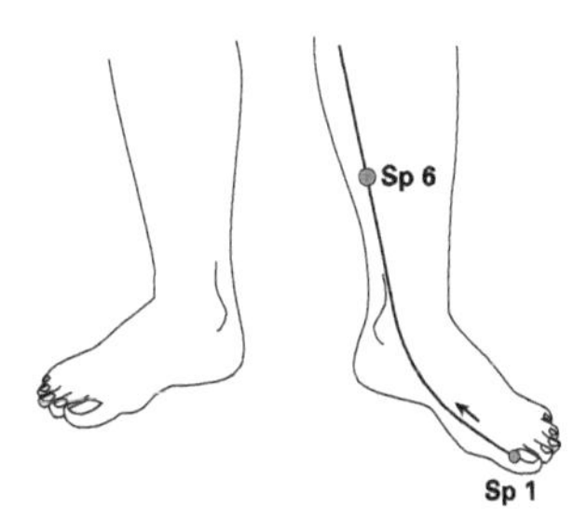

Fig 4.18a - Spleen 6

Late Summer Colors—YELLOW, ORANGE AND BROWN

These colors are seen in the changing leaves of the season. The colorful leaves are one of the most prominent indicators of transition in our environment. The foods of the season also reflect these colors with pumpkins, squash and sweet potatoes.

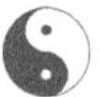 *This is a strong color palate that many respond to. We all have a boost in energy when we see the fall colors of Mother Earth in all her glory.*

Late Summer Taste—SWEET

Foods that are harvested in late summer are apples, pumpkins, squashes, sweet potatoes, and corn. These foods have a natural sweetness to them that supports balancing the blood sugars and may help prevent diabetes. On the other hand, the overconsumption of sugar can lead to autoimmune disorders and diabetes.

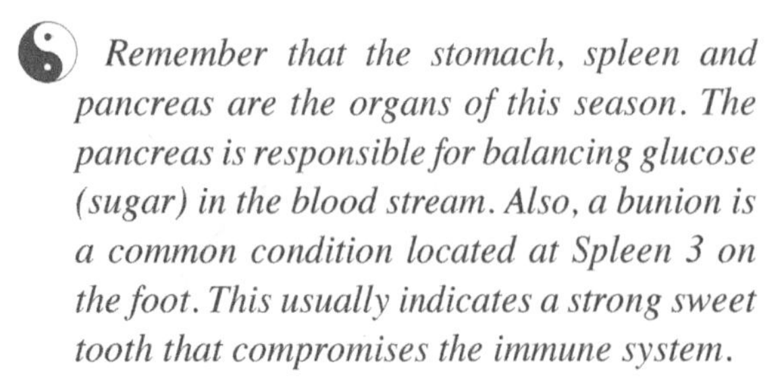

Remember that the stomach, spleen and pancreas are the organs of this season. The pancreas is responsible for balancing glucose (sugar) in the blood stream. Also, a bunion is a common condition located at Spleen 3 on the foot. This usually indicates a strong sweet tooth that compromises the immune system.

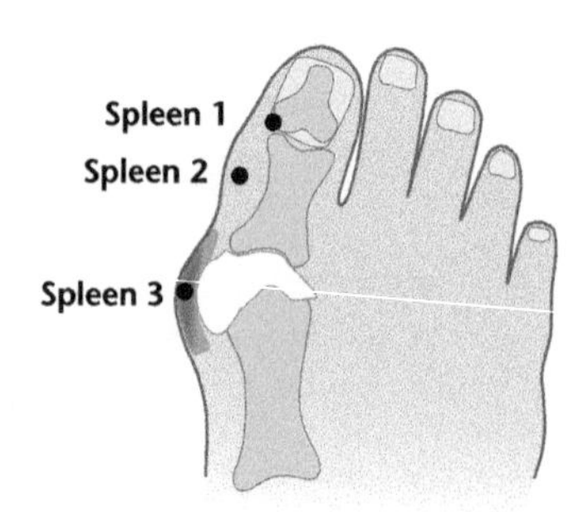

Fig 6.2
The spleen meridian points associated with a bunion

Late Summer Sense—TOUCH

The sense of touch is strong in people who are natural nurturers, like those in the hands-on healing professions such as reflexology and massage therapy. Touch is the first sense developed in utero. Studies have shown that humans and mammals, in general, will not thrive or perhaps even survive without touch.

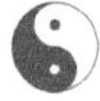 *While attending a conference, I noticed a strong trend for the massage therapists to head toward the sugary snack. As a profession of caregivers, we often need to be on the alert for how we are nurturing ourselves.*

Times of PEAK ENERGY for the Late Summer meridians

Spleen/Pancreas Meridian—9-11 am

This is the time for digesting our healthy, energy rich breakfast and establishing our energy for the day.

Stomach Meridian—7-9 am

This is when we generally have breakfast. By having a healthy, protein-rich breakfast the blood sugars tend to stay balanced, which supports a healthy functioning of the immune system for the day.

Late Summer Meridian MUSCLES

Spleen Meridian:

EXTENSOR POLLICIS LONGUS
LATISSIMUS DORSI
TRAPEZIUS
TRICEPS

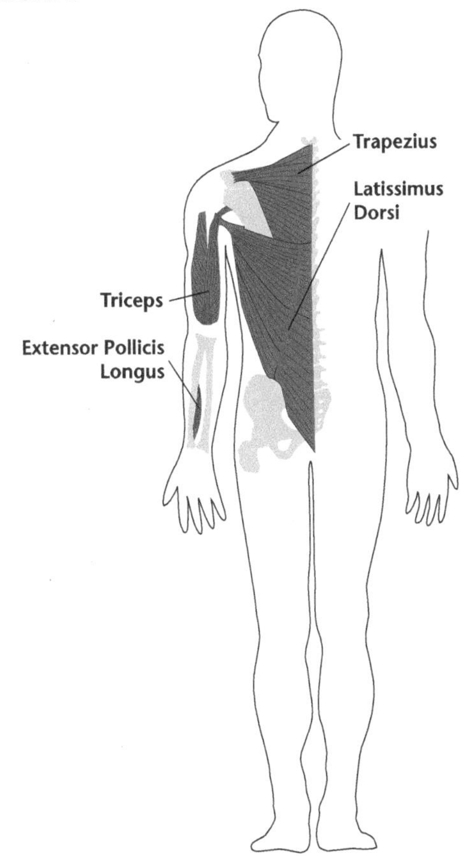

Fig 4.20
Muscles related to the spleen/pancreas meridian

For chronic neck pain, you can work the great toe with a slow gentle traction. This may bring the relief with tight neck muscles. Try it and see if this works for your client.

Stomach Meridian:

BRACHIORADIALIS
LEVATOR SCAPULA
NECK MUSCLES
PECTORALIS MAJOR

The muscles associated with the spleen/pancreas and stomach meridians are primarily in the upper body region and support much of the lymphatic system and the lymph nodes that are in the neck (200-300) and chest area. Keeping these muscle strong, flexible and relatively free of tension will support the final movement of the lymphatic fluid through the nodes and out of the body as fluid waste.

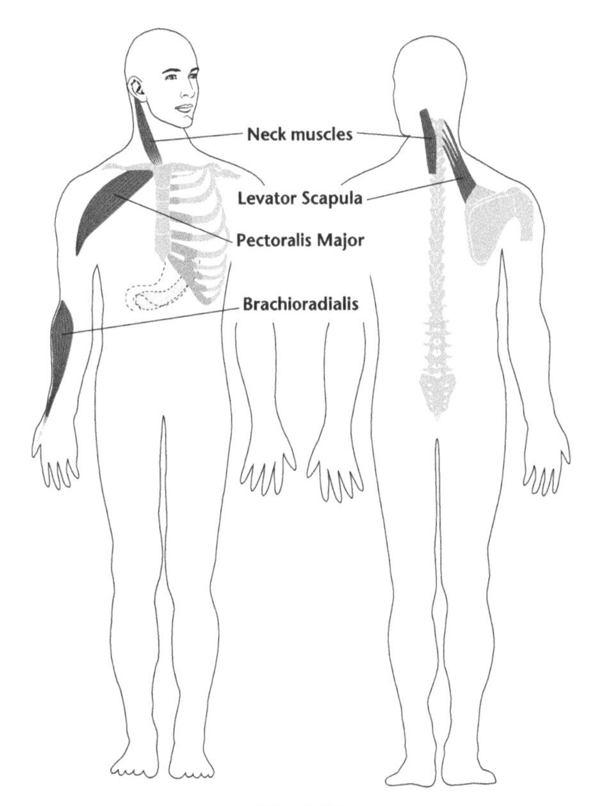

Fig 4.21
Muscles related to the stomach meridian

...clusion

...g the meridians ...our practice

...flexology® method uses the five elements approach, with the meridian system, as an observation tool to gain insight into the client's state of well-being. The first step in applying this information in your practice is to notice where this information fits for yourself, then for your family and friends, and finally, you will begin to make connections with your clients. The meridian assessment will be revealing and fascinating to help you focus on the areas in the body that need attention and to support your clients in creating greater balance and health in their lives.

In an Integrative Reflexology® session, you would observe the finger and toes as indicators of imbalances within your client's system since these are the areas where the meridians begin and end. Refer to the art and text in this book for the location of the meridians on each toe and finger. Observe the nail beds, looking for hangnails, cuts, ridges and discoloration. Consider past history of fractures, in-grown toenails, pain, swelling, malformation of the toes and/or fingers and other abnormalities. Make notes on the correlations you notice between what you observe on the hands, feet, fingers, toes and reflexology points, and what the client has shared with you about his or her health history and personal qualities. While we do not diagnose disease in their body, we can pay attention to the body's indicators of what may be out of balance. If I notice symptoms indicating a possible health concern, I usually bring this to their attention. Always remember, this is a very general assessment of observations, not a diagnosis.

Think of yourself as a detective as you give the Integrative Reflexology® session, also as an educator for your client, and finally as a facilitator for health and healing. Remember, you are finding clues to support your client's journey of balance and good health. By educating them about what you are doing, you empower them to notice these qualities in themselves, thus facilitating their ability to maintain balance within their system on a daily basis.

If the concepts of meridians and chi are new to you, I suggest that you read the books listed under Meridian Theory in Recommended Reading (page 178). As research into your own meridian system, you might consider contacting a local acupuncturist who has been trained in Chinese medicine. Receiving an acupuncture session will help you tune in to the flow of chi in your own meridians. This personal experience will help you to better communicate the meridian theory to your clients.

Meridian Exercise
Do-In

Do-In is an easy self-massage exercise that you can do as a daily routine. It is stimulating for the meridians and it can help you embody the knowledge of where the meridian pathways are located. Using simple percussion techniques along the meridians, you can start or end your day on a refreshing note.

It is recommended that this exercise be done on an empty stomach. Prepare yourself by sitting up straight in a chair or sitting on the floor. Your wrist should be loose as you gently beat along the specified lines with a loose fist. If you are confused about where to percuss for each meridian, refer to the pictures of the meridians until you are able to clarify this.

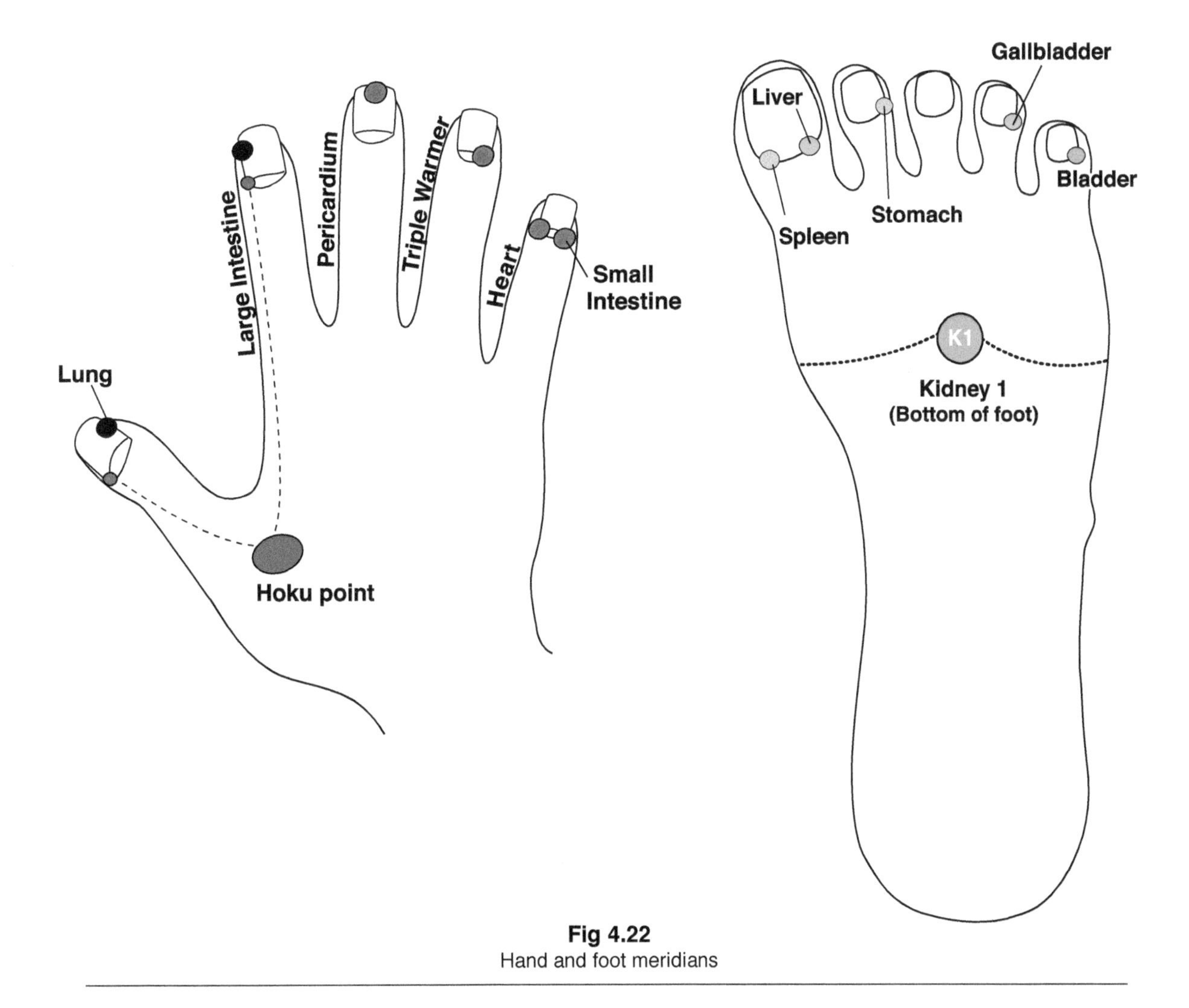

Fig 4.22
Hand and foot meridians

NOTE: This self-massage is demonstrated on the Integrative Reflexology® DVD (See products on page 181).

1. ***Lung Meridian (down the arm)***
   Your left arm is resting palm up on your knee. Begin the percussion beating at the soft depression below the clavicle, continue down the outside of the arm to the thumb.
2. ***Large Intestine Meridian (up the arm)***
   Turn the hand palm down and percuss up, beginning at the index finger, and continue up the inside of the arm to the shoulder.
3. ***Pericardium Meridian (down the arm)***
   Turn the palm up, percuss down the middle of the arm to the middle finger.
4. ***Triple Warmer Meridian (up the arm)***
   Turn the palm down, percuss up the ring finger, and continue up the middle of the arm to the shoulder.
5. ***Heart Meridian (down the arm)***
   With the palm up, percuss down the inside of the arm from the shoulder area to the inner side of the little finger.
6. ***Small Intestine Meridian (up the arm)***
   Turn the palm down, and percuss up from the outside of the little finger to the shoulder.
7. ***Shoulder***
   Support the arm that is doing the percussion with your opposite arm and continue to percuss the top of the shoulder (upper trapezius) in a relaxed manner.
   (Repeat: Switch to the right arm and repeat the entire massage sequence from the lung meridian through to the small intestine meridian and shoulder.)
8. ***Neck***
   Next, percuss up both sides of the back of the neck. This works on the bladder and the gallbladder meridians.
9. ***Head***
   Switch to fingertips and use a tapping percussion over the entire skull. Using light fingertips, tap across the forehead, cheeks and jaws.
10. ***Face***
    Press firmly with the thumbs around the orbital rim (both above and below the eyes), then lightly wash the fingers over the eyes.
11. ***Thyroid Gland***
    Very lightly tap the front of the neck. This helps to stimulate the thyroid area.
12. ***Lungs (anatomical)***
    With firm fingertips, tap between the ribs, and go over the entire chest, beating Tarzan style; you may sound "Ahhhhh" for a release in the lungs.
13. ***Gallbladder Meridian***
    Use a broad slapping percussion along the side of your torso, from the armpit to the hip. Do three times.

14. ***Large Intestine (anatomical)***

Massage the large intestine organ, not the meridian. With firm fingertips, use a tapping percussion over the entire large intestine, starting from the right lower abdomen, up the right side (ascending colon), across the abdomen (transverse colon), and down the left side (descending colon). Repeat three times.

(Move to the right foot)

15. ***Kidney Meridian (up the leg)***

Extend the right leg out and percuss with a loose fist up the back of the inside of the leg.

16. ***Bladder Meridian (down the leg)***

Rotate the leg inward and percuss down the far outside of the leg to the outer little toe.

17. ***Spleen Meridian (up the leg)***

Percuss up from the great toe along the middle of the inside of the leg.

18. ***Stomach Meridian (down the leg)***

Percuss down the top of the outside of the leg to the 2nd toe.

19. ***Liver Meridian (up the leg)***

Percuss up the top, front of the inside of the leg, from the inner side of the great toe to the top of the leg.

20. ***Gallbladder Meridian (down the leg)***

Rotate the leg inward again and percuss down the middle of the outside of the leg to the fourth toe.

21. ***Kidney 1***

Hold the foot up by the great toe to percuss the bottom of the foot.

(Repeat: Switch to the left leg and repeat from the kidney meridian through to Kidney 1)

Summary of how to use this chapter and meridian information:

- Take a complete health history.
- Include an inventory of finger and toe conditions and anomalies.
- Ask client to share strong likes and dislikes with regards to taste, time of day, seasons, elements and colors.
- Observe the client's nature: artistic, commanding, philosophical, compassionate, nurturing.
- Chart chronic muscle aches, injuries and conditions.
- Notice if you see a pattern emerging. If not at first, give it several sessions and see if you are able to correlate conditions with the meridians.
- In future sessions, focus on reflexology areas and points where indicated by the information. Be sure to chart reactions and improvements.

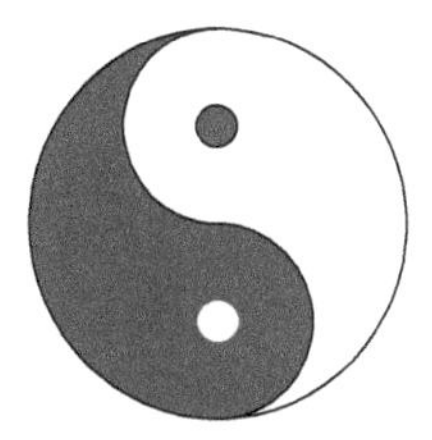

Harmony of Opposites creating Dynamic Balance

5

Psychoneuroimmunology Theory

Psychoneuroimmunology Theory of Integrative Reflexology® is based on the connection between the nervous system, the immune system and the emotions. It is now commonly agreed upon amongst the scientific community that there is, in fact, a relationship between stress and disease. In our fast-paced, performance-driven culture, people are functioning in a constant state of stress, chronically flooding their bodies with stress hormones. Many of us believe that we know how to relax, but the reality is that our bodies no longer remember how to fully relax into a state that allows for health and healing to take place. Reflexology helps to reverse the effects of chronic stress by initiating the calming mechanisms in our body, interrupting the continuous stream of stress chemicals flowing into the body and flooding the body with chemicals that support relaxation, stress relief and healing.

Psychoneuroimmunology

Psychoneuroimmunology is a field of study that investigates the interaction between the brain (psycho), the nervous system (neuro), and the immune system (immunology). The field of psychoneuroimmunology is helping us to better understand the mind-body connection and is providing us with tangible evidence that stress affects both brain chemistry and the function of our immune system. The more we learn about how the molecules in our body communicate across systems the more necessary it becomes to embrace a holistic model of health care and well-being by treating the whole client rather than one specific symptom. Reflexology is a model of holistic health care that offers stress relief and supports positive brain chemistry through nerve stimulation techniques applied to the feet.

When our body is stressed, whether by an external source or an internal, mental/emotional source, physiological reactions take place in our system. Stress hormones are released, certain metabolic functions (such as digestion and immune function) are suppressed and our sympathetic nervous system kicks into action, bracing our body to confront a perceived threat. This physiological response creates a disruption in our bodily systems and is intended to be a temporary state that shifts once the perceived

en we live with this
ical effects begin to
ms of our body,
.

d that there are
...ects of chronic stress. It is not possible to completely avoid all stress, but if we are able to notice when we are feeling stressed, we can take action to minimize its effects on our body, mind and spirit. Reflexology is one way that the therapist can help a person counteract the effects of stress on the body. Reflexology creates a state of deep relaxation that serves as a sort of "refresh" button for the body, allowing it to recover from the effects of chronic stress and replenish itself.

The HeartMath® Institute is a nonprofit that was founded in 1991 with the mission to "help people bring their physical, mental and emotional systems into balanced alignment with their heart's intuitive guidance." They offer a free Stress and Well-Being Survey that "measures your stress-management, adaptability, resilience and emotional vitality levels, then analyzes this data in relation to your 5 Aspects of Well-Being. Finally, the survey will suggest practical and easy steps for achieving your Zone of Performance." It is highly recommended that you visit their website and take this survey for yourself.

(www.heartmath.org)

The Vagus Nerve

One mechanism through which the body responds to stress is the vagus nerve. The vagus nerve is the longest cranial nerve that extends from the brain through the thorax. It contains motor and sensory fibers and, because it passes through the neck and thorax to the abdomen, has the widest distribution in the body (Tewfik, 2015). Dr. Stephen Porges, who developed Polyvagal Theory, describes the vagus nerve as a conduit—a cable with lots of fibers in it, and 80% of those fibers are sensory nerves, meaning they travel from the viscera to the brain. The other 20% of the fibers are motor nerves, which communicate from the brain to the viscera. The range of bodily functions that the vagal network commands extends from facial expressions to autonomic regulation of respiration and heart rate all the way to digestive functions (Buczynski, 2012). The fact that all of these functions are regulated by one nerve conduit becomes a valuable piece of information in the discussion of how our mental/emotional state effects our physical state.

Polyvagal Theory describes how our nervous system responds to challenges and stress in an adaptive, complex way, via the vagus nerve. It is a complex theory that bridges the gap between our physiological state and our mental and emotional state. The vagus nerve itself is the "hub" from which our body can activate calming responses when we feel safe or shut down our systems when we experience trauma or an extreme threat. This "hub" runs through the center of our thoracic cavity, branching out to communicate with the viscera. It is also associated with the area of the solar plexus. Anatomically, the solar plexus can also be called the celiac plexus, which is a nerve plexus of the vagus nerve that innervates the pancreas, spleen, kidneys, adrenals and intestines (Tewfik, 2015).

You will remember that the solar plexus point in foot reflexology is located in the same place as Kidney 1 in the meridian system. The emotion connected to the kidney is fear and anxiety. Gentle pressure on the Kidney 1/solar plexus area of the foot releases fear, anxiety and stress. It calms the vagus nerve, and by doing so, it brings ease to the organs that the vagus nerve regulates. When beginning an Integrative Reflexology® session, your first technique is to hold the area of the solar plexus. This is calming and centering for both the client and the practitioner. I call K-1 the "panic button"—it is excellent to press for stressful events.

In Integrative Reflexology®, the solar plexus and Kidney 1 represent our connection to the Earth and the breath of life through the soles of the feet. A nurse who works in the NICU (Neonatal Intensive Care Unit) once shared that when a premature baby has stopped breathing, they flick the solar plexus reflex area on the foot to stimulate their breath. This area, like the vagus nerve, can serve to calm us and to stimulate us.

The vagus nerve and Polyvagal Theory explain one mechanism through which our physical response to stress can be altered and our body can calm itself. By connecting in with the vagus nerve through foot reflexology, we can assist our client's body in utilizing this innate ability. Another mechanism through which our physical response to stress can be altered is through the emotions. The emotional aspect of Psychoneuroimmunology Theory is largely inspired and explained by the work of Candace Pert and her book, *The Molecules of Emotion*, specifically, her research into the relationship between neuropeptides and emotions.

Neuropeptides

Neuropeptides have been shown to be the primary molecule of communication throughout the brain and nervous system. By attaching to receptors on cell membranes like a lock and key, neuropeptides dictate the response of a cell. Each neuropeptide fits with a specific receptor and these receptors are located throughout the body, not only in the brain (Pert, 1986).

Initially, Candace Pert's research uncovered as many as 50-60 different neuropeptides, each specific to a particular receptor and each able to command different responses in the body. While the neuropeptides are the messengers of this communication, the receptors are the mechanism that sort out the information being exchanged and determine what is relevant for the body at any given moment. Based on this idea, Pert explored "the notion that the receptors for the neuropeptides are in fact the keys to the biochemistry of emotion" (Pert, 1986).

The limbic system, with the hypothalamus, pituitary gland and the amygdala, is the seat of emotions in the brain. Through her research, Pert found that the limbic system is highly enriched with neuropeptide receptors. This finding implies that it is a place where there is a lot of chemical action—a lot of communication between cells. Another place in the body where there is a high concentration of neuropeptide receptors is in the dorsal horn of the spinal cord—the first place where touch-sensory information is processed by the brain. This finding has huge implications for how touch effects our biochemistry and the cellular communication within our body (Pert, 1986).

During an Integrative Reflexology® session, clients often express feeling a pleasant, almost drugged like sensation wash over them. This wave of relaxation is happening at a chemical level, through the effect of endorphins. Endorphins are known to be associated with feelings of euphoria, pain relief and our ability to manage our cravings. Candace Pert is the woman who first named beta-endorphin, the body's natural version of morphine, as a neuropeptide. Receptors for beta-endorphin are found scattered throughout the brain as well as throughout the rest of the body. Beta-endorphin is only one of the 50-60 neuropeptides that are affecting biochemical responses throughout our body. Pert also discovered that some hormones, such as insulin, are actually neuropeptides. So this same lock and key mechanism of communication that takes place throughout our body with the neuropeptides is also happening throughout our body with the hormones.

Ultimately, all of these pieces can be put together to describe one pathway of communication. This pathway is initiated by physical stimulation of the feet, travels through the nervous system, and results in chemical changes in the emotional centers of our brain and in other areas of our body.

Neuropeptides and the Immune System

The work of Candace Pert has also shown that cells in our immune system have receptors for the same neuropeptides that communicate in our nervous system and brain. Monocytes are a type of immune cell that are responsible for recognizing and digesting foreign bodies, wound healing and tissue-repair mechanisms. These cells that have crucial health-sustaining functions have been found to have every neuropeptide receptor. Thus, Candace Pert asserts that the emotion-affecting neuropeptides "actually appear to control the routing and migration of monocytes, which are so pivotal to the immune system" (Pert, 1986).

We have already described how neuropeptides can create chemical changes in the brain, now we are seeing that they can also affect change in the immune system. And the implications do not stop there. Pert goes on to explain "that the cells of the immune system not only have receptors for these various neuropeptides...they also make the neuropeptides themselves." So, the immune system is not only receptive to the messages of these chemicals that are connected with our emotional centers, it is also making these chemicals that affect our mood. This discovery describes a bidirectional pathway where immune cells speak to the brain and vice versa, which gives credence to the supposition that emotions may act to enhance or suppress the immune system (Seaward, 2009).

The implications of Pert's findings are profound for those of us who work in alternative health fields. Her work leads us to the bridge that serves as the biochemical connection between body and mind. She takes her findings one step further with her suggestion that rather than there being 50-60 different neuropeptides, there may actually be only one neuropeptide molecule. This one molecule acts like a chameleon by changing its configuration as a result of our emotions, which are effecting the vibrations in our body. This indicates that there is a strong relationship between emotional responses and the biochemical changes they produce. This is especially significant in the immune system. "Before Pert's findings it was believed that cortisol played the crucial role in immunosuppression, it is now thought that structural changes in neuropeptides, influenced by emotional thought, play the most significant role in immunoincompetence" (Seaward, 2009).

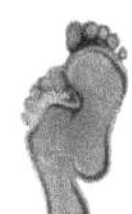

Reflexology and Post-Traumatic Stress Disorder

Reflexology is a powerful modality for use with people suffering from PTSD. Mary Middleton is a certified practitioner of Integrative Reflexology® and she works with the veterans at Walter Reed National Military Medical Center in Washington, DC. Mary has reported that the vets love Integrative Reflexology® because it is a modality that fosters a feeling of safety. The creation of a safe environment is crucial when working with clients who suffer from PTSD. Reflexology facilitates this process because the client remains fully clothed, face up or even in a seated position and they can see the practitioner the entire time they are receiving the work. Creating this sense of safety allows the client to settle into the relaxation effects of reflexology and allows their body to heal on a deeper level. The physiological effects of this state of deep relaxation support a positive emotional state, and vice versa.

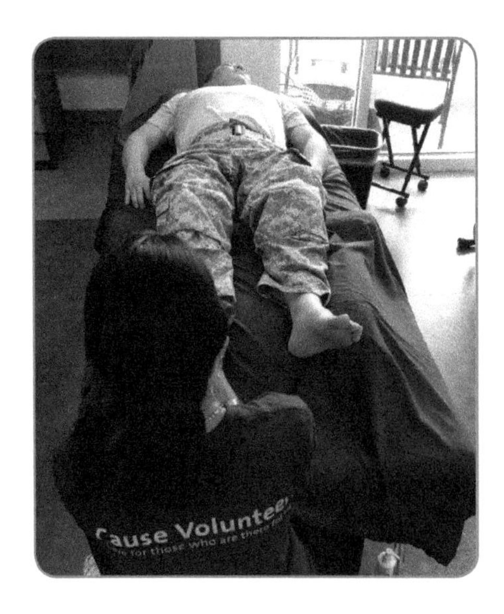

Reflexology and The Lymph System

We have investigated how reflexology can affect the chemistry of our brain and the nervous system via the vagus nerve and neuropeptides. We have also learned how the neuropeptides can communicate with and affect the immune system. Now we will learn how reflexology can affect the immune system via the lymph.

The lymph system is a part of both the circulatory and the immune system. It is comprised of the lymph vessels, lymph nodes, bone marrow, spleen, and thymus. It is a part of the body's drainage system that removes excess fluid from the body and filters out and destroys harmful material. In this way, it is one of the body's defense mechanisms that functions to keep us healthy.

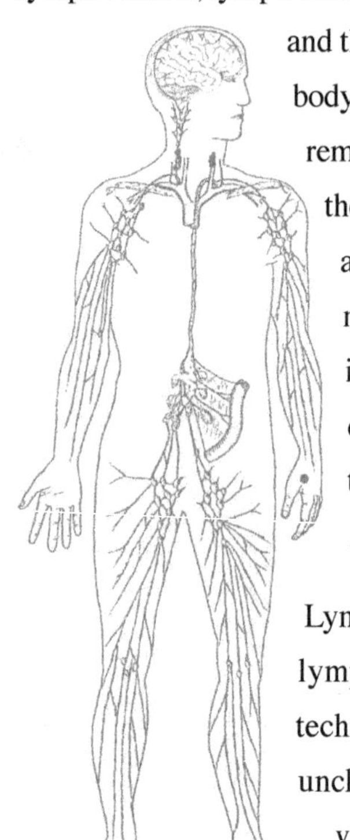

Fig 5.1
Reflexology and the Lymph System

Lymphatic massage and lymphatic drainage are techniques that support unclogging the lymph vessels and increasing optimal flow through the system. Pumping the feet, raising your legs higher than your heart and simple walking are also ways to support and increase lymphatic flow. The feet, as the most distal part of our body, are a place where fluid build-up can occur as a result of long stretches of standing, lack of activity and improper diet. The Integrative Reflexology® session is unique in its design to stimulate the lymph system and help the body remove congestion that is released during the session, as well as promote a general improvement in lymph flow.

The foot is also the most distal point of connection between the lymph system and the nerves. There are a prolific amount of tiny lymph vessels in the feet that are available to transport toxins that need to be moved out of the body. There are also 100,000–200,000 nerve endings in the feet that are constantly communicating with the brain and the body. When these channels of communication and transportation are uncongested, the body can function optimally. Unfortunately, what we find in the feet is congestion, tension and crystallized deposits that impede mobility and dull the nerves. Working to break up this congestion is one of the primary goals of reflexology.

This congestion in the feet comes from a build up of calcium and uric acid as a result of gravity and stagnation in the joints. It can be hypothesized that keeping our feet "protected" in shoes is one contributing factor. When we walk in shoes, our feet are not required to navigate uneven surfaces, especially if we are wearing hard-soled shoes and walking on flat floors or pavement. All of the many articulations of the 26 bones in our feet are not being required to adjust to different textures and shapes. These joints then become stiff and congested. If you add a sedentary lifestyle to this equation then our feet become even less mobile.

Reflexology is a way to manually stimulate and mobilize the joints in the feet. By doing this, we can break up the congestion, bringing space and mobility into the tissue. A vital factor in this process is the lymph system that removes the congestion that is broken up. An Integrative Reflexology® session begins and ends with lymph stimulation. By waking up the lymph vessels at the beginning of a session, we are activating the system. We then perform the session, breaking up the crystallized deposits and releasing toxins from the tissues and end with lymphatic pumping at the ankle and lymph strokes up the leg to encourage the removal of toxins. Eventually, the lymph fluid leaves the body via the kidneys and the urinary system. The Integrative Reflexology® session was designed to support this process—the kidney, ureter and bladder reflex points are always stimulated after the lymphatic pumping to support the full flushing of the system.

The most recent research coming out of the University of Virginia has proven that the lymphatic system extends into the brain (University, 2015). This implies that the nervous system and the lymphatic system are working together to promote health.

The neuropeptides are one point of connection between the brain and the immune system. We now see the lymphatic system as another point of connection. The feet are one place in the body that brings all of these connections together. Through a basic Integrative Reflexology® session, we can simultaneously improve brain chemistry, activate a calming effect in the nervous system and stimulate the lymph system to clear toxins out of our body. Psychoneuroimmunology Theory is the explanation for these effects. Candace Pert argues that the brain, the glands and the immune system are connected in a bi-directional network of communication with the neuropeptides as the information carriers (Pert, 1986). It is my argument that the feet are the most potent place in the body where this communication can be activated to bring healing into the system.

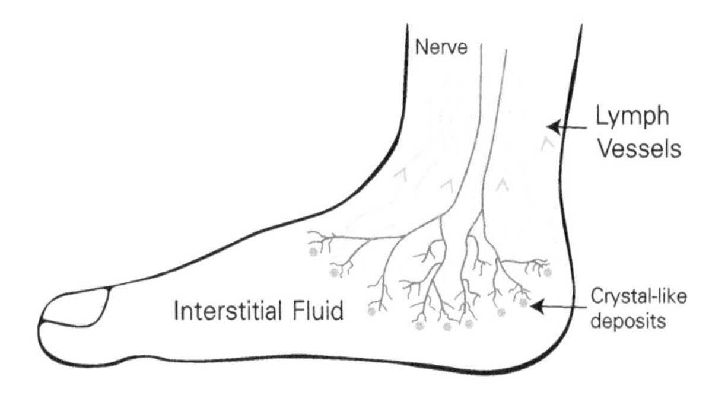

Fig 5.2
Crystal-like deposits in the feet impede optimal nerve flow. Through reflexology the deposits are broken up and the congestion is carried away via the lymph vessels.

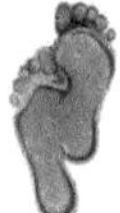

Psychoneuroimmunology Theory shows us how important it is to consider the whole body, including the emotions, when working with clients. It is important to convey positive messages to your clients when you are working with them. You might feel inspired to work with affirmations during your session. A wonderful resource for positive affirmations is Heal Your Body *by Louise Hay. This is a reference guide detailing the mental causes of physical ailments, and the corresponding positive thought patterns for reversing illness and creating health. You might create positive statements for you and your client to use during the reflexology session and also for your client to use throughout his or her day. A powerful affirmation can be a valuable mantra for a client navigating a stressful time. If this approach resonates with you, you are encouraged to do some research about how to create an effective affirmation. It is important that the statement you create resonates with your client. It will be a statement of what is and it may not feel true for them in the moment, but it represents a state of being that they want to embody, or a state of being that will bring the healing they are seeking. Using these powerful statements during your reflexology session can support the body and mind in shifting to a new place.*

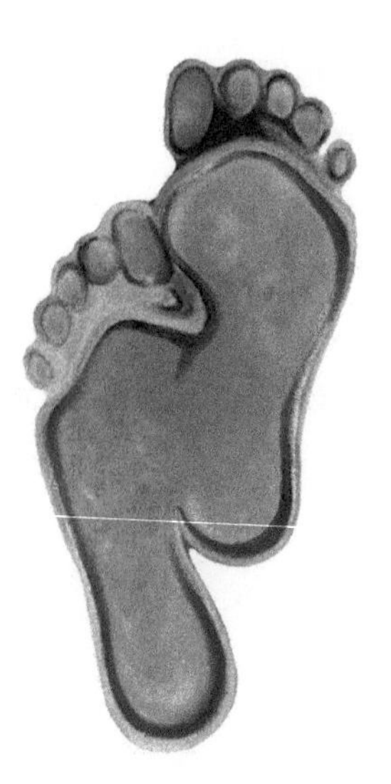

"I am perfectly balanced in my feet, in my body and in my life."

Part 2
Practice of Integrative Reflexology®

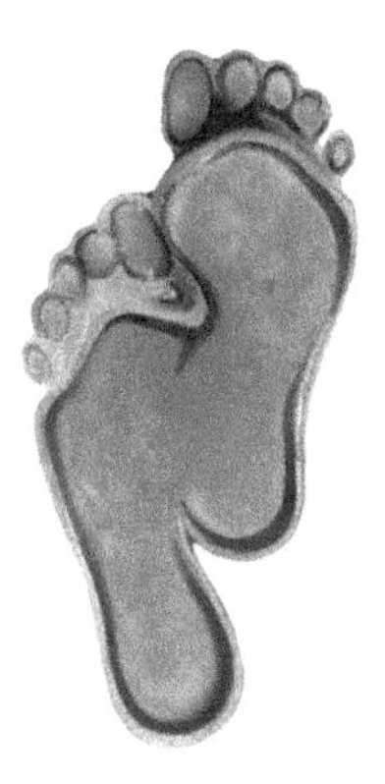

Now that we have explored the four theories of Integrative Reflexology®, we will develop a sense of how to approach a session with a client. Consider each theory as a different lens through which you can view a client's condition. You have a lot of information to work with and it is not necessary to address every theory in every session you do. With practice, you will begin to notice which lens will be the most useful for each client. The four theories are the objective lenses and you, the practitioner, are the subjective lens. Every practitioner will work with the four theories differently, so it is up to you to become familiar with them and apply them in the way that makes the most sense to you.

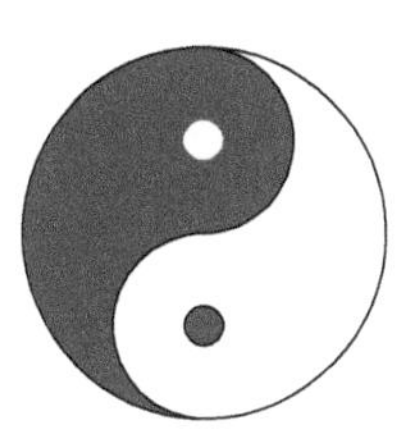

6

Putting the Four Theories Into Practice

When you are putting the four theories into practice you are listening to what the client is saying, noticing what you observe in the feet and sensing what the client's body is communicating. In this chapter, we will offer a general approach to an Integrative Reflexology® session that takes each theory into account. Then we will address four common conditions of the feet and how to treat each condition with Integrative Reflexology®.

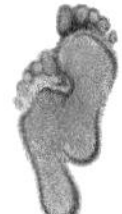

Ask yourself, is this condition rooted in the structure? The meridian? The diet? The shoes? The mental/emotional?

An Integrative Reflexology® Session

An Integrative Reflexology® session begins before you ever meet your client. One of the most valuable tools you have to share is your presence. Psychoneuroimmunology Theory taught us that safety is an essential component in activating the calming pathways of the vagus nerve and allowing the body to heal. Creating a calm, safe environment in your workspace, as well as within yourself, will allow your client to settle in more deeply during the session. It will also allow your client to trust deeply in the therapeutic touch you are offering.

Another opportunity you have, as a practitioner, is to be a positive reflection for your client. Pay attention to how you communicate with your client about what conditions they present with or what you notice during the session. By offering neutral or positive feedback, you not only help your client feel safe and heard, but you are modeling for them how to re-frame their perspective of their body. Rather than focusing on what is "wrong," find a way to be objective about your observations. For example, instead of telling a client, "your left foot is more turned out," which could be received as something that is wrong with them, you might say, "I am noticing that one foot seems to be more relaxed than the other." You might then invite them to notice what they, themselves feel, which invites them to notice their body in a new way. Perhaps you can continue to check in with them about what they notice as you rotate and rock their leg to see if there is tension in their hips. This communication engages the client and teaches them about their body. Perhaps they take this new awareness with them and use it in their daily life.

Once you have considered your treatment space and your presence, you are ready to work with your client. The first step in any Integrative Reflexology® session is to obtain a health history. This will give you an idea of what the client is presenting with in this moment, as well as anything else that is going on in their life that may affect the treatment plan. It may seem obvious how to address the client's discomfort, but it is worthwhile to be curious and ask questions, because you may uncover something unexpected that may be contributing and can be addressed. Integrative Reflexology® is a whole body approach to healing. It can be easy to get focused on the feet and forget that the whole body is a factor in what the feet are experiencing. By considering each of the four theories, you are considering the whole body's experience.

You can use the following questions as guides for how to consider each of the four theories during your intake. Your treatment plan will be based on the answers to these questions. Hopefully, you will see an overlapping of information that will point you in the direction that will best serve this client. Remember, you are not diagnosing their condition; you are offering a remedy and treatment to alleviate the symptom and address the potential cause.

Structural Alignment

- What do you notice about the structural alignment of their feet?
- Have you looked at the bottom of the client's shoes? Is there a wearing away of the surface? What reflexology area does that correlate with?
- What do you notice about the shoe quality? Could the shoe be causing stress on the feet?
- Is the arch of the foot collapsing on either side, especially the medial arch?

Zone Theory

- Where is the exact center of the pain on the foot? What area does that relate to within the body? Does that connection correlate with their health history?

Meridians

- Is there a toe that is malformed that may also be indicated in the pain the client is experiencing? What meridian is located on that particular toe?
- Is there a complimentary muscle pain associated with the particular meridian?

Psychoneuroimmunology

- What is the current emotional state of your client?
- Is there a connection to the emotions and the condition or pain presenting?

Specific Treatment Plans

Now, we will look at how Integrative Reflexology® and the four theories can be applied to specific conditions of the feet—plantar fasciitis, bunions, heel spur, Morton's neuroma. As you create a treatment plan, remember the guide questions presented above and also consider the specific questions offered for each condition.

Plantar Fasciitis

Plantar fasciitis is a common condition that many of your clients will present with. It involves the entire plantar surface of the foot. With this condition clients may experience pain on the bottom of the foot anywhere from the heel to the toes. As we have already discussed, the fascia is a continuous sheath of connective tissue that extends from the toes and the plantar fascia all the way up to the head. The pain that one experiences is a symptom that is manifesting in the foot, which may indicate tension and/or blockage in a source higher up in the body. Think of the bound up fascia as a hand towel that you are twisting and pulling at opposite diagonal corners. The twisting and pulling is happening at the corners, but bands of tension are created throughout the entire towel. In the body, it would be a point of tension or congestion that is creating stress in the entire fascial sheath and causing pain and inflammation in the plantar fascia.

With this condition it is important to ask the client exactly where they are experiencing the pain. As we will see later, the location of the discomfort can reflect a specific root cause of the issue.

Structural Alignment—Observe the alignment of the affected foot and compare it to the other foot. Plantar fasciitis will often present with a very tight and swollen area. Walking is generally painful, especially after being sedentary for a long period of time. Oftentimes, people with plantar fasciitis experience the worst pain upon first getting out of bed in the morning. The whole body will be affected due to the foot pain and the resulting compensation in gait and stance. It is hard to determine if the structure of the body is causing the pain or if the pain is resulting in changes in the structure and alignment of the body. This is part of what you will investigate in order to help unravel the pain cycle.

Meridians—When assessing plantar fasciitis, the first thing to consider is where the discomfort is located in the foot. Notice in Figure 6.1 the three major muscles/tendons on the bottom of the foot—flexor hallicus longus (in blue), quadratus plantae (in orange) and fibularis longus (in green). The locations of these structures are also the three most common areas where plantar fasciitis manifests. In Integrative Reflexology®, each of these muscles/tendons is reflective of a muscle in the body that may play a contributing role in the client's symptoms.

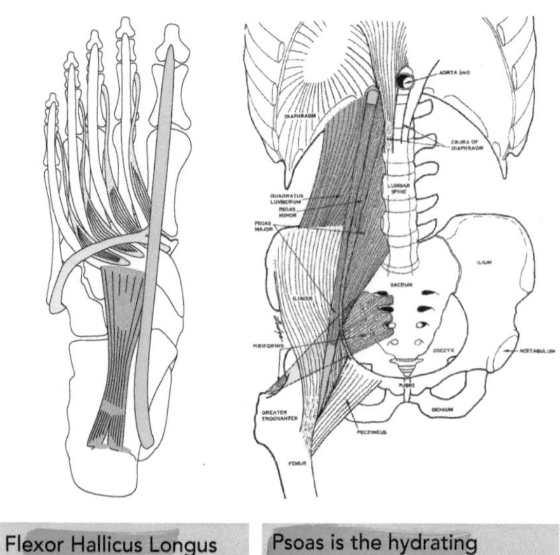

Fig 6.1
The muscles/tendons on the feet that are associated with plantar fasciitis each correspond to certain muscles in the body. And the muscles in the body correspond to certain meridians. Each of the these three relationships indicates a different potential cause for the plantar fasciitis symptoms.

The flexor hallicus longus muscle and tendon in the foot reflects the psoas muscle in the body. In *The Psoas Book,* Liz Koch calls the psoas the hydrating muscle. We can then notice that the kidney, ureter and bladder reflexes on the foot follow the flexor hallicus longus tendon. This connection between the flexor hallicus longus muscle in the foot, the psoas muscle in the body and the kidney and bladder reflexes implies that dehydration might be playing a role in the client's plantar fasciitis. The kidneys represent fear, anxiety, and exhaustion in Meridian Theory. All of these emotions can cause us to forget or overlook some of the basics of nourishment. If your client's plantar fasciitis manifests in this area, you might suggest that they be sure to consume a certain quantity of water every day and notice if their symptoms improve.

The quadratus plantae in the foot is associated with quadratus lumborum in the body, which is associated with the large intestine in the meridian system. If a client has both plantar fasciitis and digestive issues, and the pain shows up in the middle of the foot toward the heel, look to the meridians for a remedy and treatment plan. The large intestine is related to grief, depression, and a sense of melancholy in Meridian Theory. You might inquire as to whether there are emotions or life circumstances that are challenging for your client to digest right now. It could also be that their diet is causing a chemical shift in their body that is irritating the tissue and playing a factor in the inflammation. Digestive challenges to consider include irritable bowel syndrome, Crohn's disease, celiac disease, ulcerative colitis, constipation and diarrhea.

The fibularis longus tendon in the foot reflects the piriformis muscle in the body. Plantar fasciitis discomfort in this area can reflect something going on in the relationship between the hip and the sacrum, or in the piriformis muscle specifically. In this instance, notice if there is any swelling in the sacrum reflex area of the foot or if the hip reflex point is tender. You might also use the "Roll" leg release technique on page 138 to feel how freely the leg moves. This movement extends into the pelvis and can be an indicator of tightness between the sacrum and the hip, specifically in the piriformis muscle. Tightness in the piriformis can reflect overall freedom to move in the body. The piriformis is one of the muscles that is associated with the pericardium meridian, which is about the heart muscle. The muscles associated with this meridian are about moving and getting the heart pumping.

Psychoneuroimmunology (PNI) — The emotional aspect of plantar fasciitis is mostly related to the meridians, as described above. Based on the meridian you isolate as being related to the client's plantar fasciitis, you might ask your client if the associated emotion is relevant to them. That question may provide them with a surprising insight. You do not need to have a conversation about their life if it is not appropriate, but you may simply offer that association as a piece of information for them to take with them after the session.

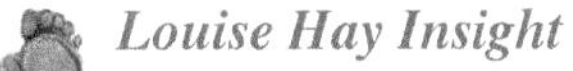

Louise Hay Insight

Louise Hay describes the feet as representing our understanding of ourselves, our life and others. Often, when we have a condition that is causing us pain, there is confusion as to what is the cause, which may reflect confusion about our self and our life. This condition may be presenting an opportunity to change something in our life or come into better connection with our self and others. Louise Hay relates issues of the feet with fear of the future and not stepping forward in life. Having a new understanding of a situation, and of ourselves, can free up our energy in new ways and allow us to overcome our fears (Hay, 1984).

Affirmation: *With ease and grace I move forward in full acceptance of my life.*

Affirmation: *I fully and lovingly accept and understand my SELF.*

Treatment Plan — Your treatment plan for plantar fasciitis will be based on where the symptoms are presenting in the foot.

- Work the reflexes in the foot where the pain is presenting.
- If you are licensed to do massage, work the corresponding muscles in the body.
- Address the meridians associated with the area of pain.
- Have a conversation with your client about the underlying cause of the symptoms and the emotions associated with the meridian you isolated.

Bunion

A bunion is a thickness or increase in the bony area at the first joint at the base of the great toe. The toe will consequently be bending in toward the second toe and may also create a hammer-toe—lifted and bent second toe. The joint is often painful, swollen and red.

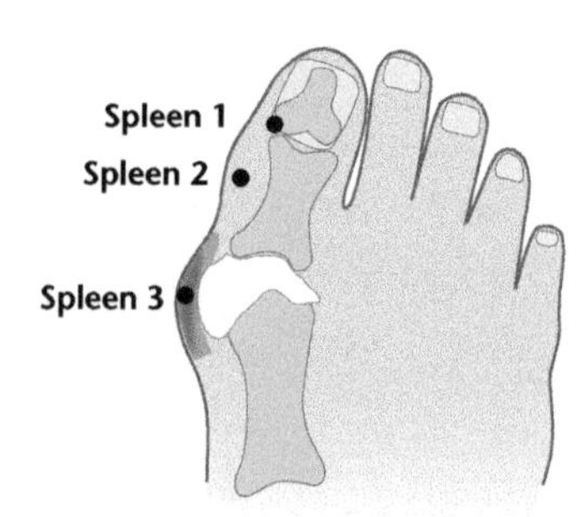

Fig 6.2
The spleen meridian points associated with a bunion

Structural Alignment—Structure plays a large role in this condition. A bunion can be caused by shoes that are too tight and narrow, one leg being shorter than the other, or a lateral imbalance in the feet or hips. All of these conditions create tension and instability on the joints and tendons of the feet. Over time, this tension creates a deformity of the first metatarsophalangeal (MTP) joint of the great toe. It may also occur with weight gain or fallen arches and may have a genetic tendency due to foot shape.

There are a variety of factors to pay attention to when assessing how structure plays a role in your client's bunion. Remember that this area of the toe is the reflex area for the neck, specifically the 7th cervical vertebra. Perhaps you notice that your client holds a lot of tension in their neck. If you are a massage therapist, you can be sure to address this area in the bodywork portion of your session. You might notice that your client stands with their weight more on one leg than the other. Pay attention to their shoes and ask to look at the wear on the soles of their shoes. Also, consider their daily activity and their job. This may give clues to the position the foot is in for extended periods of time. The body can get stuck in particular standing postures out of habit if we do not bring attention to these patterns.

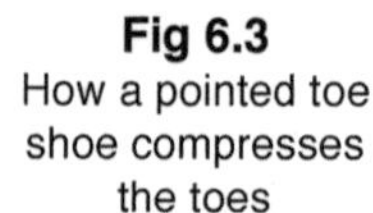

Fig 6.3
How a pointed toe shoe compresses the toes

Zones—As you observe your client in a relaxed, standing posture see if the neck on the same side as the bunion is tight or leaning to one side. The observations that are relevant for zones will align with the observations you noted with regards to structure.

Meridians—The meridian associated with a bunion is the spleen/pancreas meridian. Its paired meridian is the stomach meridian, which is associated with a hammertoe. A hammertoe is often a byproduct of a bunion. The taste associated with these two meridians is sweet, and the pancreas is involved with balancing the blood sugar levels. If your client consumes a lot of sugar, they may notice that the bunion area becomes tender and achy. Many of the neck muscles are associated with these meridians. This further indicates working with the neck itself to relieve tension.

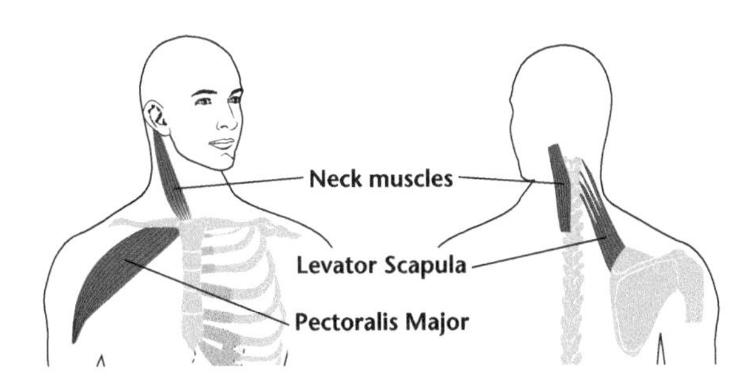

Fig 6.4
The muscles related to the spleen/pancreas meridian

Psychoneuroimmunology—When you consider the meridian information discussed above, and the association between the location of the bunion and the meridians associated with sweetness, you may be able to see the correlation between a bunion and stress. We all know that sugar can be an emotional crutch for stress. Stress eating is a proven coping mechanism and sugar is the #1 taste craving when under stress. We also know that sugar can weaken the immune response. It is considered one of the most damaging foods that we consume in excess. Sugar, in any of its forms, is the #1 cause of arthritis, and a bunion is arthritis. This condition of having a bunion may run in the family, perhaps due to learned eating habits and stress behaviors, rather than actual genetics.

Louise Hay Insight
In her book, Heal Your Life, Louise Hay suggests that the cause of bunions is: "Lack of joy in meeting the experiences of life."
Affirmation: *I move forward with great joy in all that life's experiences bring to me.*
Affirmation: *I choose to feel the sweetness of life.*

Treatment Plan—Depending on the cause of the bunion and how long the client has had it, you may not be able to make it go away. However, educating your client to the potential causes or contributing factors can empower your client to make changes that will minimize the stress on the bunion and ensure that it does not continue to grow or become inflamed.

- Work the bunion area as deeply as the client can receive. Do toe stretches in all directions.
- Work deeply on both the neck area of the foot and the actual neck to release the tightness that is pulling on the fascia.
- Suggest shoes with a wide toe box such as Altra zero drop shoes.
- You may suggest toe separators, such as Correct Toes®, to help with realignment. These will require that your client be willing to wear shoes to accommodate the use of the toe separators.

Heel Spur

A heel spur is a build up of calcium deposits on the plantar surface of the calcaneus. This will be painful for the client when standing or walking, adding more stress on the entire body as it compensates for the discomfort. The heel spur may be associated with plantar fasciitis that is manifesting at the tendon attachment on the calcaneus (see Fig 6.5).

Structure—A heel spur may occur due to improper shoes or shoes that are worn out and allow for the foot to roll inward. The constant irritation and friction creates a thickening in the bone that hardens and calcifies. As a practitioner, you would want to assess your client's standing posture.

Zones—The heel is the reflex area for the entire pelvic zone. Notice where the heel spur is located and see if there is any related tension in the pelvis.

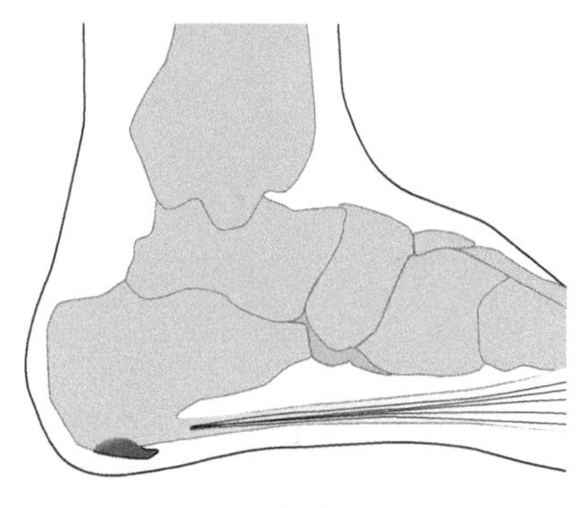

Fig 6.5
Heel Spur

A student in an Integrative Reflexology® workshop had developed a heel spur after traveling and trekking though India. As a result of the three day Integrative Reflexology® course and the combination of relaxing the whole body, loosening the ankles and working the heel spur with castor oil cream, the heel spur disappeared. This was a mild heel spur that had developed quickly and was treated in a timely manner. Some heel spurs require laser treatments, which can be painful and expensive. Reflexology is certainly worth a try first!

Meridian—Heel spurs are associated with the gluteal muscles. The meridian associated with the gluteal muscles is the pericardium meridian. This meridian is about movement, walking and getting the heart muscle pumping. If a heel spur occurs, it may be due to weakness or tightness in the gluteal muscles. Consider how your client spends his or her day. Perhaps the client has a sit-down job or a long commute in the car; or perhaps they are simply a couch potato. If this is the case, encouraging your client to include more activity in their day may help loosen and strengthen the gluteal muscles and alleviate the discomfort of the heel spur. You might suggest stretches that address this area of the body, as well as activity that will not further irritate the heel spur or require that they neglect their alignment to compensate for the discomfort in the heel.

Psychoneuroimmunology—The emotional aspect of a heel spur may be resistance to change, to moving or to being in the physical body. You may consider the reflex connection between the heel and the pelvis and how the pelvis holds our emotions related to feeling safe and present in the world. Remember that not every theory will apply to every condition. It may be that your client simply has worn out shoes.

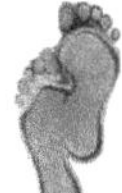

Affirmation: I am balanced in my life. I am supported by both the masculine and feminine aspects of myself.

Treatment Plan—You might suggest that your client treat their heel spur with castor oil as part of their daily self-care regimen, especially in the evening, after a long day of using or not using their feet.

- Work the heel spur area as deeply as the client can receive.
- Do ankle stretches in all directions.
- Cross-fiber friction over the heel spur if the client is able to handle the discomfort. Use castor oil in some form while you work directly on the heel spur. Castor oil has a wonderful ability to hydrate and break up congested tissue.

Morton's Neuroma

Morton's neuroma is a cyst that occurs around a nerve in the foot and causes pain when standing or walking. It most often occurs between the 3rd and 4th toes on the ball of the foot. Most people report that it feels like having a pebble in your shoe. It may also feel like a sharp, stabbing pain in the area of the cyst.

Structure—This condition is most likely due to improper shoes. High heel shoes and narrow, pointed toe shoes are the type to cause this condition. The constant compression across the widest part of the foot, combined with the pressure placed on the ball of the foot as it holds the body weight in high heel shoes, can contribute to this condition.

Zones—The Morton's neuroma would occur in the zone with the chest and lung reflex area. You may ask the client if they have any breathing challenges or feel tightness across the chest or diaphragm. If the client is a woman, it might even be the wearing of a tight underwire bra that correlates with the tightness in the foot.

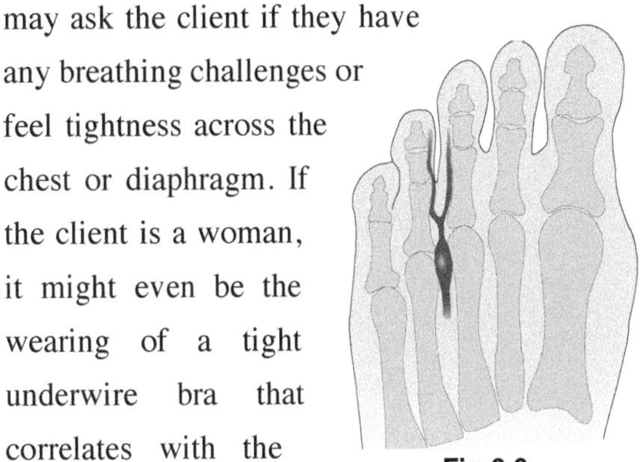

Fig 6.6
Morton's Neuroma

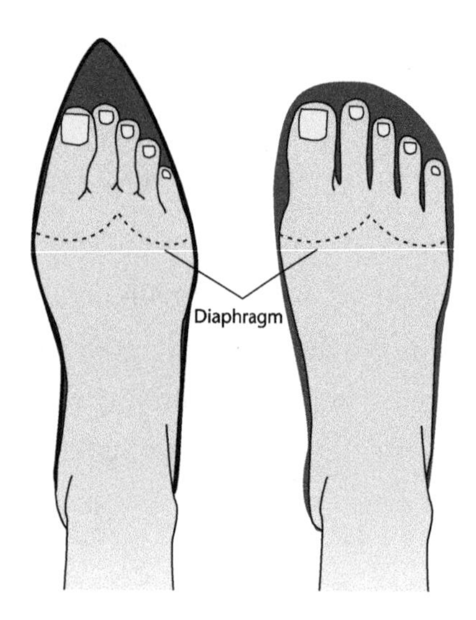

Fig 6.7
Notice what tight shoes do to your foot and toe alignment

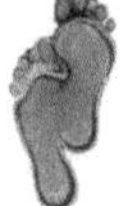

Women who have daily dress codes to adhere to often report that the first thing they do when they get home is take off their shoes, then take off their bra and take a deep breath. It is interesting to notice the connection between the constriction on the feet and the constriction on the ribcage.

Meridians—The meridian that flows near the 3rd and 4th toe is the gallbladder meridian. When your client presents with a Morton's neuroma it is recommended that you check both the gallbladder reflex area and the gallbladder meridian on the fourth toe for any tenderness or congestion. This meridian is also associated with the commander personality. Perhaps a client with this condition is striving to embody a strong, commanding presence.

Psychoneuroimmunology — A Morton's neuroma seems to be associated with constriction, whether it be in our clothing and footwear, or in our body and our ability to breathe in the breath of life. Constriction of any kind is stressful. Wearing high heel shoes conveys a certain personality, which may or may not be reflective of how a person truly feels. It is important to notice our motivations for wearing the clothes we wear and if those clothes are aligned with who we truly are. When we are comfortable in our clothes, we are comfortable in our bodies, and vice versa. This is something for you to keep in mind when working with a client who presents with this condition.

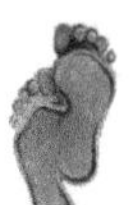

Affirmation: I am free to be who I am. I am free to dress for me.

Treatment Plan:

- Work the toes very gently—the neuroma may be very painful.
- Do gentle toe stretches in all directions.
- You might suggest toe separators, such as Correct Toes® and shoes with a wider toe box.

With all conditions described in this section, have your client consult with a physician if the problem persists or becomes unbearable. These treatments are a suggestion and are not intended to take the place of medical care.

7

Anatomy of the Feet and Hands

Anatomy of the Feet

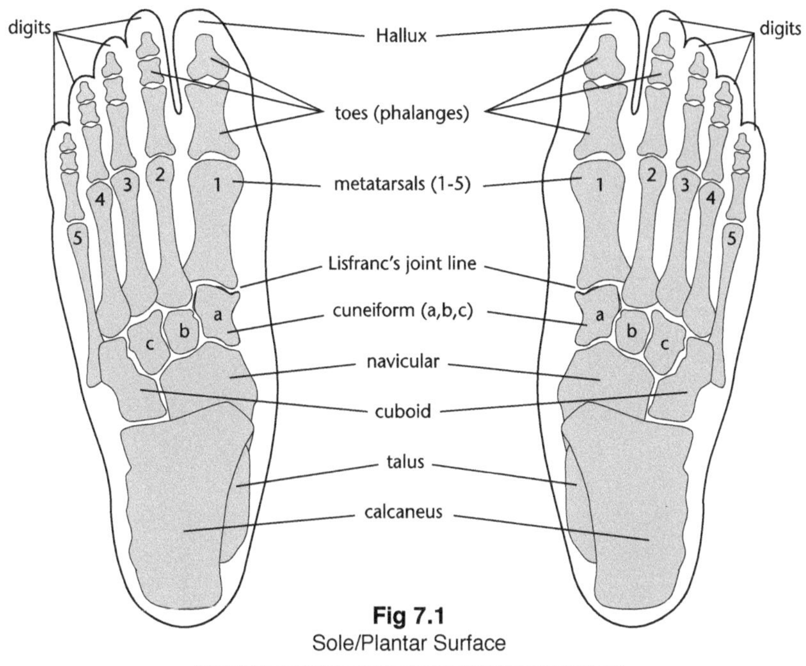

Fig 7.1
Sole/Plantar Surface

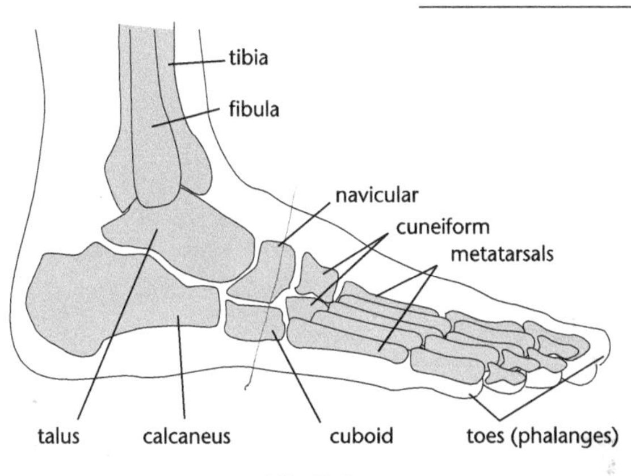

Fig 7.2
Outer/Lateral Aspect

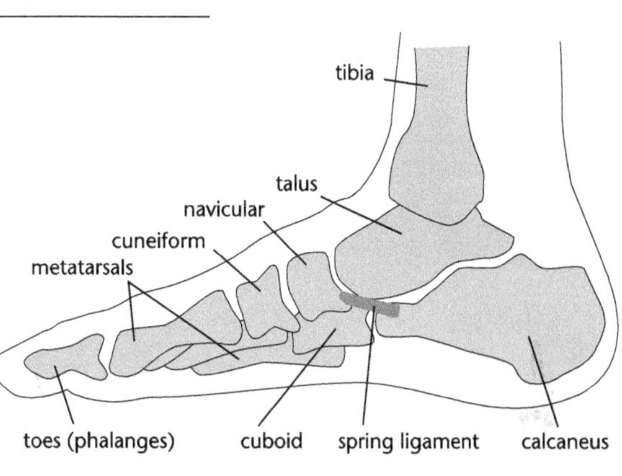

Fig 7.3
Inner/Medial Aspect

Muscles of the Lower Leg

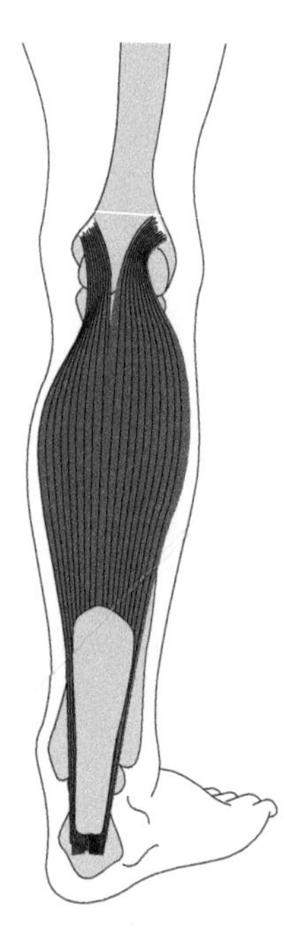

Fig 7.4
Gastrocnemius

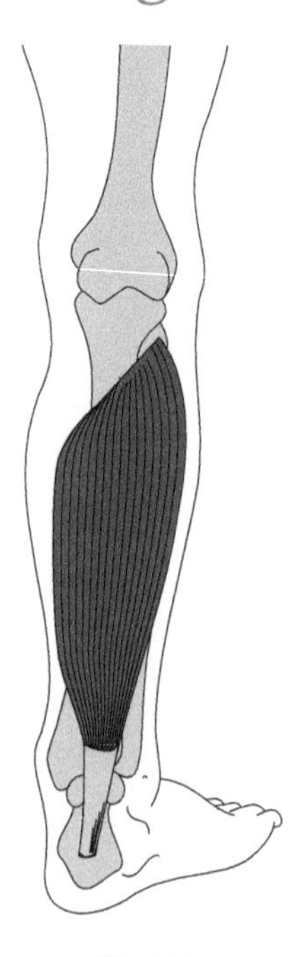

Fig 7.5
Soleus

Flexor Compartment (Posterior) of the Lower Leg

Gastrocnemius originates at the medial head (medial epicondyle) of the femur and the lateral head (lateral epicondyle) of the femur. It inserts on the calcaneus via the Achilles tendon. The muscle actions are plantar flexion of the ankle and assistance in flexion of the knee. You may palpate via the upper half of the posterior calf. The tendon is palpated as part of the Achilles tendon.

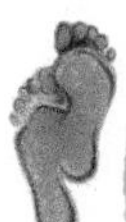

Gastro is the Greek term for belly. This muscle can act on the knee or the ankle separately, but not simultaneously.

Soleus originates at the soleal line of the tibia as well as the posterior and upper shaft of the fibula. It inserts on the calcaneus via the Achilles tendon. Its action is plantar flexion of the ankle. You may palpate the upper half of the posterior calf. The tendon is palpated as part of the Achilles tendon.

Soleus is Latin for sole, a flat fish. Deep to gastrocnemius, soleus is the stronger plantar flexor. Considered a heart pump muscle. May assist in preventing blood clots by point and flex exercises utilizing this muscle. Foot rolling also helps.

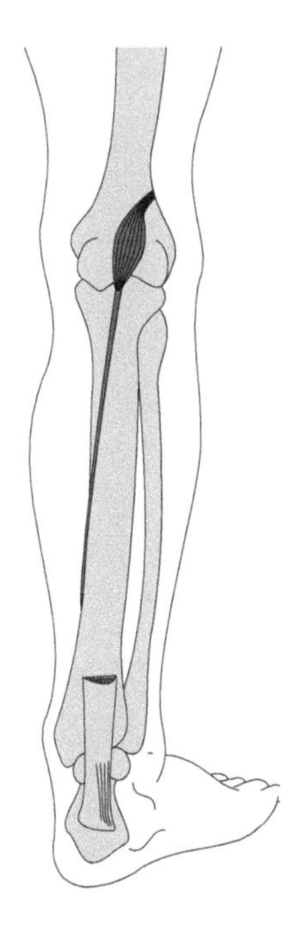

Fig 7.6
Plantaris

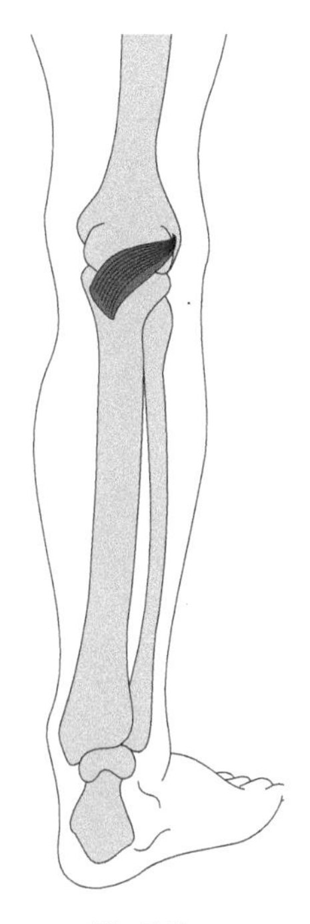

Fig 7.7
Popliteus

Plantaris originates at the lateral epicondyle of the femur. It inserts on the calcaneus via the Achilles tendon. Its actions are assistance in both plantar flexion of the ankle and flexion of the knee. It cannot be palpated.

Plantaris is the lower extremity counterpart of the palmaris longus and lies between the soleus and the gastrocnemius. Gastrocnemius, soleus, and plantaris share a common insertion, the Achilles tendon.

Popliteus originates at the lateral condyle of the femur. It inserts on the posterior proximal tibial shaft. The muscle action is to initiate knee flexion by medial rotation of the tibia to "unlock" the extended knee. It cannot be palpated.

Because of its action, popliteus is remembered as "the key that unlocks the knee." It is the deepest muscle at the back of the knee.

You will feel a thickening in the back of the knee in people who chronically lock either one or both knees.

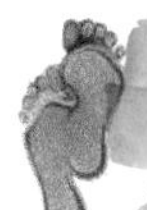

Remember which meridian is associated with the popliteus and knee locking? It is the gallbladder meridian.

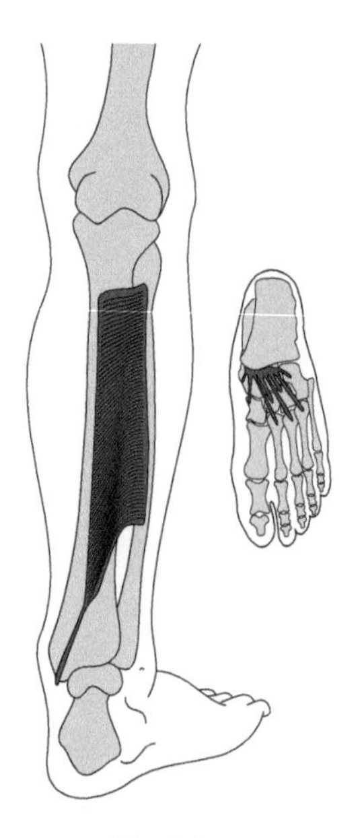

Fig 7.8
Tibialis posterior

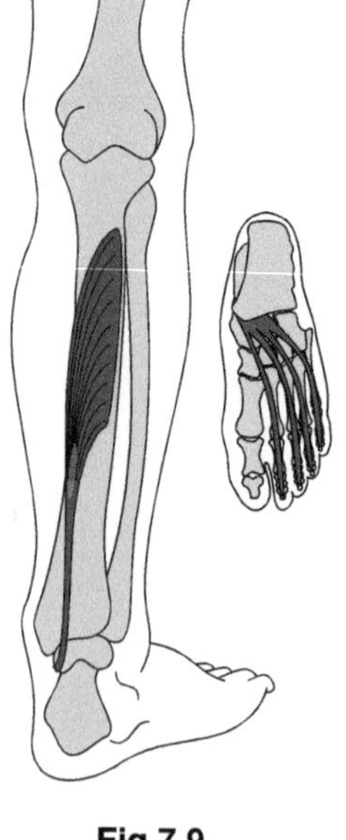

Fig 7.9
Flexor digitorum longus

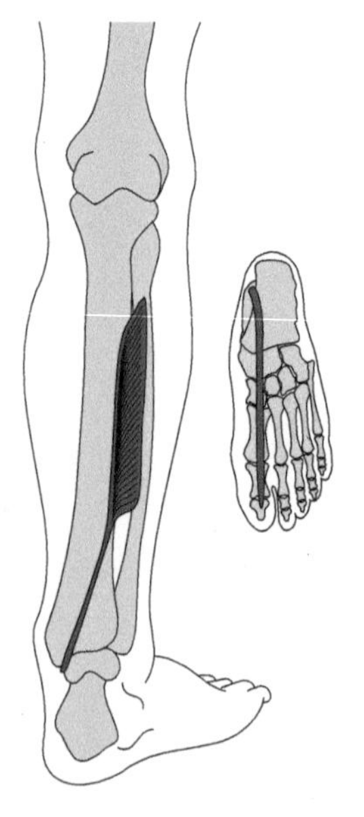

Fig 7.10
Flexor hallucis longus

Tibialis posterior originates at the posterior tibia, fibula and the interosseous membrane. It inserts on the navicular bone, and adjacent metatarsals on the plantar surface. Its actions are inversion of the foot and assistance in plantar flexion of the ankle. You may palpate the tendon on the medial malleolus.

Three deep posterior calf muscles have tendons which course around the medial malleolus, with the tendon of tibialis posterior being the most anterior and superficial, flexor digitorum next, and flexor hallucis longus the most posterior and deep in relation to the medial malleolus. Tibialis posterior is the deepest of the three muscles.

Flexor digitorum longus originates at the posterior tibia. It inserts on the distal phalanges of the four lateral toes on the plantar surface. Its actions are flexion of the four lateral toes at the distal interphalangeal joints (DIP) and assistance in plantar flexion of the ankle. You may palpate via the medial aspect of the distal calf.

The tendon is palpated by going around the medial malleolus just posterior to tibialis posterior tendon. (Alternate inversion and toe flexion to differentiate them).

Flexor hallucis longus originates at the posterior fibula. It inserts on the distal phalanx of the great toe (plantar surface). Its actions are flexion of the great toe and assistance in plantar flexion of the ankle. The palpation of the tendon is difficult to differentiate from flexor digitorum longus. However, the tendon may be palpated just medial and slightly deep to the Achilles tendon.

This muscle connects to the flexor hallucis longus tendon. You will see this tendon when the foot is fully flexed. This is near the kidney, adrenal, ureter, and bladder reflexes. Be gentle when working this area.

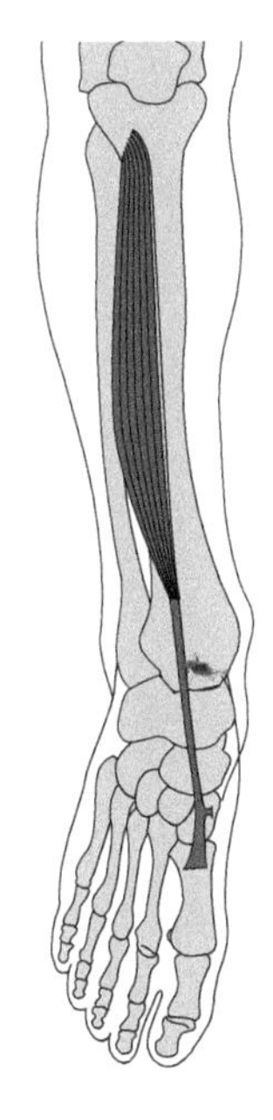

Fig 7.11
Tibialis anterior

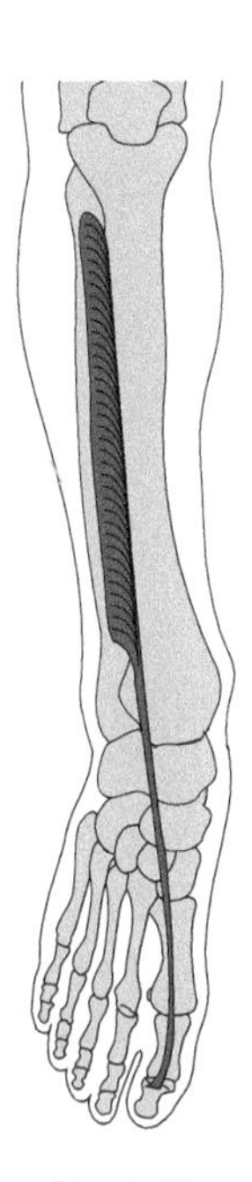

Fig 7.12
Extensor hallucis longus

Extensor Compartment (Anterior) of the Lower Leg

Tibialis anterior originates at the lateral shaft of the tibia and the interosseous membrane. It inserts on the base of the 1st metatarsal and the 1st medial cuneiform. Its actions are dorsiflexion of the ankle and inversion of the foot. You may palpate via the lateral side of the tibia on the anterior surface. The tendon is palpated on the medial side of the anterior surface of the ankle.

Extensor hallucis longus originates at the anterior shaft of fibula interosseous membrane. It inserts on the base of the distal phalanx of the great toe. Its actions are extension of the great toe and assistance in dorsiflexion of the ankle. You may palpate the tendon lateral to the tibialis anterior tendon on the anterior surface of the ankle and also on the dorsum of the foot near to the great toe.

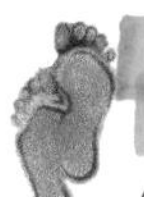

*Paralysis of the tibialis anterior causes "foot drop" which can be an indicator of having had a stroke. If you notice this condition in your client, time is of the essence to get this person medical attention. FAST is the acronym used by medical personnel in a stroke-related emergency: **F**acial drooping, **A**rm weakness, **S**peech difficulties, **T**ime to take action. Receiving medical attention as soon as possible reduces the severity of the stroke side effects.*

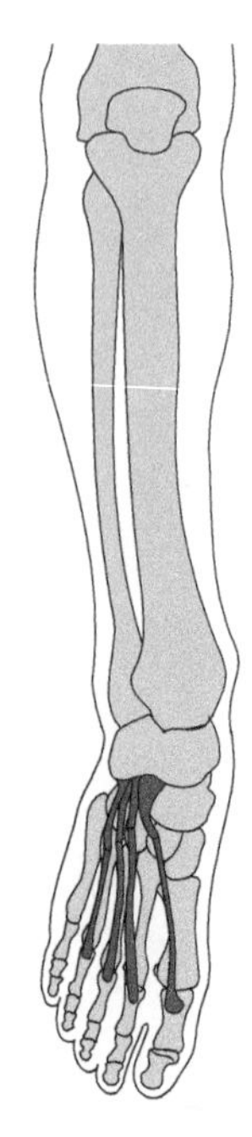

Fig 7.13
Extensor digitorum brevis

Extensor digitorum brevis originates at the anterior calcaneus. It inserts on the extensor expansion of the four medial toes. Its actions are assistance in extension of the four medial toes. You may palpate anterior to and slightly below the lateral malleolus on the dorsum of the foot.

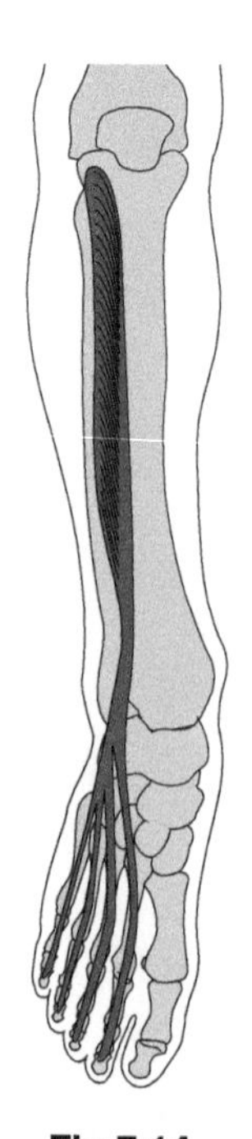

Fig 7.14
Extensor digitorum longus

Extensor digitorum longus originates at the lateral condyle of the tibia and the proximal 2/3 of the anterior shaft of the fibula. It inserts on the middle and distal phalanges of the four lateral toes. Its actions are extension of the four lateral toes and assistance in dorsiflexion of the ankle. You may palpate the common tendon on the anterior surface of the ankle, lateral to the extensor hallucis longus tendon. The divided tendons palpate on the dorsum of the foot.

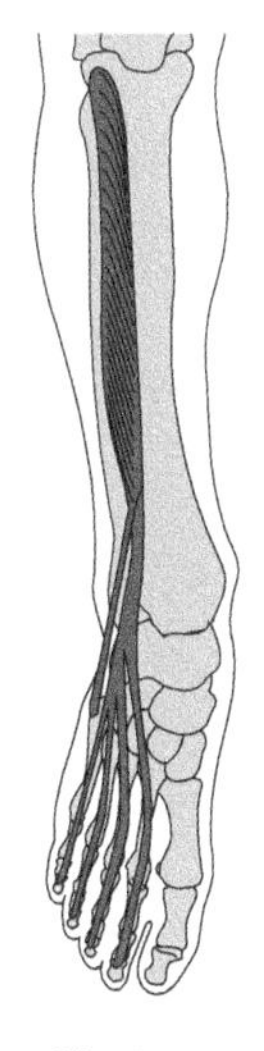

Fig 7.15
Fibularis (peroneus) tertius

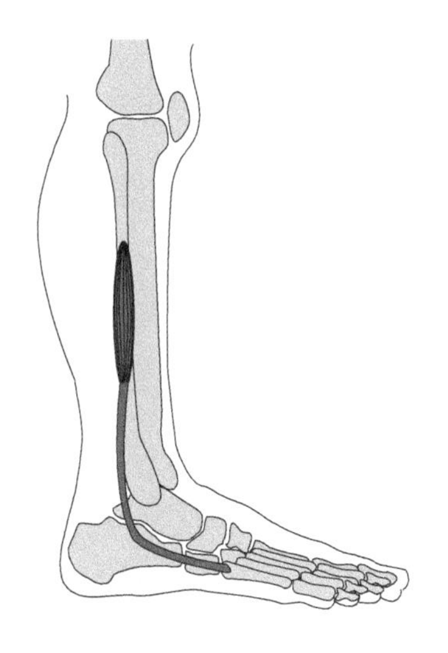

Fig 7.16
Fibularis (peroneus) brevis

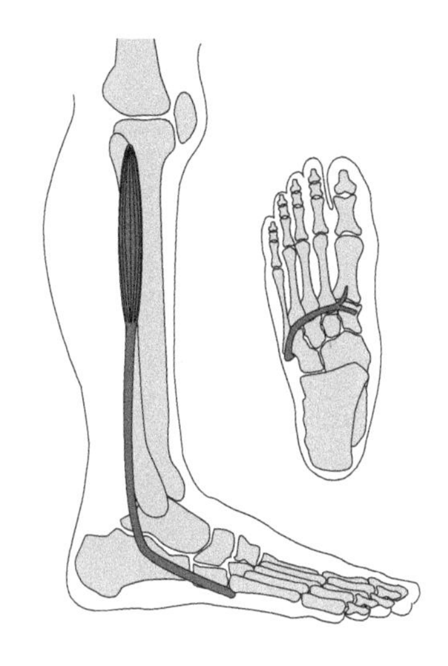

Fig 7.17
Fibularis (peroneus) longus

Lateral Compartment of the Lower Leg

Fibularis (peroneus) tertius originates at the anterior distal fibula (with extensor digitorum longus). It inserts on the base of the 5th metatarsal. Its actions are eversion of the foot and assistance in dorsiflexion of the foot. You may palpate the tendon lateral to the extensor digitorum longus tendon on the dorsum of the foot at the base of the 5th metatarsal. This muscle functions to place the foot flat on the ground by raising the lateral border.

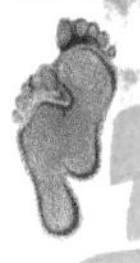

Current thinking is to be consistent using the Latin word, so peroneus is changed to fibularis.

Fibularis (peroneus) brevis originates at the lateral shaft of the fibula (the lower 2/3). It inserts on the base of the 5th metatarsal. Its actions are eversion of the foot and assistance in plantar flexion of the ankle. You may palpate the tendon on the lateral dorsum of the foot where it inserts on the tuberosity at the proximal end of the 5th metatarsal. It is closest to the malleolus and stands out more than the fibularis longus tendon.

The action of the foot evertors (as well as invertors) is especially helpful when walking or running on uneven surfaces. Sometimes the muscles "give out," and a sprained ligament can result.

Fibularis (peroneus) longus originates at the lateral shaft of the fibula (upper 2/3). It inserts on the base of the 1st metatarsal and the 1st (medial) cuneiform (plantar surface). Its actions are eversion of the foot and assistance in plantar flexion of the ankle. You may palpate via the lateral surface of the proximal half of the lower leg. The tendon is palpated just above and behind the lateral malleolus, slightly posterior to the fibularis brevis tendon.

Fibularis longus traverses the sole of the foot to meet the tibialis anterior tendon to form a stirrup for the foot.

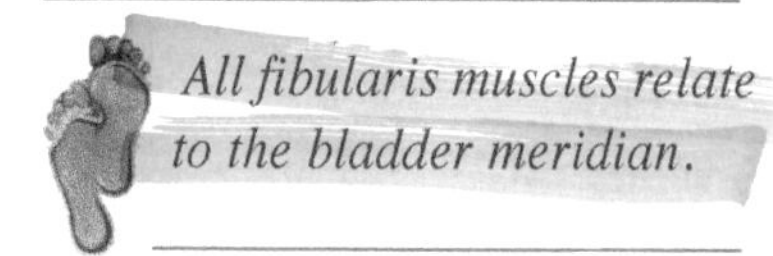

All fibularis muscles relate to the bladder meridian.

Muscles of the Foot

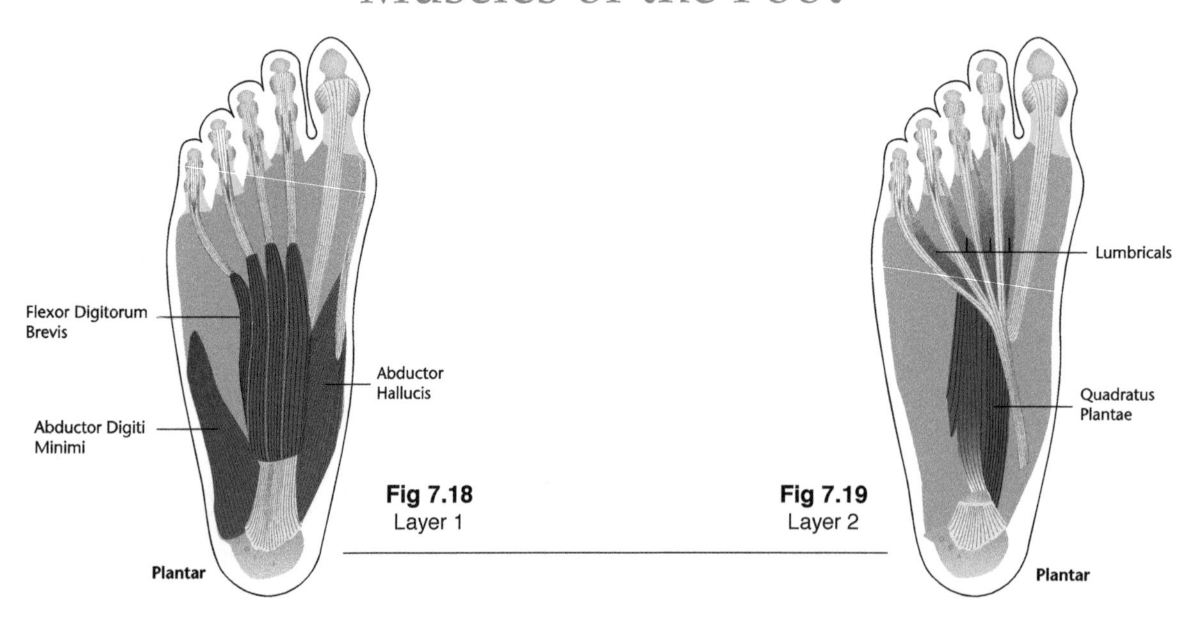

Fig 7.18
Layer 1

Fig 7.19
Layer 2

From the superficial layer to the deepest layer

Layer 1—Most Superficial

Abductor Hallucis originates at the calcaneus. It inserts on the base of the proximal phalanx of the great toe. Its actions are flexion and abduction of the great toe at the metatarsophalangeal (MTP) joint. It cannot be palpated. Abductor hallucis allows you to spread your big toe away from the other toes.

Flexor Digitorum Brevis originates at the calcaneus. It inserts on the middle phalanges of the four lateral toes. Its actions are flexion of the proximal interphalangeal (PIP) joints of the four lateral toes. It cannot be palpated. This muscle allows you to lift and spread the other toes.

Abductor Digiti Minimi originates at the calcaneus. It inserts on the base of the proximal phalanx of the little toe. Its actions are flexion and abduction of the little toe at the MTP joint. It cannot be palpated. This muscle allows you to spread your little toe.

Layer 2—Deep to Layer 1

Lumbricals originate at the tendon of the flexor digitorum longus. They insert on the extensor expansion to the four lateral toes. Their actions are flexion of the MTP joints and extension of the DIP and PIP joints.

Quadratus Plantae originates at the calcaneus. It inserts on the tendons of the flexor digitorum longus. It acts to assist the flexor digitorum longus in the flexion of the DIP joints.

The quadratus plantae muscle has a relationship to the quadratus lumborum muscle in the body. Quadratus lumborum is also associated with the large intestine meridian. The Integrative Reflexology® approach is to work both areas (quadratus lumborum and quadratus plantae) and the large intestine.

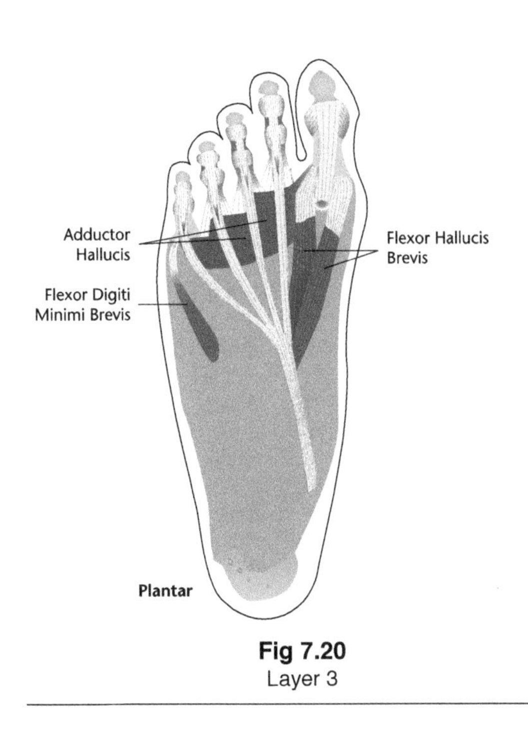

Fig 7.20
Layer 3

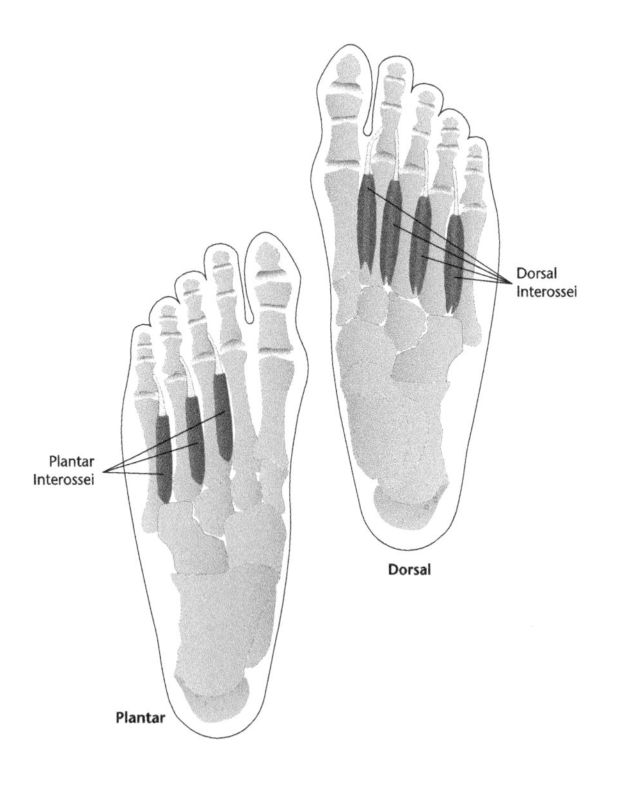

Fig 7.21
Layer 4

Layer 3—Deep to Layer 2

Flexor Hallucis Brevis originates at the base of the metatarsal of the great toe. It inserts on the base of the phalanx of the great toe. Its actions are flexion of the MTP joint (great toe).

Adductor Hallucis originates at the oblique (base of the 2nd and 3rd metatarsals) and the transverse (the 3rd, 4th, and 5th) MTP joint capsules. It inserts on the base of the proximal phalanx of the great toe. Its actions are adduction and flexion of the great toe. These actions allow you to lift and cross your big toe over the second toe. With the adductor hallucis, you may be able to pinch and pick up things with your toes.

Flexor Digiti Minimi Brevis originates at the cuboid and base of the 5th metatarsal. It inserts on the base of the proximal phalanx of the 5th toe. Its action is flexion of the MTP joint.

Layer 4—Deepest

Dorsal Interossei originate at the adjacent metatarsals. They insert on the extensor expansion of the 2nd, 3rd, and 4th toes. Their actions are abduction of the 2nd, 3rd, and 4th toes.

Plantar Interossei originate at the medial side of the 3rd, 4th, and 5th metatarsals. They insert on the extensor expansion to the three lateral toes. Their actions are adduction of the three lateral toes.

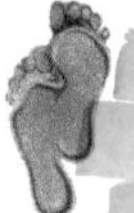

The Interossei muscles between the metatarsals are the deepest muscles in the foot. Giving gentle manipulations to the bones will stimulate these muscles.

Anatomy of the Hands

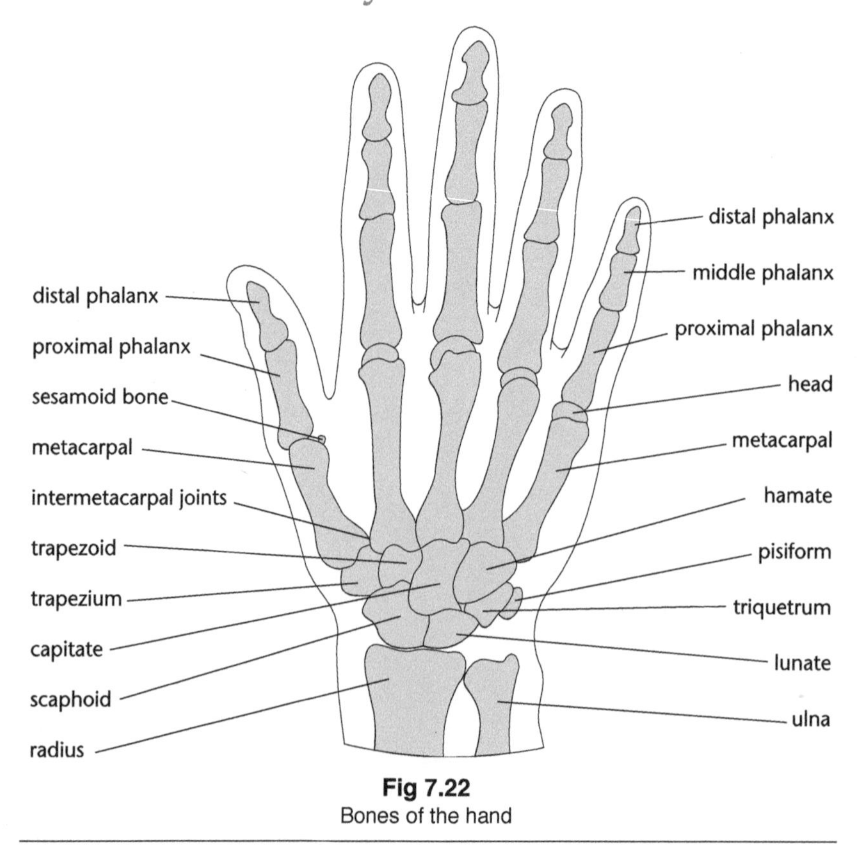

Fig 7.22
Bones of the hand

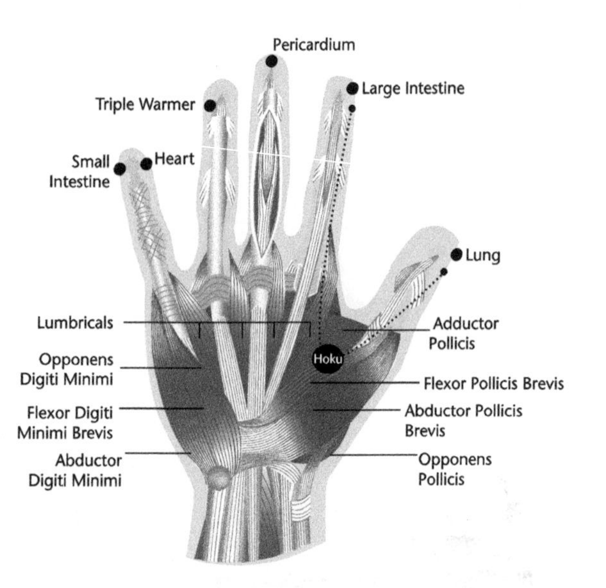

Fig 7.23
Palmar superficial view

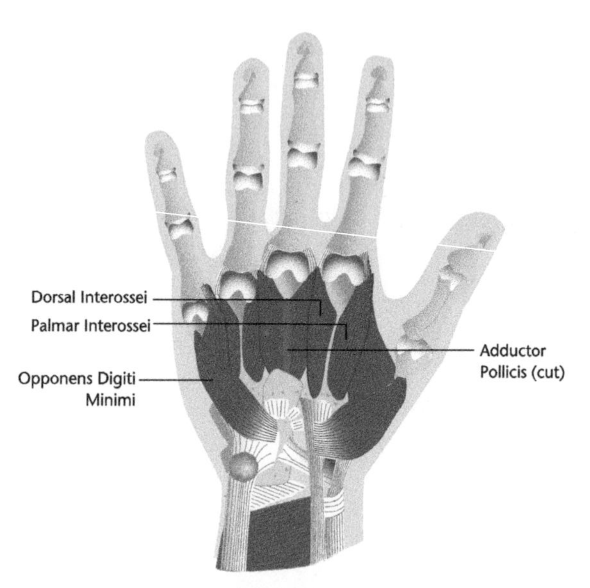

Fig 7.24
Palmar deep view

Muscles of the Hands

The hands are responsible for daily activities that involve gripping, precision skills (including typing) and pinching.

The hand muscles are divided into three areas.

Lateral Aspect of the palm includes the muscles that make up the thumb pad also called the thenar eminence.

- **Adductor Pollicis**—adducts the thumb, brings it closer to the fingers (this would help with the massage technique cupping).
- **Flexor Pollicis Brevis**—flexes the thumb and helps hold onto things (I use it in knitting).
- **Abductor Pollicis Brevis**—abducts the thumb, opening and stretching the thumb out. Good for hitch-hiking, which is not recommended.
- **Opponens Pollicis**—brings the thumb across the palmer surface to meet the little finger (used in making a scout pledge).

Midpalmer muscles are in the deep areas between the fingers. They allow for the flexion and extension of the fingers. We certainly could not play music without these magical fingers.

- **Lumbricals**—flex and extend each finger.
- **Palmar Interossei**—flex and spread the fingers, all but the 3rd finger.
- **Dorsal Interossei**—flex and extend the 2nd, 3rd and 4th fingers.

Medial Aspect of the palm is also called the hypothenar eminence. This is the raised mount by the little finger.

- **Abductor Digiti Minimi**—abducts the little finger, spreading it out.
- **Flexor Digiti Minimi**—flexes the little finger.
- **Opponens Digiti Minimi**—brings the little finger toward the thumb (good for the girl scout pledge).

8

Client Observations, Reactions and Contraindications

Observing the Feet

Arches

Fallen arches are also called "flat feet." This condition may be congenital (from birth), or may occur with age. Regardless of the onset of the condition, it can be improved through exercising the foot. One specific exercise is the "Tiger's Mouth" exercise described in Chapter 2 (page 22). Picking up small, smooth, round stones or marbles with the toes is another exercise that can help strengthen the arch. People with fallen arches may need to wear arch support in their shoes. If their condition is causing knee and hip problems, a referral to a podiatrist or chiropractor may be indicated.

High arches are an inherited structural imbalance and the condition may cause spinal alignment problems. Women's high heeled shoes can increase the severity of the condition. Shoes with good arch support are often needed for persons with high arches, but it is best for them to see a professional concerning footwear. One beneficial foot exercise for this condition is rolling on a foot log (information on ordering this product is on page 182), which stretches the arch and allows it to lengthen and flatten. The exercise of actively spreading the toes and bones of the feet—stretching or elongating the tight muscles as often as possible, is also beneficial. Rolfing, structural integration, and deep connective tissue massage may help to open up the tight foot muscles.

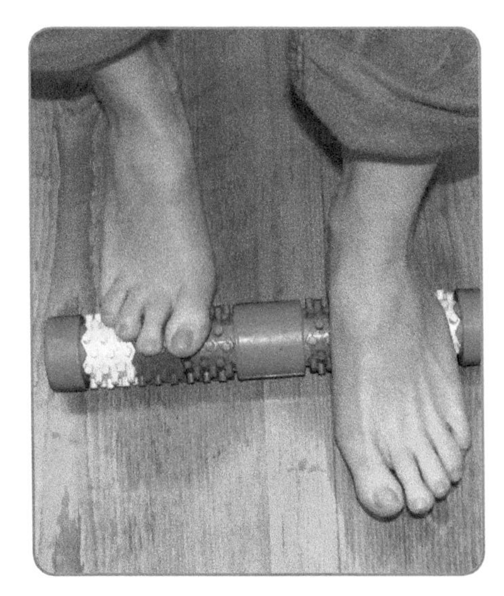

Fig 8.1 - Foot roller

Calluses and Corns

Calluses are a build-up of tissue on the surface of the skin and can be formed by wearing shoes that are old or worn, exercising (such as runner's callus,) or even going barefoot a lot. Calluses may be pumiced as part of your treatment for your client. You may have a pumice stone for each individual client or simply use an emery board, which you would discard after the session. An Epsom salt foot soak will soften the callus. A foot scrub, as used in the spa sequence, will also reduce the callus.

Corns are calluses that grow into the skin and are often the result of wearing too-tight shoes. This can be very painful for the client. If the condition is severe, professional attention may be indicated. Note where the corn or callus is located and design your treatment to correspond with the associated reflex point or meridian.

Edema and Lymphatic Congestion

Notice any swelling around the ankle and the top of the foot. Check to see if it is pitting edema by pressing your finger into the swollen area. If it leaves an indentation, a pit, then it is pitting edema and you need to ask your client if they have any conditions that are related to the swelling in their feet and ankles. Swelling may occur due to any of the following conditions: general lymphedema, kidney imbalances, congestive heart failure, pregnancy and injury. If the edema is due to these conditions, then reflexology is contraindicated unless medical approval is given.

Once the cause has been determined, and it is not a contraindication, you may begin the session. You would design your treatment plan to include all of the Integrative Reflexology® lymph techniques and repeat them at various times throughout the session, including the beginning and end. If you are a massage therapist trained in additional, more comprehensive lymphatic massage, you can add those techniques into the session as well. Your client might need a bathroom break during the session due to all of the fluids that will be moved.

Toenails

Infected toenails will be red and swollen. This may be due to an ingrown or involuted toenail, injury or other conditions. Avoid any work in those areas whether the client is being treated for the condition or not. If they are not receiving treatment, refer them to a professional, as needed.

Ingrown toenails occur when the nail is growing under the skin. This may lead to inflammation and infection. If the condition is severe, the client should be advised to seek professional help. One natural remedy is to let the nail grow with cotton placed between the skin and the toenail. You can advise your client that toenails need to be trimmed straight across the top and then smoothed out with an emery board. This method can help prevent ingrown toenails. Most ingrown toenails occur on the great toe. If you notice that either the spleen meridian (medial border of the great toe) or the liver meridian (lateral border) is involved, design your treatment to include stimulation and balancing for those meridians.

One of my clients, whom I worked with for years, had a recurring ingrown toenail on the liver meridian side of her great toe. This client also presented with a story of being angry with her family in almost every session (anger is the emotion for the liver meridian). Unfortunately, it was not appropriate for me to discuss this correlation with her, but when she and I parted ways in our therapeutic relationship, I did suggest that she see a podiatrist about her "festering" ingrown toenail.

Involuted toenails occur when the curve of the nail is so exaggerated that it may actually grow back into the top of the toe. This results from not cutting the toenails for long periods of time. Proper toenail trimming on a regular basis is the remedy. Nail trimming is not within the scope of practice for a reflexologist or massage therapist. When this is needed in a treatment situation, please refer clients to a podiatrist.

Nail fungus is a common condition. Most types are not contagious. You will have to rely on the client's knowledge of the condition. You may want to avoid those areas or use gloves. Tea tree oil is a natural remedy for this condition.

Other Conditions of the Feet

Athlete's foot is a fungus that is contagious and should be avoided. It is best to suspend reflexology treatments until the condition is successfully treated. A natural remedy for treatment of athlete's foot is thyme in olive oil and tea tree oil. Getting the feet out in sunshine also may help. This fungus likes moist, sweaty feet.

Blisters, Cuts and Bruises should be avoided.

Cracks and fissures are places where the skin has broken open. A fissure is a very deep crack; usually the skin is dry and thick. Pumicing and using skin softening creams may help. The area most often affected is the edge of the heel. This corresponds to the hemorrhoid reflex area, and the bladder meridian. You may wish to discuss this with your client and see if this fits with his or her health history.

Plantar warts are common and treatable. Both natural and over-the-counter remedies are beneficial in treating this condition. If the condition does not respond to these remedies, then the client should seek professional help. If the wart is exposed, broken, open or bleeding, it may be contagious and contact should be avoided. You might take note of where the wart appears and see if there is an imbalance in that reflex area or meridian.

Varicose veins are usually in the lower leg. In my practice, I have never seen a large one in the feet. The little red or blue spider veins are not dangerous to work on. The large swollen blue veins should be avoided. You could go around them or above them, but do not massage into them.

Observing the Client

Physical

Notice, is your client

- In a robust state of health?
- Recovering from recent illness?
- Dealing with chronic illness?
- Of an age that you need to take care when providing treatment?

Your observations will determine the depth of your pressure and which reflex points you may choose to work or avoid.

Mental/Emotional

Before and during a session, clients will often offer insights to their current emotional state, which may or may not be related to their body. They might be experiencing difficulties at work, family-related stress or maybe they are worried about their own health. Listening to the verbal clues they offer can give you insight into how to proceed with their session.

- **Stress** is known to affect the spleen and the immune system.
- If your client is **depressed**, Meridian Theory would indicate stimulation of the lung and large intestine reflexes.
- If the client expresses **anger**, I would focus on the liver reflex.
- If the client expresses **fear or anxiety**, then hold the Kidney 1 point (also the solar plexus reflex).

Let your intuition guide you as you listen to your client.

Spiritual

It is a common belief in most energy work modalities that illness begins in the spiritual body. This approach is a basic tenet in chakra balancing, polarity therapy and healing touch. Most states recognize reflexology as energy work rather than bodywork; therefore, the spiritual state is an important observation to include in your therapeutic approach. Your client's spiritual state will overlap with their emotional and physical states; all are intertwined and must be considered as a part of the client's whole being.

Observing Client Reactions

The effects of a reflexology session usually last for 24-48 hours. These effects can be immediate or delayed.

Common Reactions

Your client may experience one or more of these reactions after their session. Assure them that it is common to experience a mild detoxifying effect.

Increased urination (darker and stronger smelling than normal)—This will decrease swelling in general and specifically in the feet and legs. They may report less pain and easier mobility.

Flatulence and more frequent bowel movements — The colon work is very effective in stimulating peristaltic movement in the bowels.

Sweating—It is not uncommon for the client to experience an outbreak of sweating in the palms of the hands, feet or other areas of the body. This is often thought of as a toxic release. There are some who sweat due to hormonal imbalances. You might inquire if this is a recurring symptom for your client.

Increased secretion of the mucous membranes—The sinuses may start to drain during the session. Coughing up phlegm is also a reaction.

Increased vaginal secretions and discharge—If your client notices this, it may be that she has some yeast imbalances. This is very common with the increased use of birth control pills and sugar in our diets.

Disrupted sleep patterns—If the client slept more or deeper, then continue the sessions as before. If your client has a fitful night's sleep, then lighten up your pressure, reduce the number of stimulations to each endocrine point, and do more calming nerve strokes in future sessions.

Tiredness—This may be due to the cleansing effect. The body needs rest in order to rejuvenate.

Feeling refreshed, relaxed, and energetic— This means your client is in a state of good health.

Less Common Reactions

These reactions may occur with less frequency and may require some additional attention on your part.

Headaches—As the practitioner, you will want to determine if the headaches are due to allergies, sinus infection, hormonal imbalance or a detox release. You would have to question the client to see what is the reason behind the headache.

Dizziness—This rarely occurs, but if it does, then do more calming nerve strokes and grounding strokes at the end of the session.

Emotional release, tendency to weep—This may occur due to the deep relaxation effect. The client may feel emotions on a deeper level and feel relaxed and safe enough to release them.

Temporary outbreak of suppressed diseases—The relaxation effect of the reflexology can allow colds, flu symptoms and other common conditions that are already brewing within the body to surface.

Aggravated skin conditions (pimples)—The skin is the largest organ in the body. It is an organ of elimination. Skin eruptions are the body detoxifying.

Chilliness and shivering—This can be an indication that the client has been over stimulated. This can also be a detoxifying release. I would suggest that the session be terminated, and a warm blanket and a warm drink be offered. Stay with the client until they feel well enough to go home. Suggest an Epsom salt bath when they get home.

Increased appetite—This occurs due to stimulation of the digestion system.

Swelling—This is a rare reaction since the lymphatic system is stimulated during the session. This reaction would suggest that there are conditions present that may not benefit from the reflexology; or it may be that the pressure was too deep, causing the lymph to fill up.

As the practitioner, you never want to exceed the tolerance level of the client. Each client's sensitivity to the treatment will vary. It is necessary to maintain verbal communication between yourself and your client throughout the session. If some of the less common reactions occur and require a change in the treatment plan, or some additional attention, you can respond based on the guidelines below.

Addressing Client Reactions

The following are suggestions for how to respond when your client has a therapeutic release during the session.

1. Remain calm and observant.
2. Apply less pressure and work at your client's tolerance level.
3. Take the heels in the palm of your hands and apply gentle traction to the legs. This will help the legs relax and will calm the nerves and help ground the client's body.
4. Instruct the client to breathe deeply and slowly while you gently and simultaneously stimulate the solar plexus points on both feet.
5. If the client feels chilly, cover them with a warm blanket. Getting cold is a sign that the body is releasing toxins and the blood pressure may be decreasing.
6. Stay with the client and hold the intention of calmness and support.
7. Have the client rest for at least 30 minutes before leaving.
8. Suggest that the client increase intake of water.
9. Suggest that the client take a warm or hot Epsom salt bath.
10. Suggest that the client eat lightly for 24 hours.
11. Suggest that the client wait at least one week until the next appointment.
12. Contact the client 24-48 hours after the session to check on further reactions.
13. Decrease pressure in the next session.

Cautions and Contraindications

Acute Flare of Various Chronic Diseases

If a client's chronic condition is in a state of acute flare, it is advisable to allow their body to rest and return to a non-inflamed state before doing reflexology. Examples of conditions that can be in a state of flare are lupus, rheumatoid arthritis, cancer, Lyme's disease, multiple sclerosis and other autoimmune disorders.

Acute Inflammation

Acute inflammation is a contraindication for reflexology. The inflammation could be due to a variety of conditions such as rheumatoid arthritis, gout, lymphadenitis (inflamed lymph nodes) or an inflamed spleen. Allow the tissue to return to a less inflamed state before working on the feet.

Athlete's Foot

This is highly contagious and a contraindication for reflexology.

Atrophy of the Feet

This condition could be due to long-term bed rest, paralysis, severe congestive heart failure or age. This condition is a contraindication for reflexology since circulation and nerve response is impaired.

Blood Clot (Thrombosis)

This condition is an **absolute contraindication** for reflexology. As the practitioner, you should be aware of unilateral swelling (only one leg) especially above the knee, with associated redness, heat and pain in that leg. This may be an indication of a blood clot and you would not offer any bodywork. You would advise your client to seek medical attention. If your client has a history of blood clots, but has been on blood thinners for at least six months, they may receive reflexology with a physician's approval.

Chemotherapy

There are multiple considerations to take into account when your client is receiving chemotherapy. Reflexology is contraindicated if the cancer is located in a place that may be directly affected by reflexology (e.g., bone cancer in the leg), if the client's overall health is depleted and over stimulation is a concern, and if the chemicals used are harsh and cause sweating. In the latter scenario, the practitioner can absorb the chemicals sweating out through the pores in the feet.

Diabetes

Diet-controlled—Reflexology is indicated in this condition. You would want to stimulate the pancreas reflex area as well as the stomach and spleen reflex points.

Medication-controlled—Reflexology is indicated in this condition. You can still stimulate the pancreas reflex, but be aware of any tenderness in that area. The stomach and spleen reflex points are also beneficial.

Insulin-controlled—As long as the diabetes is controlled, and the tissue quality and circulation are healthy, reflexology is indicated. If the feet are experiencing numbness or neuropathy, and are red or blue, then reflexology is contra-indicated. Reflexology is also contraindicated if there are any cuts, bruises or ulcers on the feet as a result of the diabetes. Avoid the pancreas reflex area when the client is insulin dependent.

Fever

It is better to wait until the fever passes so as not to over stimulate the body.

Gangrene

This indicates that there is a severe breakdown of the circulation system and that the client should be under a physician's care. The only beneficial massage indicated in this circum-stance is gentle lymph drainage.

High-Risk Pregnancy

Be cautious about over stimulation due to possible early delivery. Energetic support may be indicated.

Infections of the Feet

This condition is a contraindication for reflexology. A responsible professional would not risk spreading the infection.

Infectious Disease

Infectious diseases include colds, the flu, tuberculosis, hepatitis, etc. There are two things to consider with infectious disease: (1) could you, as the practitioner, catch this condition and (2) could the session be too much stimulation for the client's body, which is already fighting an infection. If you have any concern about either factor, reschedule your session.

Lymphedema

This would be a contraindication if the swelling is extreme and full-body and the lymph fluid is not moving easily.

Multiple Medications

If your client is on multiple medications, you will want to research why the client is taking the medications and how each medication affects the organs. The website www.drugs.com may be a good place to review the medication and its side effects. For example, antibiotics affect the digestive system; you may find that stimulation of the digestive reflexes supports your client. Some medications can affect the liver, so gentle stimulation of the liver reflex may be beneficial or it may be too detoxifying, leaving the client feeling nauseated or with general malaise. You will need to determine if reflexology is supportive based on your client's reaction to the session.

Open Wounds, Bruises, Rashes, Broken Bones

Acute injuries and open wounds are contra-indicated for reflexology.

Osteoporosis

This condition is most often seen in elderly ladies whose bones are very fragile. Any stretches or manipulations of the feet could result in a fracture. It is fine to do gentle reflexology on clients with mild osteoporosis, but advanced osteoporosis is a contraindication.

Peripheral Neuropathy

If the client is unable to give feedback about the pressure, you may do the session using light pressure and listening to the tissue as you work. Work with caution.

Pitting Edema

This exists when pressing into the swollen area creates an indentation that remains when you remove your finger. You will need to determine the reason for the edema. If the cause for the condition is related to heart failure, kidney disease, liver disease, a local infection or blockage in the circulatory system, reflexology is a contraindication. If you are able to move the fluid first, then you may proceed with the reflexology session.

Pregnancy-Related Contraindications

The uterus reflex, spleen 6 and Hoku points, as well as all endocrine points, are all contraindicated for pregnant clients until the time of delivery or within a week before the due date. Stimulation of these points can cause the uterus to contract and labor to begin. It is my experience that even when these points are worked, a baby comes when it is ready, but as a professional, you must err on the side of caution. For pregnant clients who are at or beyond their due date, I have found that stimulation of these points has been helpful in promoting labor.

Sprains and Strains of the Ankle (acute)

These acute injuries are a contraindication for reflexology until the bruising and swelling has subsided.

Surgery is Indicated

It is best to check with your client's health care provider.

Varicose Veins

Avoid the veins if they are raised and swollen. If there is an extreme amount of varicosities in the lower leg, reflexology is contraindicated.

(Here are two suggested books for you to use as reference for any conditions not listed above: Mosby's Pathology for Massage Therapists, by Susan G. Salvo; A Massage Therapist's Guide to Pathology, by Ruth Werner)

9

Preparing for your Integrative Reflexology® Session

Health History

Name: ______________________________

Phone (home): ______________ (work): ______________

Address: ______________________________

Email: ______________________________

Occupation: ______________________________

Hobbies/Physical Activities: ______________________________

General State of Health: ______________________________

Are you currently taking medications? ❑ Yes ❑ No

If YES, please list ______________________________

For what condition ______________________________

List any allergies: ______________________________

Have you had any surgeries? ❑ Yes ❑ No

If YES, please describe ______________________________

Are you currently being treated for any conditions by a physician? ❑ Yes ❑ No

If YES, please describe ______________________________

Are you receiving care by a holistic health practitioner (acupuncture, chiropractic, bodywork, etc)? ❑ Yes ❑ No

If YES, please describe ______________________________

Have you ever received foot and/or hand reflexology? ❑ Yes ❑ No

If YES, when? ______________________________

For how long? ______________________________

Any reaction? ______________________________

Do I have your permission to contact you 48 hours after the treatment to record your reaction? ❑ Yes ❑ No

Fig 9.1
Sample Health History Form

Always have your client fill in a basic health history form that will provide you with initial information as you prepare to offer them a therapeutic session. You will want to collect contact information, information about their daily activities, and any health conditions that may affect the treatment you provide.

Observations:
(corns, calluses, bunions, and other foot deviations)

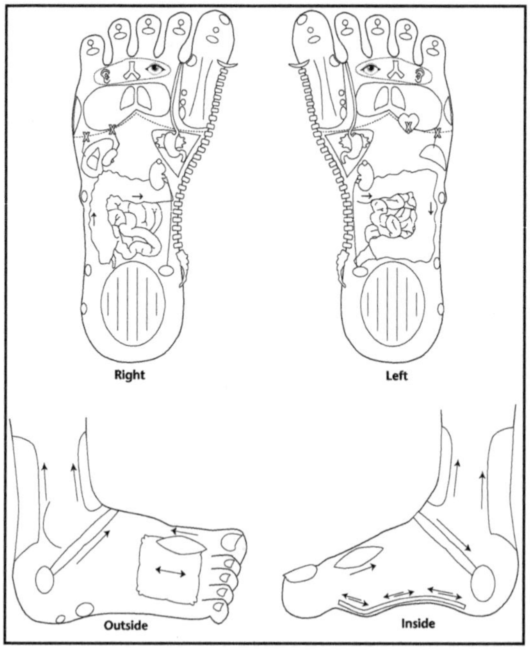

Label Tender Areas 1–5:
1—Very slight tenderness
5—Extremely tender
* Best to work at Level 3

Reactions During Session:

Reactions Immediately After Session:

Right

Left

Outside

Inside

Reactions 24–48 Hours After Session:

Client Overall Experience of Session:

*Disclaimer: Foot Reflexology does not claim to treat or diagnose physical conditions. Please refer clients to physician for medical treatment.

Fig 9.2
Sample Note Taking Form

You would use a note-taking form to record your observations of your client's conditions, your assessments of the degree of tenderness they experience during the session, as well as the reactions they experience during and after the session. These notes will allow you to keep a record of the treatment you provide and how the client responds to it. It will also guide you in creating future treatment plans.

It is always important to include a disclaimer on your health history form that expresses to the client that you are not diagnosing physical conditions and that reflexology is not a substitution for medical treatment. For conditions outside the scope of your practice, you will need to refer them to a physician for diagnosis and treatment.

In addition to your health history and notes, you might also question your client more specifically about information related to the four theories of Integrative Reflexology®. The following are examples of questions that you might ask your client directly, in order to facilitate a deeper understanding of the condition(s) they are presenting with. The questions are divided up as related to each of the four theories:

Structure

- What style of shoe do you wear? For exercise, for work, at home?
- Do you go barefoot? How often and what type of surface do you walk on?
- Do you need or use orthotics?

Zones

- If there is pain in the foot, do you have pain in that location in the body?

NOTE—If you are a massage therapist, you might want to palpate that area of the body and see if there is a connection between what you find in the feet and what you find in the body.

Meridians

These questions relate to information provided in the meridian table on page 32.

- What is your favorite/least favorite time of the year?
- Do you prefer certain climates? Hot, cold, windy, dry?
- What emotion is dominant at the moment?
- What is your dominant personality type? Are you a caretaker, an artist, a commander or a lover?
- What foods do you tend to desire/avoid? Pungent, salty, sour, bitter or sweet?
- Do you have recurring muscular pain? In what muscles?
- What time of day do you have the most energy? The least energy?
- Do you wake up at certain times in the night? Is this recurring or random?
- Have you ever broken any toes or fingers?
- What element is strong in your life, and your personality? Are you fiery and passionate, watery and emotional, grounded and earthy, or airy and intellectual? Combinations apply, too. (The client may not be able to answer this directly; you will have to observe it for yourself.)

Combine the answers to these questions and notice if a pattern emerges that directs you to work with a specific pair of meridians and their associated reflex areas.

Psychoneuroimmunology

- Have you had any significant stressful events in the past 12 months? This could be related to a personal loss, relationships, jobs, family, health, finances, world events, etc.

NOTE—You might refer your client to the stress assessment on the HeartMath Institute's website (www.heartmath.org) to help them understand their stress and learn how to reduce it.

Working With Your Client

Client Communication

Communication is an important factor in your session. Clear, confident and comforting communication can be accomplished by maintaining eye contact with your clients. Some clients may feel nervous about their first session and, as the practitioner, you may be nervous about your first session with them. Explain to the client about feedback and the importance of client/practitioner communication. The entire session relies on the client letting you know which areas are tender and to what degree of tenderness.

During the session, notice if your client winces, or if facial muscles tighten. These can be indications that the pressure is too much in that reflex area. Many clients hesitate to voice their discomforts, thinking that a painful treatment is a more effective one, or that you are the professional and you know better. Some clients may need your reassurance and inquiry to feel comfortable expressing what they are feeling during the session. It is more effective to work at a level of pressure that the client can tolerate. A gentle but firm treatment is best and most effective.

It is also important for you to record the tender areas that your client experiences in the session. It can help to have your client provide a number for the degree of tenderness they are experiencing: 1 (slight)—5 (tender). Keeping a record of this will allow you to track changes in the tenderness of the reflexes from session to session.

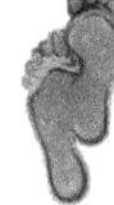

When the reflex point/area is tender it can indicate either a slight imbalance in the associated organ or a significant imbalance. The reflex point can range between 5x to 25x more sensitive than the actual organ. This is why we do not diagnose based on what we notice during the session.

Client Positioning

After the optional foot soak, position your client so that their back, neck, hips and knees are comfortable. You may use a massage table or a reclining style chair. The popular chair used for reflexology today is the LaFuma (Fig 9.3) — a French lawn chair that easily reclines.

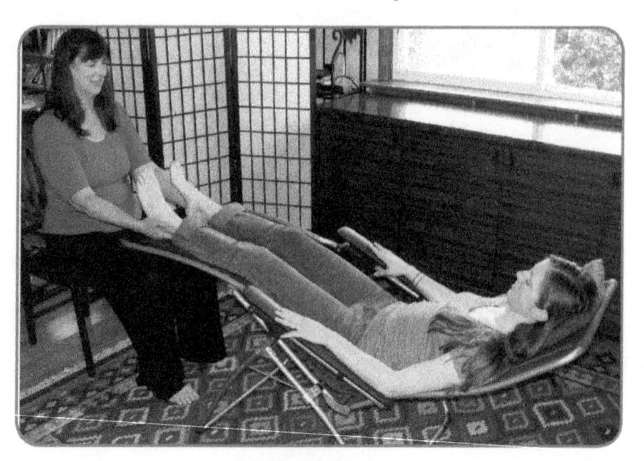

Fig 9.3
LaFuma chair

Massage tables (Fig 9.4) are my preferred method of positioning because I feel that the client fully relaxes onto the table, and I am able to work other areas easily. Be sure to have a pillow under the knees to release the knees and lower back. Using the traction of the body by pulling the heels may also allow the client to fully relax into the table and the session.

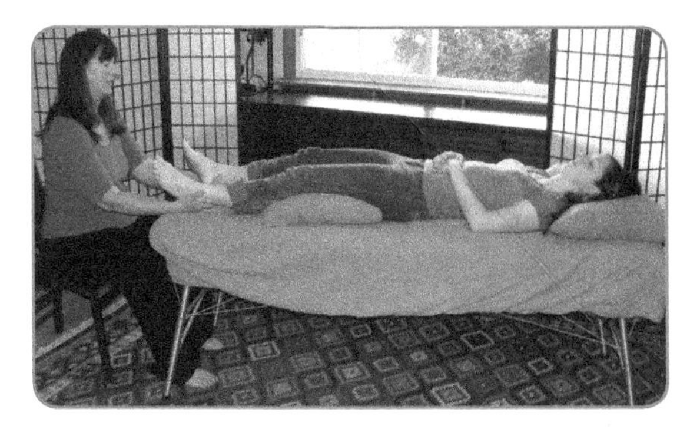

Fig 9.4
Massage table

Grades of Pressure

You will want to use different grades of pressure during your treatments. Different levels of pressure are necessary for different clients and also for different reflex areas. You might think about it on a scale of 1-5, with 1 being a light touch and 5 being deep pressure. Most clients will appreciate work in the 3-4 range and that will be effective. Notice what areas require less pressure and what areas can handle deeper pressure.

Planning Sessions

Duration of Sessions

The duration of your sessions will vary according to the intention and the client's needs. In an average 60-minute session, approximately 45-50 minutes is spent on the feet, with 5-10 minutes on the hands. This book includes sequences and suggestions for 30-minute spa sessions, a basic 60-minute session, and a 90-minute session that includes additional techniques and the opportunity for other bodywork.

Frequency of Sessions

Sessions can occur as frequently as once a week. In acute situations, reflexology may be performed every third day. It is best to rest the endocrine glands for at least two days. The reflexes such as the spine, sinuses, lungs, and large and small intestines can be stimulated daily.

Setting Intentions

Once you have positioned your client comfortably and settled into your position at their feet, you will be starting with the solar plexus hold. This is the time to set your intention for this session with your client. This is a mental exercise that focuses on what the client needs and allows you to clear your thoughts and become fully present in the moment. You may have a personal ritual or affirmation that you say to yourself at this point, or perhaps you and your client have come up with an intention you can both hold in your mind as you begin.

When the session is over, take a moment to consciously disconnect from your client. The scientific community is beginning to prove how energetically connected we are. It is truly possible for you to go home with aches in the same area as your client. Therefore, it is important for you to release your client's energy to them and claim your own energy as yours.

Opening Intentional Statements:

- "I affirm good health for (insert client's name)."
- "I affirm a strong and balanced body for (insert client's name)."
- "I affirm openness to all that is good and healing for (insert client's name)."

These are a few suggestions. Find statements that resonate with you and your client.

Closing Intentional Statements:

- "I release all negativity and all toxins from both (insert client's name) and myself."
- "We are surrounded by healing light and all is well."
- "Divine Healing light surrounds and protect us all."

In closing, you want to have your statement to speak to releasing anything that was brought to the surface, supporting continued healing light and protection and creating closure for the session in a way that is balancing for both the client and yourself.

Foot Soaks

You may choose to begin your treatment session with a therapeutic foot soak. The foot soak (Fig 9.5) can be a nice way for the client to transition from the world outside and into the treatment space. It supports their body by relaxing and preparing them to receive your therapeutic touch. It is also a nice way to cleanse their feet in preparation for you working on them.

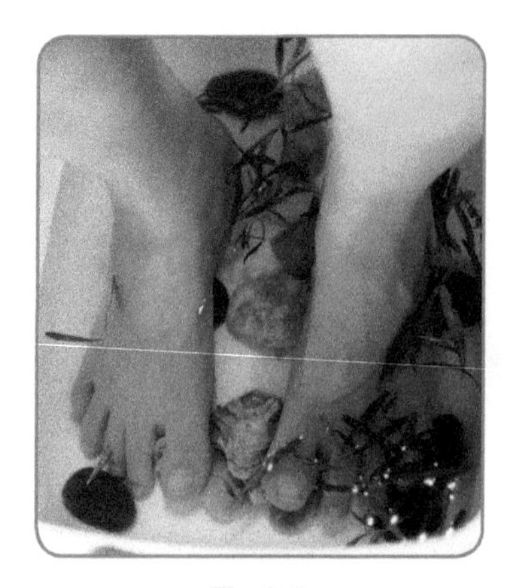

Fig 9.5
Sample foot soak with rocks and herbs.

I suggest a simple Epsom salt soak. This magnesium salt is known to help with tired, achy muscles. The heat of the water opens the pores in the soles of the feet and draws the moisture out of the tissue.

Generally, you will use about ¼–½ cup of Epsom salt added into a basin of warm to hot water, according to your client's preference. You might start with hot water and add cold water to achieve the desired temperature. Soaking for 3-5 minutes is enough. Adding in essential oils or medicinal herbs will enhance the experience of the foot soak as well as the effect of the Integrative Reflexology® session.

You might add any of the following herbs into the foot soak to achieve the desired effect. This is a suggested list of additions; you may come up with your own fun and therapeutic concoction.

- ***CAYENNE PEPPER***—A pinch will help clear out the sinuses; use with caution, as it can be an irritant.
- ***CHAMOMILE***—For calming and relaxing. Steep enough for a cup of tea for 5 minutes, then add to the soaking basin with warm/hot water.
- ***EUCALYPTUS***—Helps with breathing and sinus congestion. Use fresh or dried leaves—3 tablespoons in muslin or cheesecloth to soak in the water.
- ***GARLIC***—For infections, colds or flu that are mild or already in the healing phase (no fever). Do not disregard the cautions and contraindications for these conditions. You can press 2-3 cloves into cheesecloth then soak it in the water.
- ***GINGER***—Used to heat and detoxify the body. Use 2-3 tablespoons of grated ginger in muslin or cheesecloth to soak in the water.
- ***LAVENDER***—For calming and relaxing. Use 2-3 tablespoons of dried or fresh flowers in muslin or cheesecloth to soak in the water.
- ***LEMONS***—Add one fresh lemon, sliced, into the foot soak for a refreshing and cleansing treatment. Massaging the feet with the lemon slices is also a nice way to wrap-up at the end of the reflexology session.
- ***MUSTARD***—To heat and warm the body. For infections, colds or flu that are mild or already in the healing phase (no fever). Do not disregard the cautions and contraindications for these conditions. Use therapeutic grade mustard powder (from a health food store) and sprinkle it into the water for the foot soak.

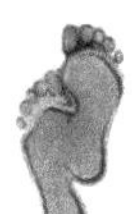

Mustard plasters were an old-time remedy for lung congestion due to colds or chest infections. You can find recipes online for your own use or to recommend for clients.

Foot Scrubs

Simple foot scrubs will add a relaxing and luxurious quality to your session.

Basic recipe:

¼ cup Epsom salt

4-8 drops essential oils (Choose one or use up to three in combination.)

Carrier oil—enough to make the scrub spreadable

The carrier oil can be any cold-pressed oil, such as olive, almond, jojoba, fractionated coconut, sesame or avocado oils.

Castor Oil Cream

This Sweet Feet© cream was designed specifically for Integrative Reflexology®. It combines only two ingredients—Shea butter and castor oil. It takes only ½ teaspoon to cover the entire foot

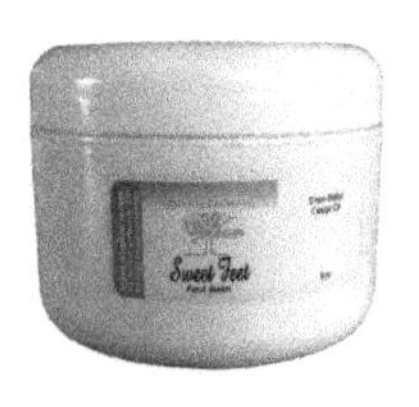

Fig 9.6
Sweet Feet© Cream

with a smooth emulsifying quality that allows the practitioner to easily work the reflexology areas. It is best applied after the opening toe work.

Aromatherapy

Aromatherapy can be used in both the foot scrubs and as an addition to the Sweet Feet© cream. The following are the eight essential oils that I currently work with.

Cypress (Cupressus sempervirens)

Cypress is clearing, strengthening and refreshing. It is anti-infectious, antibacterial, antimicrobial and antispasmodic. It is also an astringent, decongestant, deodorant, diuretic, liver tonic and nervous system tonic. It arrests bleeding and increases perspiration.

Benefits include:

- Treatment of varicose veins, edema, hemorrhoids, venous blood congestion.
- Restoring calm to an over-burdened nervous system.
- Regulation of menstruation and relief of painful menses.
- Management of acute and chronic bronchitis and whooping cough.
- Drawing out impurities from the skin.
- Movement and elimination of excess fluid.

Geranium (Pelargonium graveolens)

Geranium is balancing, elevating, cooling and supportive. It is antifungal, anti-inflammatory and antiseptic. It arrests bleeding and acts as an antidepressant, astringent, diuretic, deodorant, sedative and circulatory/liver tonic.

Benefits include:

- Diuretic action and stimulation of the lymphatic system.
- Facilitating the healing of wounds, burns, and bruises.
- Regulation of fluid levels—edema and cellulite
- Reducing stress, nervous tension, depression, headaches, and anxiety.
- Regulation of the entire endocrine system.
- Stimulating the adrenal cortex.
- Stabilizing fluctuating hormones related to conception, PMS and menopause.
- Balancing the production of sebum (our body's natural oils).

Lavender (Lavandula angustifolia)

Lavender is balancing, renewing and strengthening. It is antibacterial (wide-ranging), anti-inflammatory, antimicrobial, antispasmodic and antiviral. It is an analgesic, antidepressant, decongestant, diuretic, fungicide and sedative. It balances menstrual flow, lowers blood pressure and promotes wound healing. This is one of the safest and most versatile of the eight essential oils. It is so safe that we can use it with small children.

Benefits include:

- Treatment of burns—it eases the pain, prevents infection, promotes rapid healing and lowers the potential for scarring.
- Treatment of acne, dermatitis, eczema, psoriasis, boils and wounds.
- Pain relief associated with muscles, rheumatism, sciatica, arthritis, menstruation and childbirth.
- Harmonizing the nervous system – it balances the sympathetic and parasympathetic components of the nervous system.
- Treatment of insomnia and headaches, including migraines.
- Preventing and treating colds, flu, bronchitis, throat infections and mucus membrane inflammation.
- Balancing the feminine and masculine natures.

Lemongrass (Cymbopogon citratus)

Lemongrass is invigorating, clearing and refreshing. It is analgesic, antibacterial, antifungal, anti-inflammatory, antimicrobial (wide ranging) and antiseptic (airborne). It is an antidepressant, antioxidant, astringent and deodorant. It lowers fevers and acts as a sedative (boosts parasympathetic nervous system). It is better to avoid using this on hypersensitive or damaged skin, as well as on children under the age of 2.

Benefits include:

- Deodorizing the air.
- Eliminating airborne MRSA bacteria (staph) via diffusion.
- Improving thymus and spleen functions.
- Improving menstrual flow.
- Stimulation of the lymphatic system and detoxification.
- Treatment of acne, athlete's foot and excessive perspiration.
- Relieving arthritis and muscular pain.
- Improving concentration/focus.
- Elevating mood.

Peppermint (Mentha piperita)

Peppermint is refreshing, invigorating and mentally clearing. It is analgesic, antibacterial, antifungal, anti-infectious, antispasmodic and antiviral. It is a decongestant and expectorant. It increases bile production, thins mucus secretions and reduces fevers. It is the most effective essential oil for the digestive system. It should not be used on or near infants and small children, on the face, or on some people with G6PD liver enzyme deficiency.

Benefits include:

- Relief of indigestion, nausea, vomiting, travel sickness, obstruction of bile ducts, gallbladder inflammation and digestive challenges, such as irritable bowel syndrome and spastic colitis.

- Reducing pain associated with menstrual and muscle cramping.
- Stimulating lymphatic flow.
- Relief of headaches.
- Aiding memory and improving mental fatigue.
- Cleansing and decongesting the skin.

Ravensara (Ravensara aromatica)

Ravensara is fresh, revitalizing, clearing and uplifting. It is analgesic, antibacterial (for staph bacteria), antifungal, anti-infectious, anti-inflammatory, antiseptic, antispasmodic and powerfully antiviral. It is a detoxifier, expectorant, immune balancer and tonic for the nervous system.

Benefits include:

- Being a powerful preventative and treatment for colds, flu, bronchitis, rhinitis and sinusitis.
- Mental and physical stimulation in cases of fatigue.
- Stimulation of the circulatory, lymphatic and cardiovascular systems.
- Relief of pain and irritation associated with shingles blisters (in combination with lemongrass).
- Pain relief for a wide range of muscular and joint restrictions.
- Aiding in the treatment of autoimmune disorders.

Rosemary (Rosmarinus officinalis)

Rosemary is clearing, stimulating and refreshing. It is analgesic, antimicrobial, anti-rheumatic, antibacterial, antispasmodic and antifungal. It is an antidepressant, antioxidant and decongestant. It promotes the flow of bile, the production of white blood cells, circulation, menstruation and the break down of mucus. It serves as a memory aid and muscle relaxant. It should not be used in large quantities during pregnancy or with people who have dangerously high blood pressure or epilepsy.

Benefits include:

- Being a heart tonic by reducing palpitations and improving low blood pressure, cardiac fatigue and circulation to and from the extremities.
- Improving gallbladder infections, biliary colic and helping dissolve gall stones.
- Treatment of tired muscles, rheumatism, and arthritis.
- Stimulating the central nervous system.
- Improving concentration and memory.
- Treatment of bronchitis and sinusitis.
- Stimulating hair growth and preventing baldness and dandruff.

Rosewood (Aniba rosaeodora)

Rosewood is grounding, enlivening, uplifting and angelic. It is called the oil of the angels. It is antibacterial, antiparasitic, antifungal and antiseptic. It is an antidepressant, aphrodisiac, deodorant, stimulant, general tonic and immune system modulator.

Benefits include:

- Gently elevating the mood and is excellent in post-pump depression (depression after having heart surgery).
- Treatment of nausea and digestion-related headaches.
- Prevention and treatment of coughs, colds and the flu.
- Supporting the healing of dermatitis, scars and wounds.
- Nourishing dry, sensitive, inflamed and aging skin.
- Providing energetic support when feeling anxious, lethargic, weary, overburdened or sad.
- Aiding in meditation.

(This information about essential oils was composed by master aromatherapist Cynthia Loving.)

10

Integrative Reflexology® Sequences

This chapter teaches you all of the hands-on techniques for Integrative Reflexology®.
The **Basic Sequence** is a suggested protocol for a 60-minute session.
The **Variety of Techniques** is a comprehensive list of all of the Integrative Reflexology® techniques.
The **90-Minute Protocol** is a suggested session that includes ways to incorporate bodywork if you are licensed in massage therapy.
The **Spa Protocol** is a suggested sequence for a 30–minute session.
The **Hand Reflexology Sequence** can be added to any of the longer sessions.

Before you begin, locate the **landmarks of the feet**. You need to be familiar with the physical landmarks of the feet as reference points for finding the reflex areas that you will be massaging. The main areas to be able to locate are the great toe and the ball of the great toe, the ball of the foot, the arch of the foot and the heel. Notice in Figure 10.1, each of these corresponds to one of the four anatomical cavities of the body. The great toe and the ball of the great toe correspond with the head and neck. The ball of the foot corresponds with the thoracic cavity. The arch of the foot corresponds with the abdominal cavity, and the heel corresponds with the pelvic cavity.

These primary landmarks are defined by color changes in the sole of the foot. The ball of the foot and the heel are both darker as compared to the arch of the foot. The line where the color changes between the ball of the foot and the arch is the diaphragm reflex. The line where the color changes between the arch and the heel is the line joining the hip and sacrum reflexes which also corresponds to the piriformis muscle.

The toes are obvious landmarks that serve as references for the vertical zones of the feet. Note that the toes are counted from the great toe out to the little toe; the great toe as one and the little toe as five.

Finally, note the location of the prominence of the cuboid notch along the outside edge of each foot; this is important for establishing the waistline as a reference for other reflexology areas. The cuboid notch is actually the proximal condyle of the 5th metatarsal, and is the reflex for the elbow. It is interesting to note that dress makers determine your true waistline by where the crease of your elbow lines up with your torso.

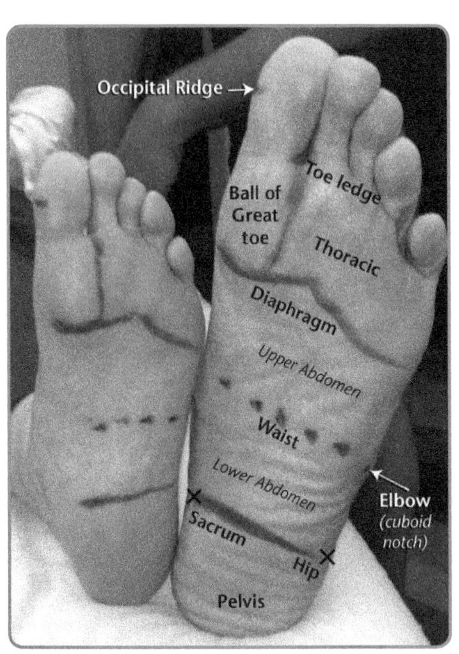

Fig 10.1 - Physical landmarks of the feet

Integrative Reflexology® Basic 60-Minute Sequence

1. **Leg Release Techniques**

   a. ***Traction both legs***—Holding from the back of the ankle, lift legs, only 4-6 inches off the table and gently pull both legs, giving a traction. Do this 2-3 times.

   b. ***Side to side***—Next rock legs from side to side, while still holding and lifting the ankles. This move will help release the hips. (Be aware of your own body mechanics—sit into your pelvis, spine lifted, bend your knees, and plant your feet.)

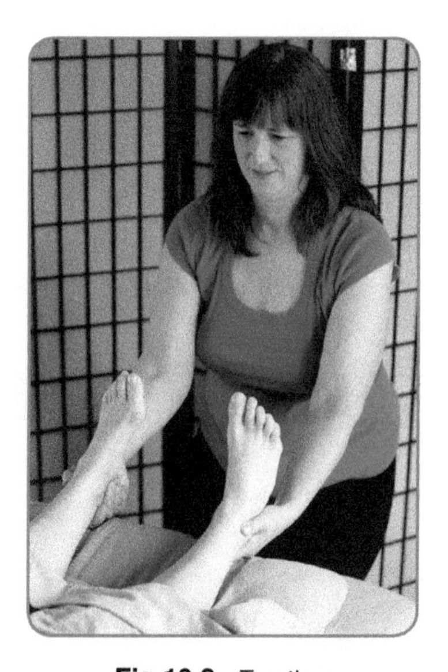

Fig 10.2 - Traction

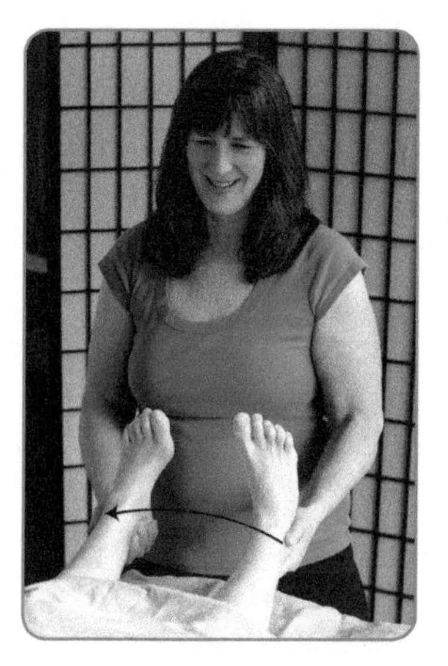

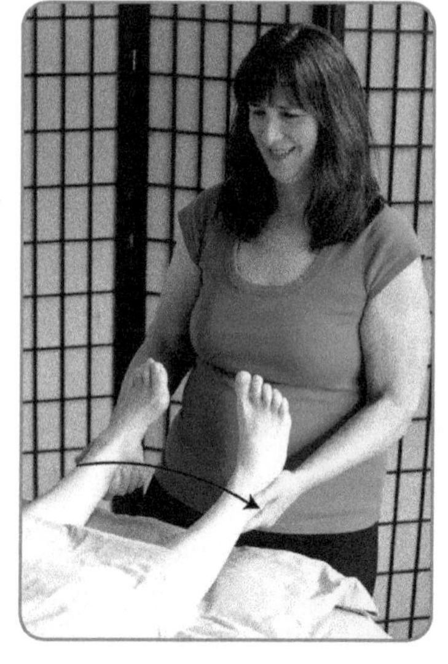

Fig 10.3 - Hip release - side to side traction

2. **Solar Plexus**—Begin with holding solar plexus/ Kidney 1 on both feet. This is when you center yourself and set your intention. Hold this point for 3-5 deep breaths.

3. **Opening Lymph Drainage**—Stimulate the lymph points between the great toe and the second toe by lightly stroking toward the heart. This area is the reflex for the right and left thoracic lymphatic ducts. (Anatomically, these ducts are located above the clavicle. It is here where the lymph is moved into the vena cava and mixed with the returning blood to exit via the kidneys.)

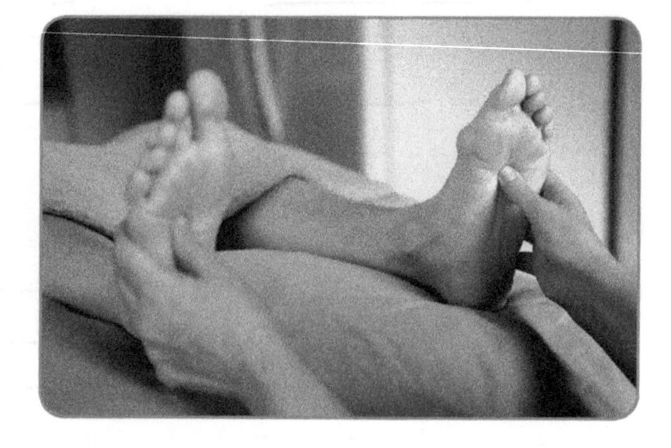

Fig 10.4 - Opening solar plexus hold

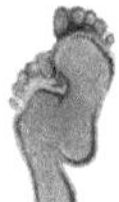

As an X-ray tech, I helped with the lymphangiograms performed in the 1970s. The doctor would put a tiny needle in this area to inject a radio-opaque dye for the procedure. Additionally, this is also Liver 3 in the acupressure system.

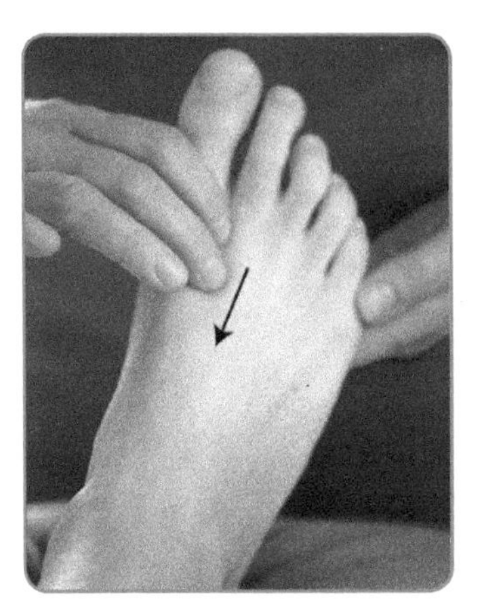

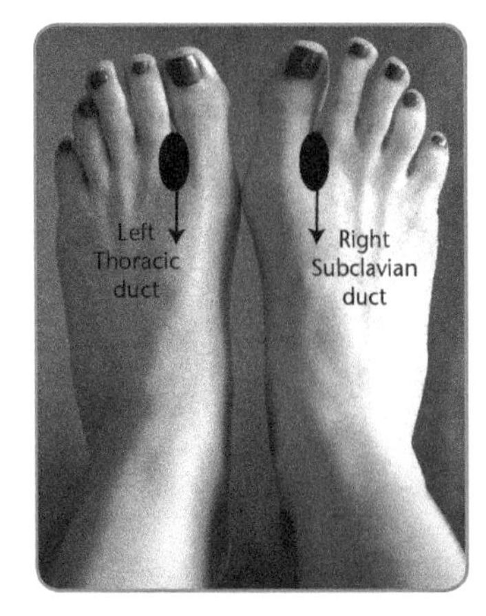

Fig 10.5 - Lymph drainage of feet

4. **Toes**—Circumduct and milk each toe. Feel the quality of each toe. Apply a gentle traction to each toe—a toe may pop, but do not force it to pop (some people have an aversion to this, so you may want to ask them before you put traction on their toes). Repeat on other foot.

NOTE: Apply lotion or cream to whole foot but NOT toes. You may apply to toes after you work the sinuses. As you continue the Integrative Reflexology® session, go back and forth between both feet on each step.

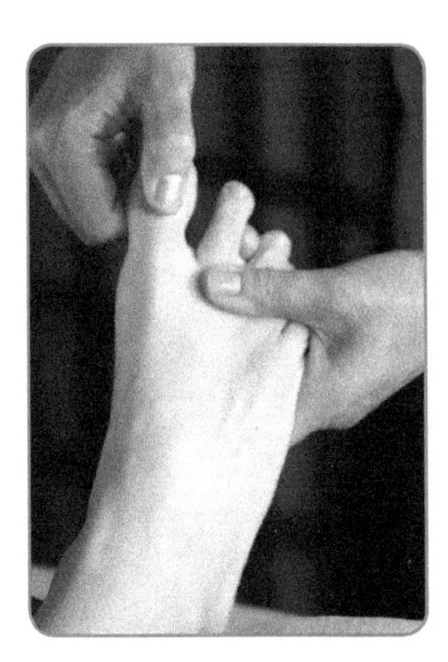

Fig 10.6 - Full circumduction

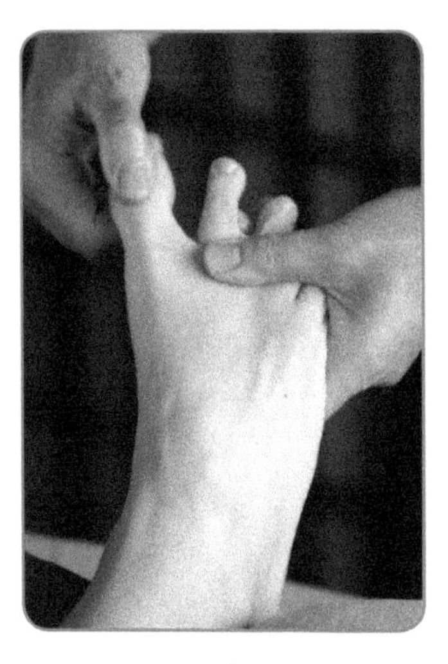

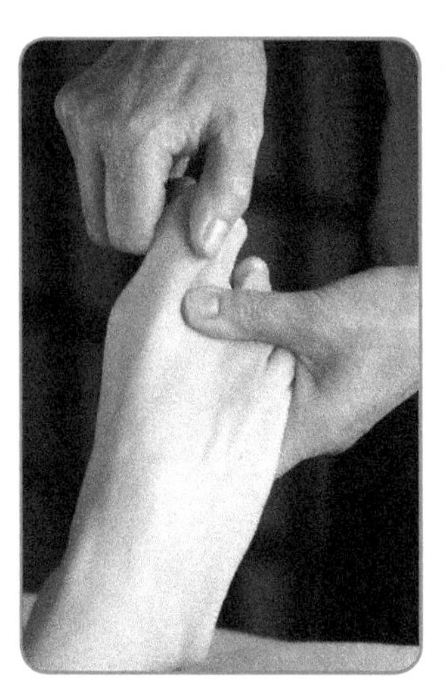

Fig 10.7 - Traction as you circle

5. **Warm Up the Feet**

   a. ***Toothpaste squeeze***—With hands on either side, compress the foot with fingers and thumbs as you slide up from the heel to the toes. The squeezing out to toes, should feel like squeezing toothpaste. Don't grip too hard. This is best done sitting.

   b. ***Wringing***—With hands held around the foot, wring back and forth and up and down, as if you were wringing out a towel.

NOTE: Pressing and circling on a reflex point is one of your basic techniques, along with pressing and holding. Press and circle is more stimulating while press and hold is calmer for the nervous system to receive. I like to start with press and circle. If that is too much for the client, I will revert to press and hold. You can choose which you prefer and which achieves the results you desire.

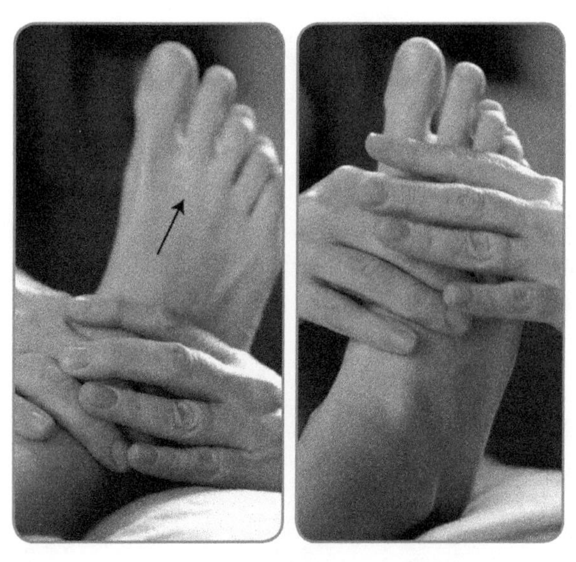

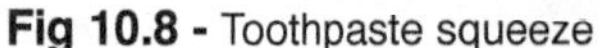

Fig 10.8 - Toothpaste squeeze

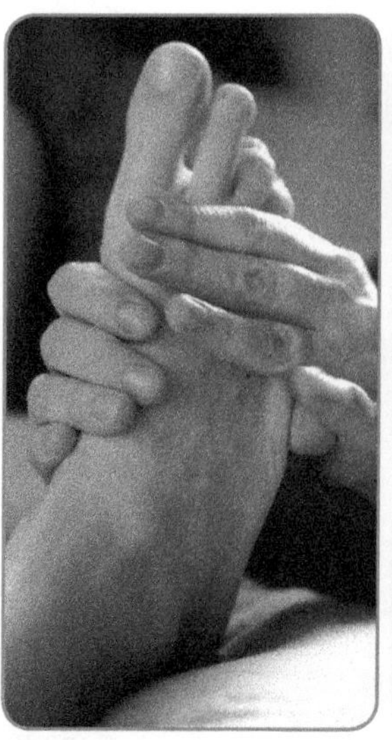

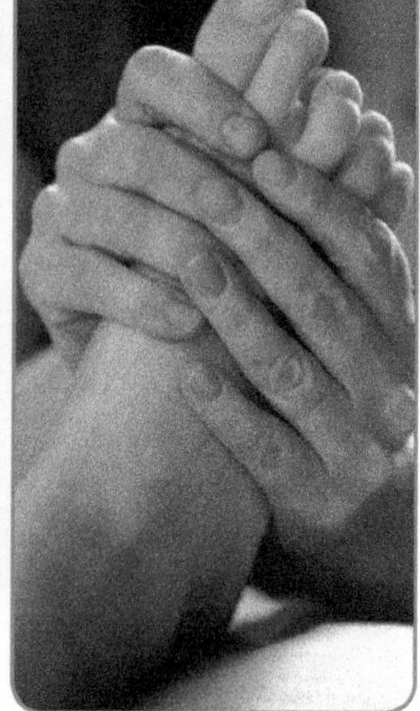

Fig 10.9 - Wringing

6. **Pineal Gland**—Press the top medial corner of the great toe. This is best done sitting. You may not feel an exact point. Just try to be in the general area, using intention. You can press and circle on the point or just press and hold (Fig 10.10).

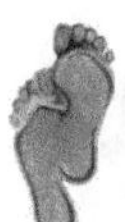

The pineal gland secretes melatonin that is needed for healthy sleep rhythms. Serotonin is also created in the pineal and the small intestine. We need this to feel good. This is a light sensitive gland. It needs total darkness at night and natural light during the day.

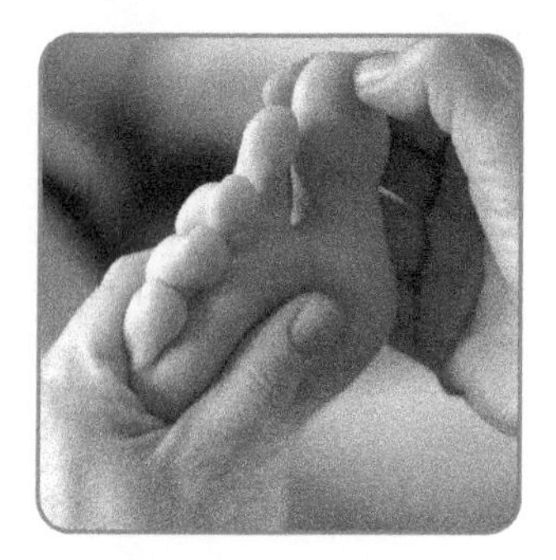

Fig 10.10 - Pineal

7. **Pituitary Gland**—Press into the center of the great toe. You should feel a bony area. Clients often react to this point. You may circle friction on the point or just press and hold. Some describe it as an electrical sensation (Fig 10.11).

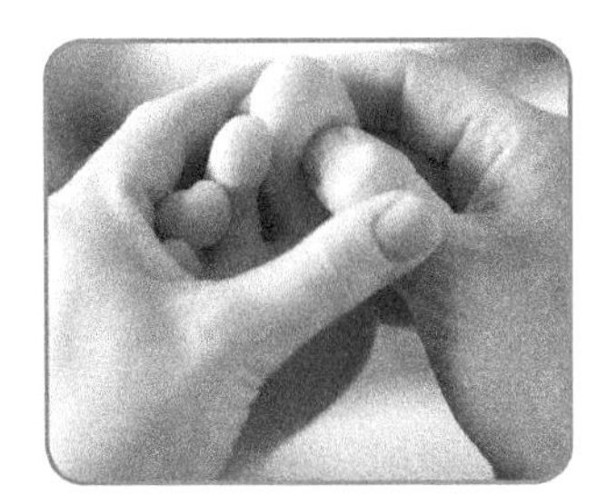

Fig 10.11 - Pituitary

The pituitary, along with the hypothalamus, secretes 16 different hormones. The pituitary is called the master gland. It is also light sensitive and can be the cause of seasonal affective disorder (SAD). Oxytocin, a major pituitary hormone, is often called the love hormone, due to its release in both love-making and childbirthing. By stimulating the pituitary reflex point, it may bring pain relief during labor.

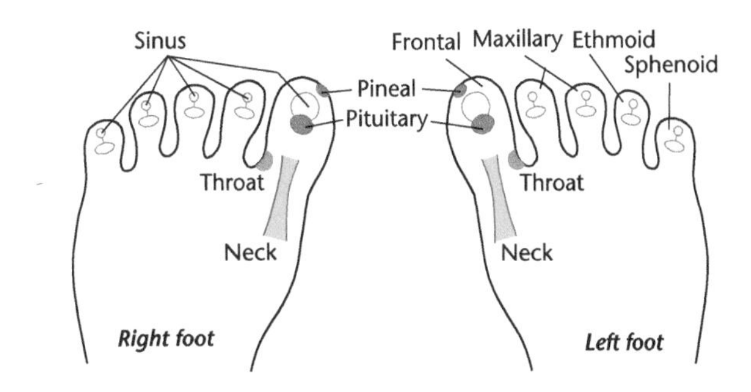

Fig 10.12 - Pineal, pituitary, sinuses, and throat

8. **Sinuses**—Press and hold the tips of each toe. Notice which ones are tender. This may indicate a blockage in that specific sinus.

   a. ***Squeezing***–squeeze the tops of each toe.
   b. ***Scratching***—scratch the tops of the toes.
   c. ***Brushing***—smooth across the tops of the toes with your fist.
   d. You may even try the ***"This Little Piggy"*** rhyme with children!

*****Apply lotion or cream to the toes if you haven't already*****

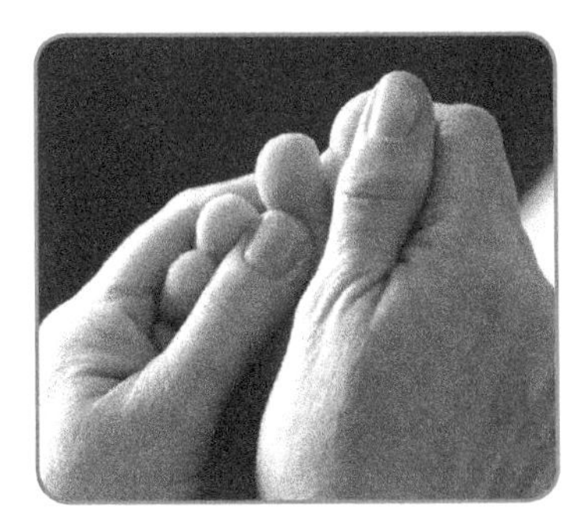

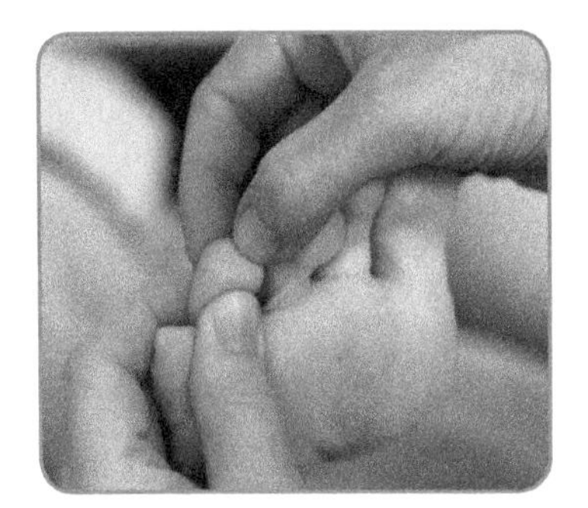

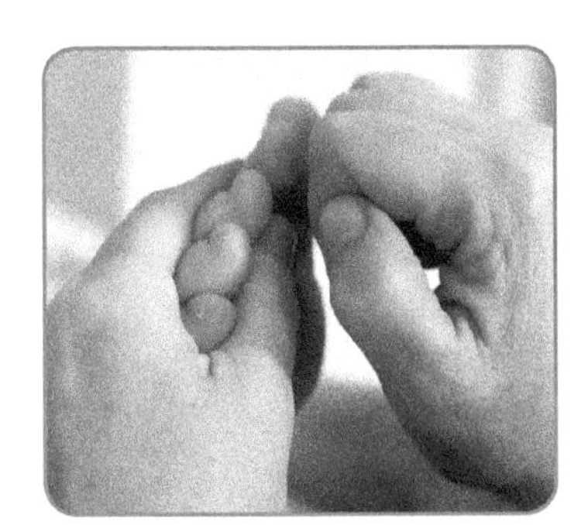

Fig 10.13 - Squeezing, scratching and brushing sinus points

9. **Throat**—Press and circle on the throat reflex at the inside base of the great toe.

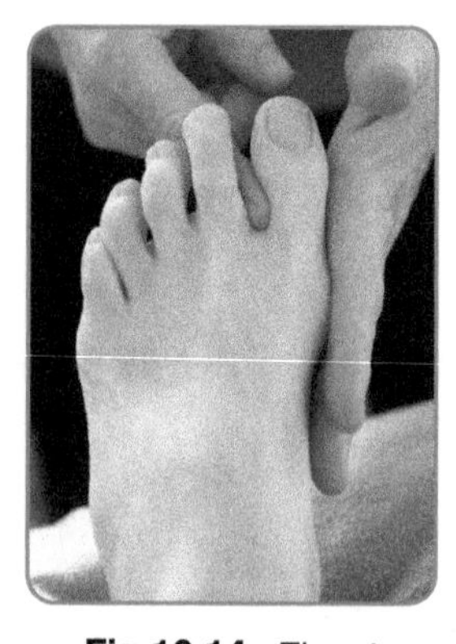

Fig 10.14 - Throat

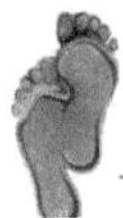

Traction the great toe gently. This correlates with traction of the neck.

10. **Neck**—Massage around the entire base of the great toe. Include the full ball of the toe (front, side, back). This area may be tender if they have a bunion.

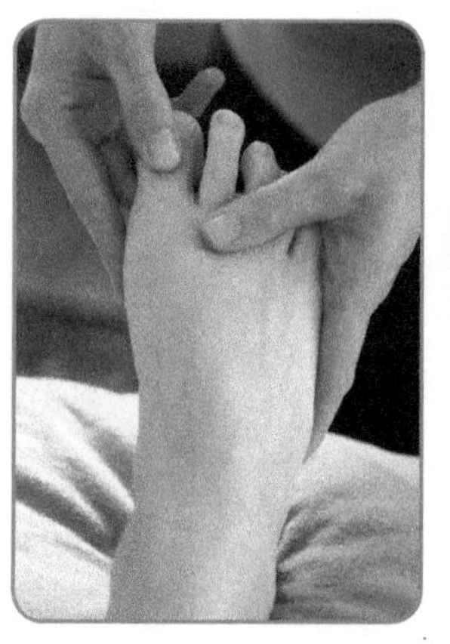

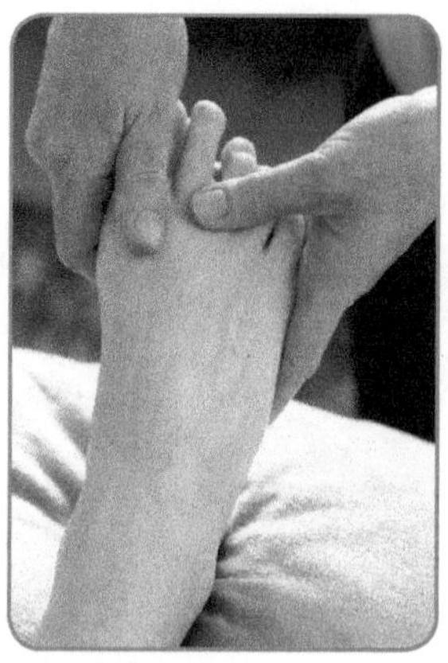

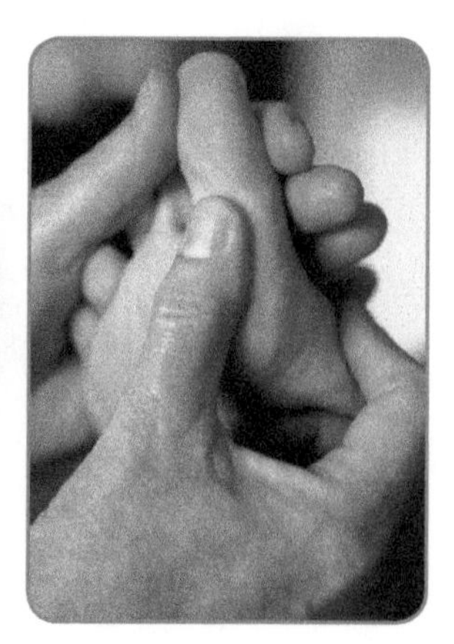

Fig 10.15 - Neck

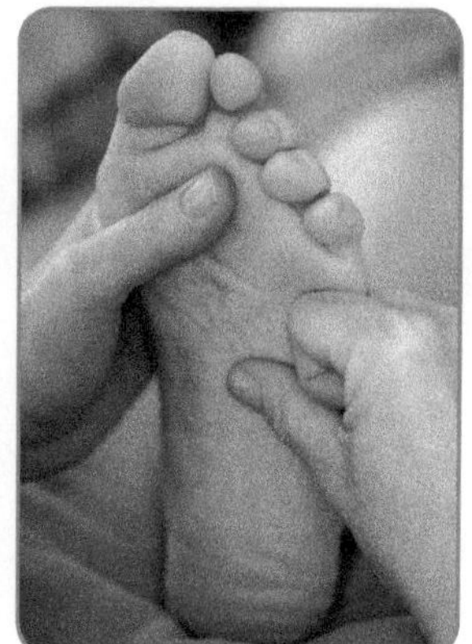

Fig 10.16 - Neck/ Shoulder Combo

11. **Neck and Shoulder Combo**—Work these areas simultaneously and back & forth between both feet.

12. **Shoulder**—Located on the edge of foot below the 5th toe. Use a pinch and twist technique. Also use your knuckles on the area, front, side and back.

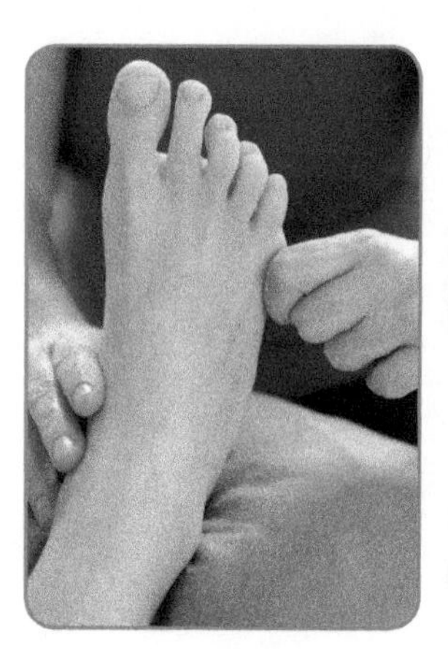

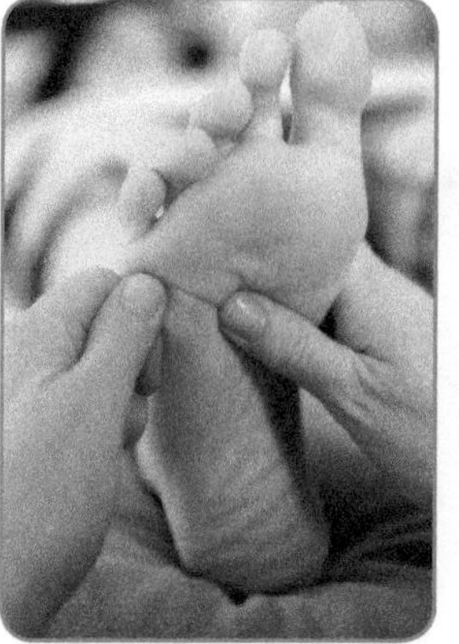

Fig 10.17 - Shoulders

13. **Ear**—Press and circle on the toe ledge between the 4th and 5th toes. May help in ear infections. May help with ear congestion and release crackling noises in the ear.

14. **Bronchial Tube**—Press and circle on the toe ledge between the 3rd and 4th toes. May assist in chest colds, bronchitis, and asthma.

15. **Eye**—Press and circle on the toe ledge between the 2nd and 3rd toes. May help improve vision. May assist in dissolving cataracts.

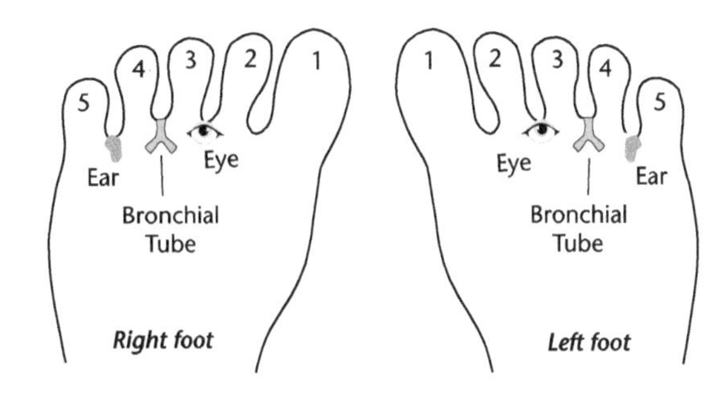

Fig 10.18 - Ear, eyes, bronchial tubes, and shoulders

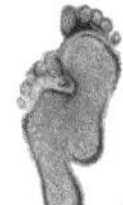

If the sinus points on the 4th and 5th toe are tender, then the ear point might also be tender, because the ethmoid (4th) & sphenoid (5th) sinuses drain into the ear. It helps to give all three some extra attention if one is tender.

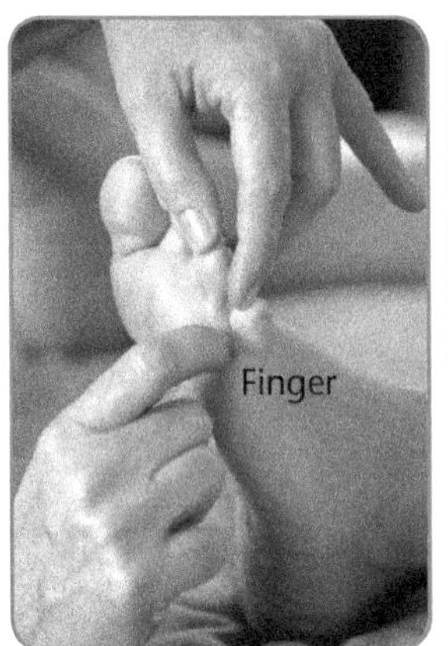

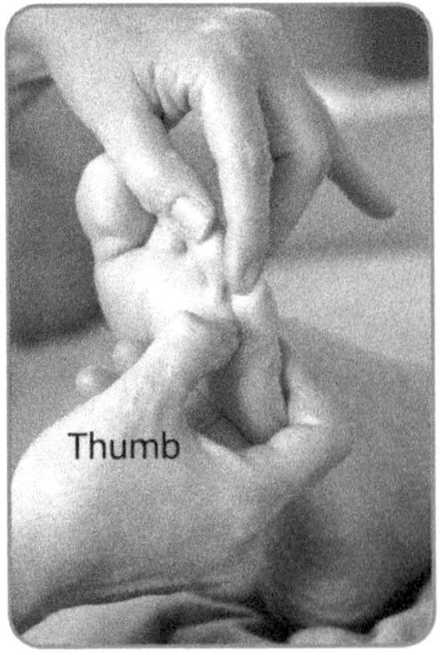

Fig 10.19 - Ear

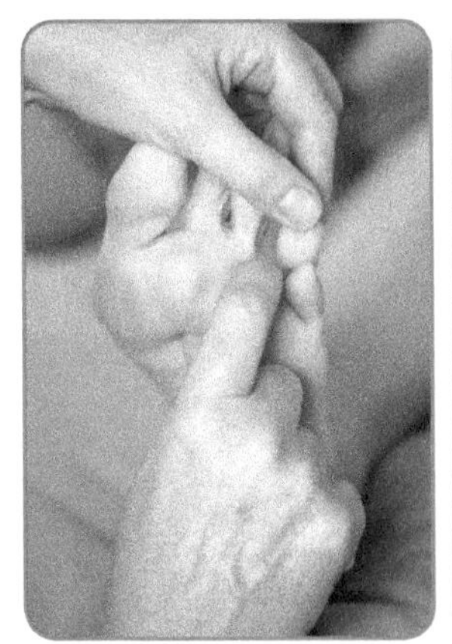

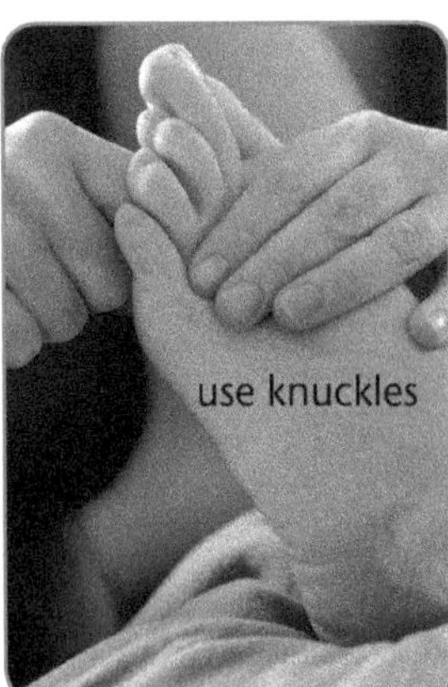

Fig 10.20 - Bronchial

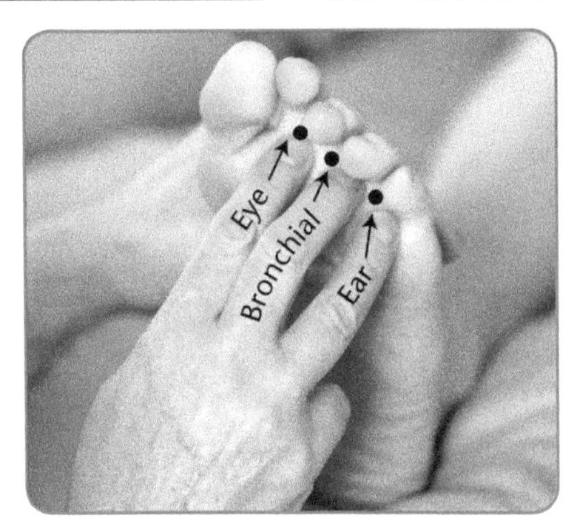

Fig 10.21 - Trumpet–Stimulating all three points simultaneously

16. **Thyroid Reflex**—Hook into the sesamoid bone on the ball of the great toe and gently press the thumb in a medial direction. Apply pressure to the inside corner. You should feel that you are on the condyle (bump) of a bone. You may hold and repeat 2 more times. This is often a sensitive point on women. It regulates metabolism and the menstrual cycle. Avoid if client is pregnant. Be cautious with clients on thyroid medication.

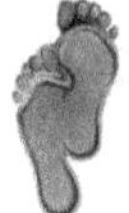

The thyroid has been called the mother gland. It rules many of the female hormones. It rules metabolism, heat regulation, and the electrical system of the heart.

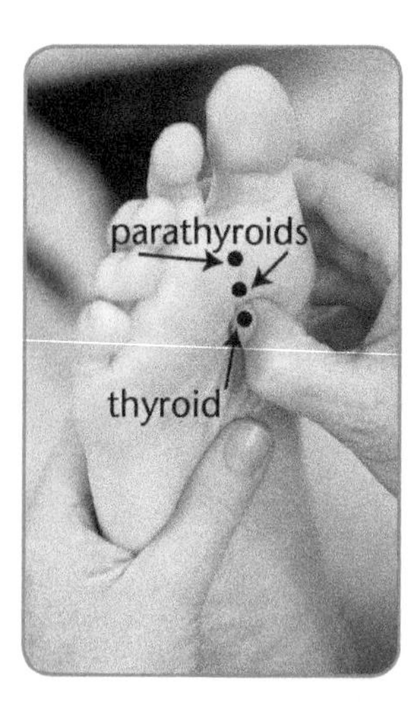

Fig 10.22 - Thyroid hook into the bone. Press parathyroid after thyroid hook

17. **Parathyroid Points**—Press the two points above the thyroid gland.

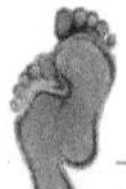

Parathyroids assist in calcium metabolism.

18. **Lungs**—Techniques can include knuckle twist, pinch and twist and thumb walking. Be sure to cover the entire lung pad area. Alternating between the diaphragm spread and chest spread makes a great combination for opening and expanding the lungs.

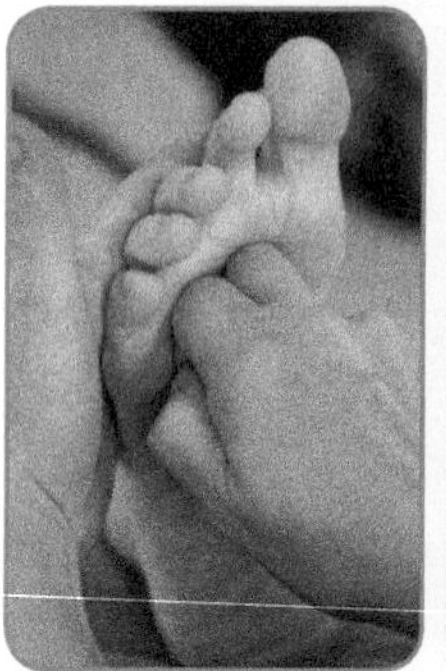
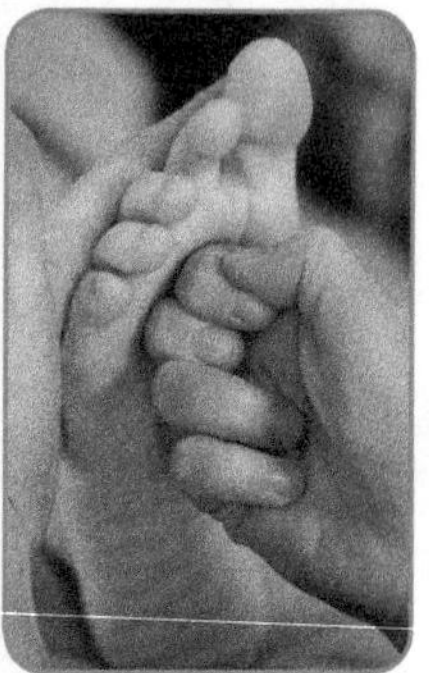

Fig 10.23 - Knuckle twist

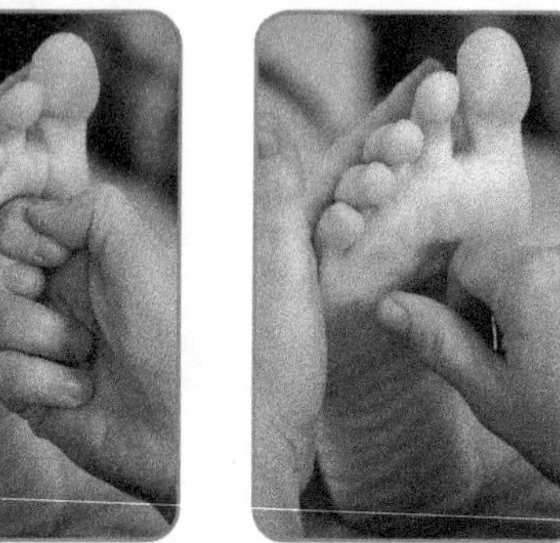
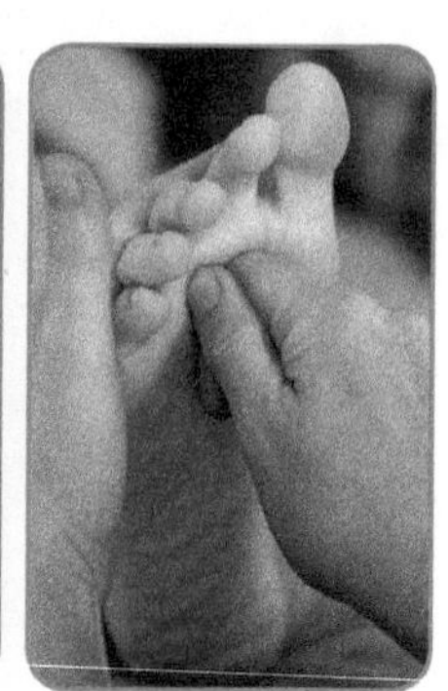

Fig 10.24 - Pinch & twist

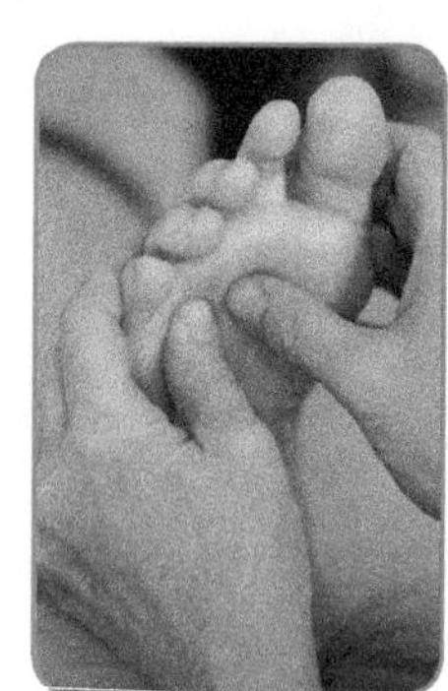

Fig 10.25 - Thumb walking on lung pad

a. ***Diaphragm Spread***—Stretch the thoracic area using thumbs at the solar plexus point and smoothing out to the sides.
b. ***Chest Spread***—Using both hands, grasp the thoracic area and spread out.

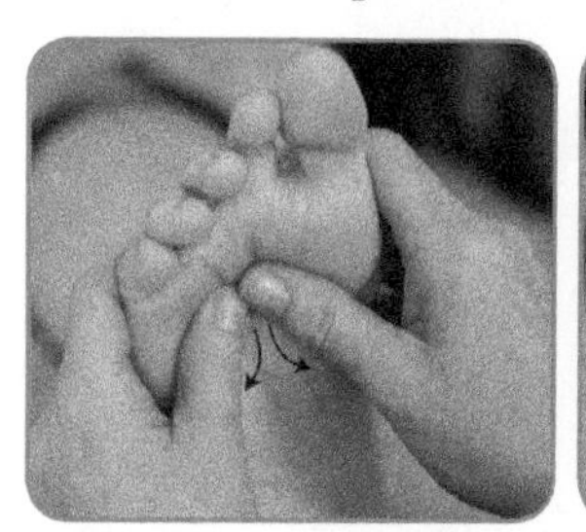
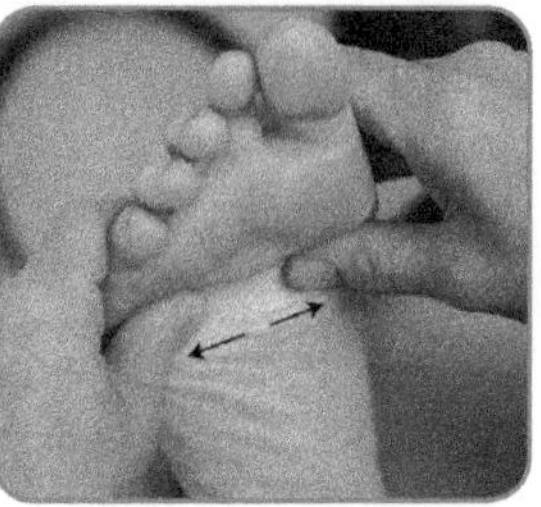

Fig 10.26 - Diaphragm spread

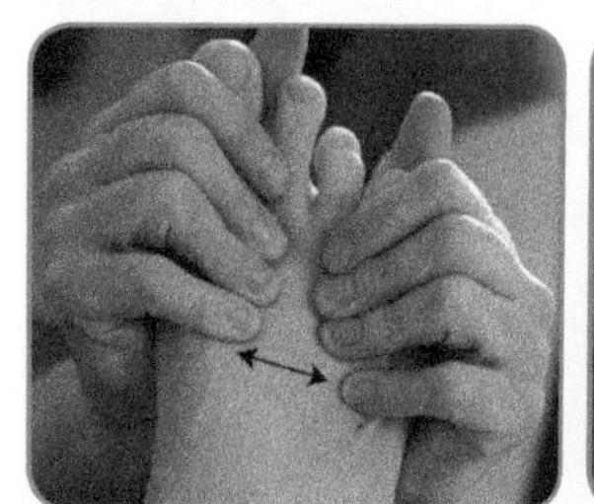
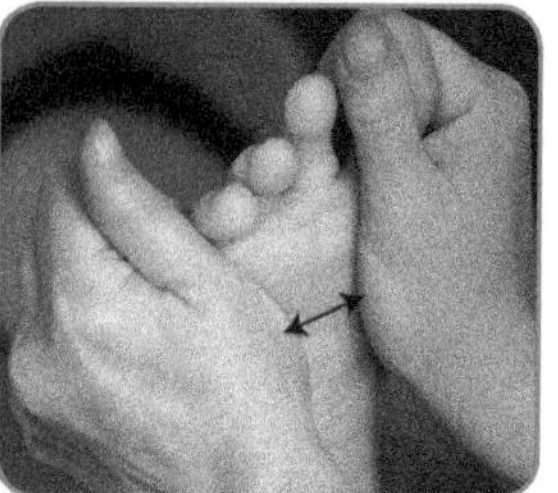

Fig 10.27 - Chest spread

19. Solar Plexus—Locate the solar plexus point just under the diaphragm line. Hold both feet simultaneously. On the exhale (both client's and yours) press into the point while flexing the foot. Do this 3 or more times. This may help with anxiety attacks, shallow breathing and even hiccups.

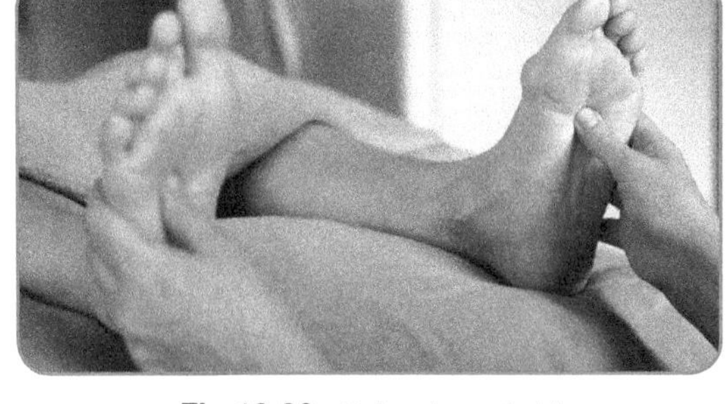

Fig 10.28 - Solar plexus hold

20. Esophagus and Stomach—Slide down between the great toe and the second toe for the esophagus. Gently circle the stomach area as if you were rubbing a child's tummy. Note, you may circle in either direction. Repeat several times. May help with acid reflux.

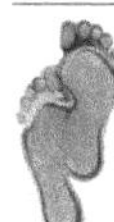

The stomach cooks your food. You may stir in either direction.

21. Pancreas—Sits below the ball of the great toe. Press the top of the thumb deeply into the middle of the stomach area. Use caution with diabetics. If they have been diabetic for a long time and are insulin dependent, do not stimulate.

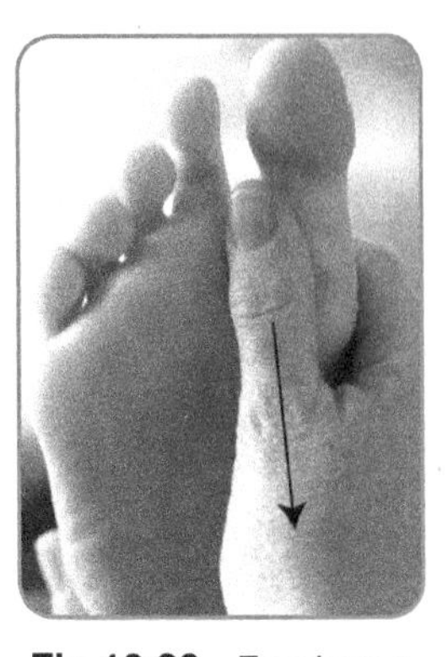

Fig 10.29 - Esophagus

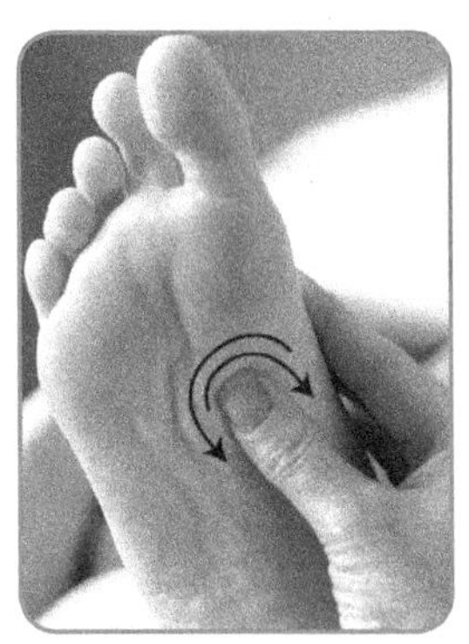

Fig 10.30 - Stomach

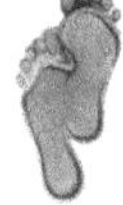

The pancreas sits behind the stomach. It is a large gland that regulates the breakdown of fats, proteins, and carbohydrates so that body cells may absorb them as sugars.

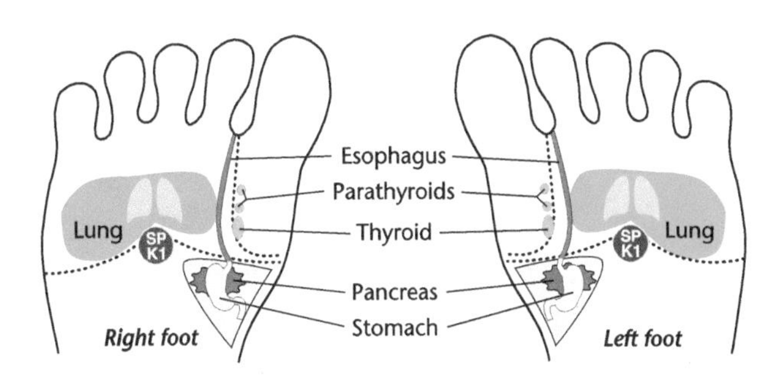

Fig 10.31: Lungs, solar plexus, esophagus, stomach and pancreas

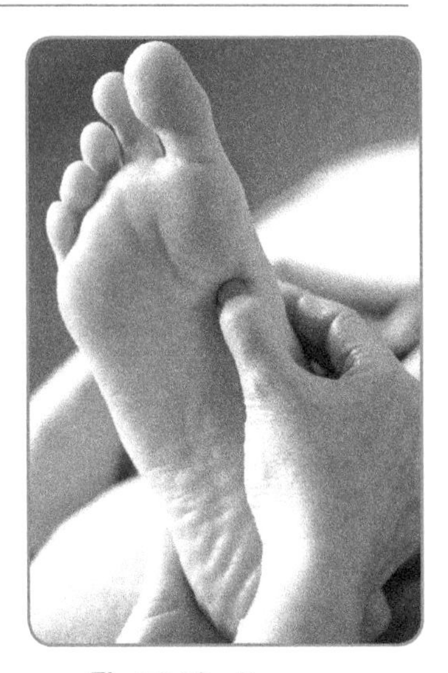

Fig 10.32 - Pancreas

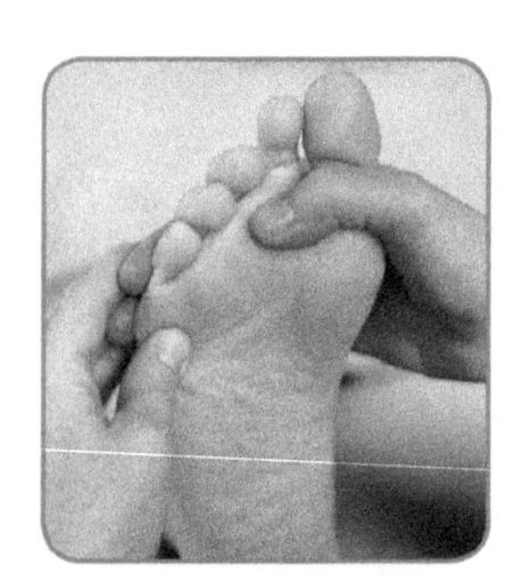

Fig 10.33 - Liver

22. Liver—At the joint of the 5th toe and metatarsal on the right foot. Press deeply on the condyle of the underlying bone to stimulate the reflex point.

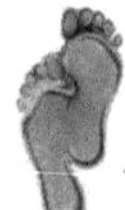

The liver is the great filter of the body. It helps metabolize and eliminate various toxins, including many medications.

23. Gallbladder—At the joint of the 4th toe and metatarsal on the right foot. Press deeply on the condyle of the bone to stimulate the reflex point.

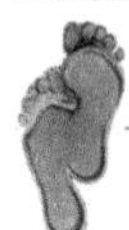

The gallbladder produces bile which aids in the digestion of fats.

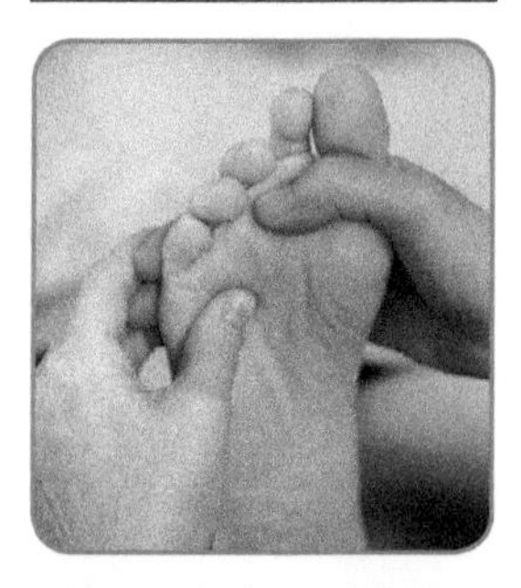

Fig 10.34 - Gallbladder

24. Spleen—At the joint of the 5th toe and metatarsal on the left foot. Press deeply on the condyle of the under-lying bone to stimulate the reflex point.

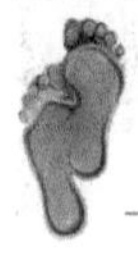

The spleen plays a role in autoimmune regulation and the regulation of red blood cells.

25. Heart—Press down onto the point from above the diaphragm at the joint of the 4th toe and metatarsal on the left foot.

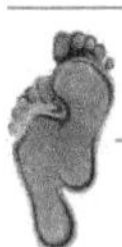

Physical and emotional imbalances may be reflected in the heart.

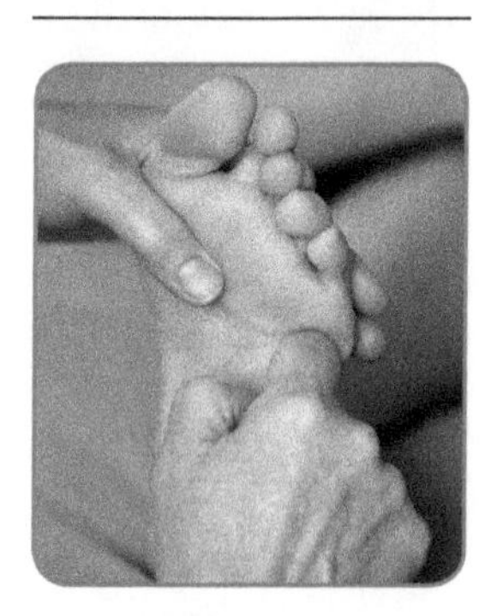

Fig 10.35
Knuckle on spleen

NOTE: Use the C-clamp with your opposite hand to protect the top of the foot as you apply pressure to each point.

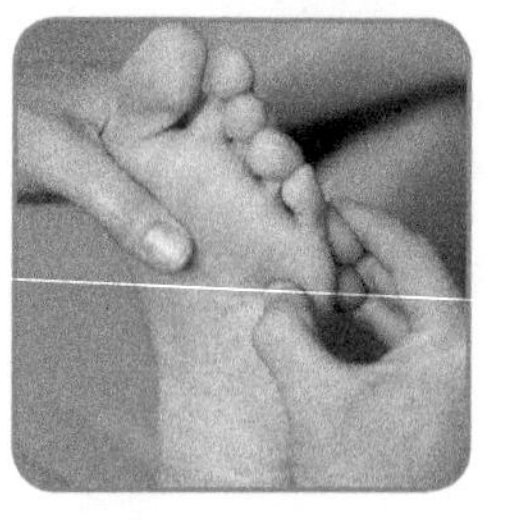

Fig 10.37
C-clamp for spleen

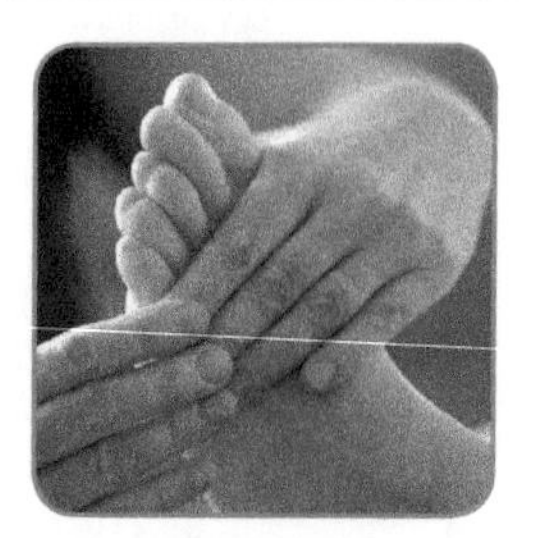

Fig 10.38
C-clamp for all 4 points

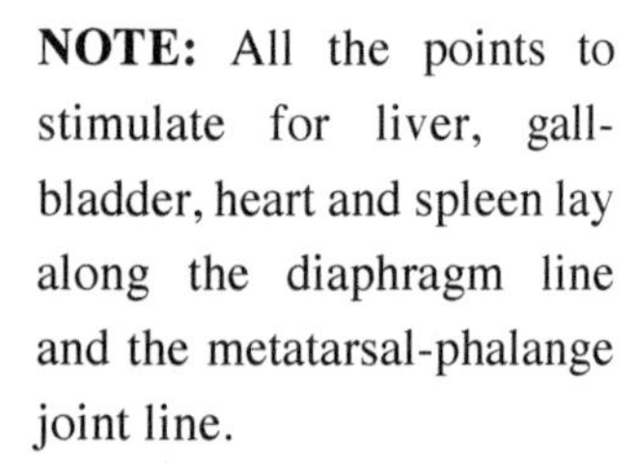

NOTE: All the points to stimulate for liver, gall-bladder, heart and spleen lay along the diaphragm line and the metatarsal-phalange joint line.

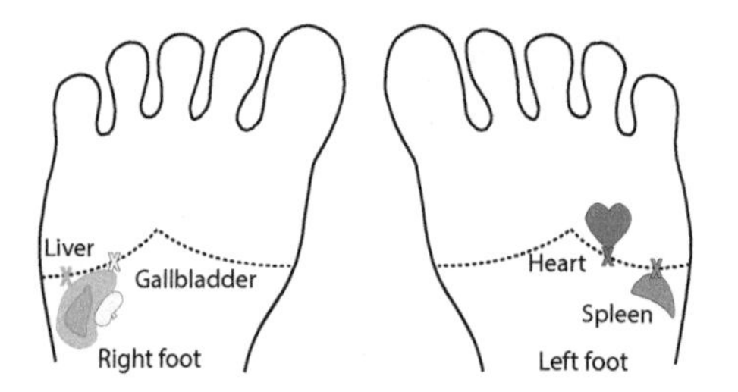

Fig 10.39 - Liver, gallbladder, spleen, and heart

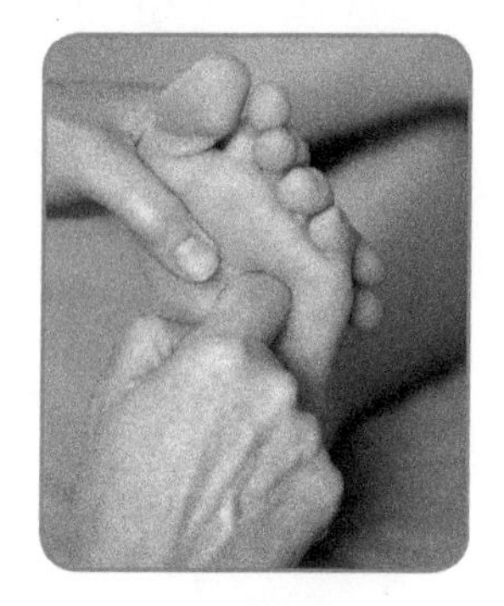

Fig 10.36
Knuckle on heart

26. Large Intestine—Different segments are located on each foot. Try to break up any crystal deposits that are metabolic waste.

- Starting on the left foot, massage down the outside for the DESCENDING COLON. Continue massaging and circle toward the inside to massage the SIGMOID FLEXURE.
- Massage across the arch from the inside to the outside for the TRANSVERSE COLON. This is above the waistline (defined by the cuboid bone). Repeat down the descending and sigmoid colon areas.
- Move to the right foot and massage across the arch from the outside to the inside for the TRANSVERSE COLON
- Work up the outside of the right foot on the ASCENDING COLON, using thumbs or knuckles, and repeat all previous strokes. Repeat this series several times for an effective LARGE INTESTINE massage. Pay special attention to the APPENDIX and ILEOCECAL VALVE area. Use your intention to define the points.

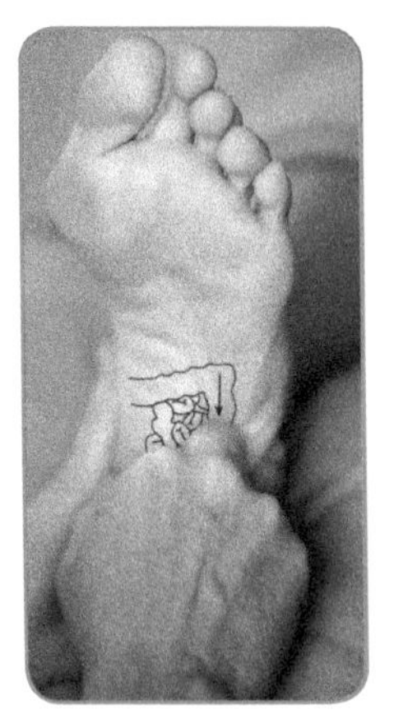

Fig 10.40
Descending colon

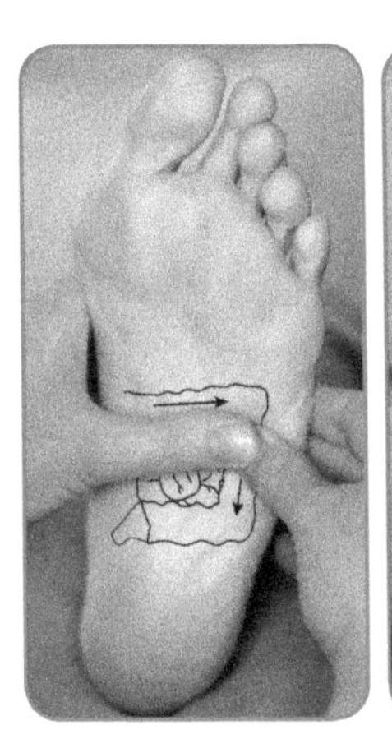

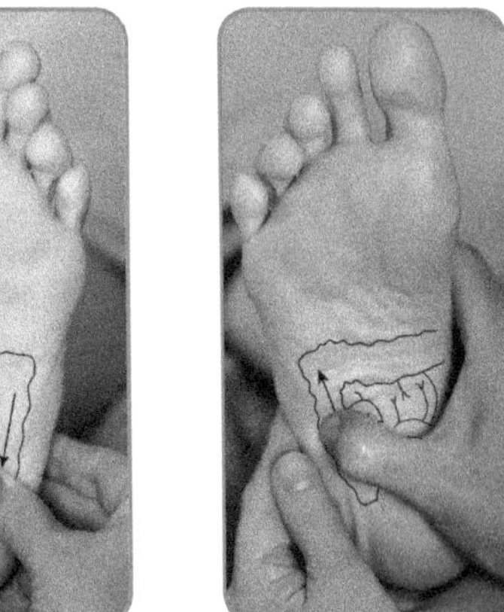

Fig 10.41 - Transverse & descending colon, sigmoid flexure

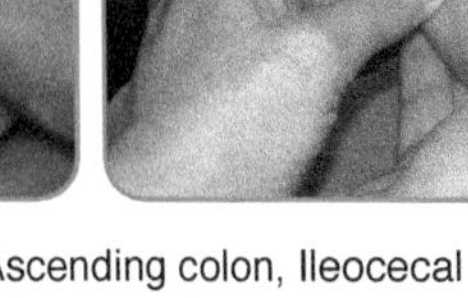

Fig 10.42 - Ascending colon, Ileocecal valve & appendix area

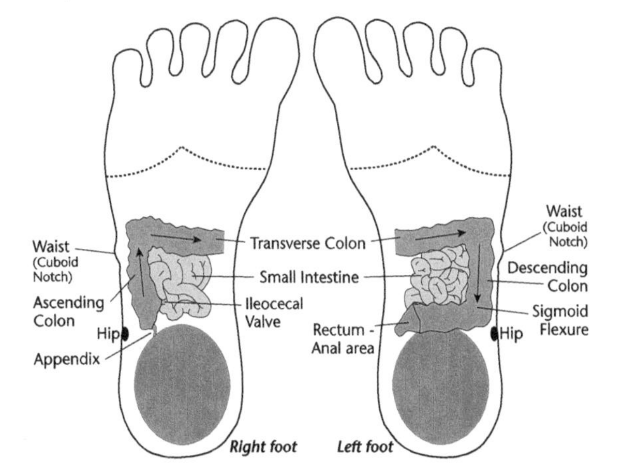

Fig 10.43 - Large and small intestines and their components

27. Small Intestine—Using a knuckle-twist, massage the entire inner arch of the foot.

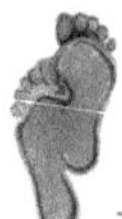

The small intestine is about 23 feet long, and is where the absorption of nutrients takes place.

28. Elbow—Circle and pinch the elbow point.

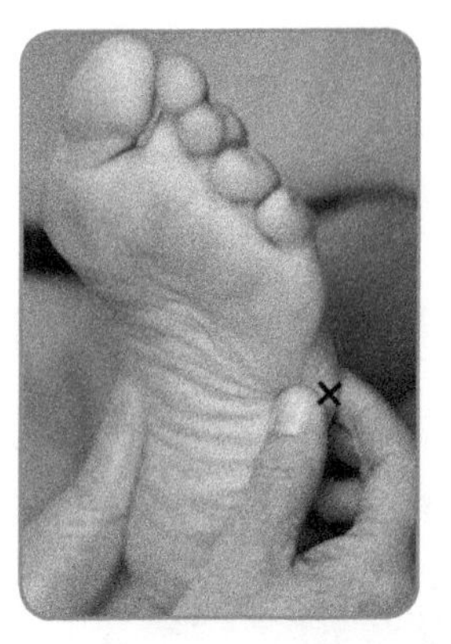

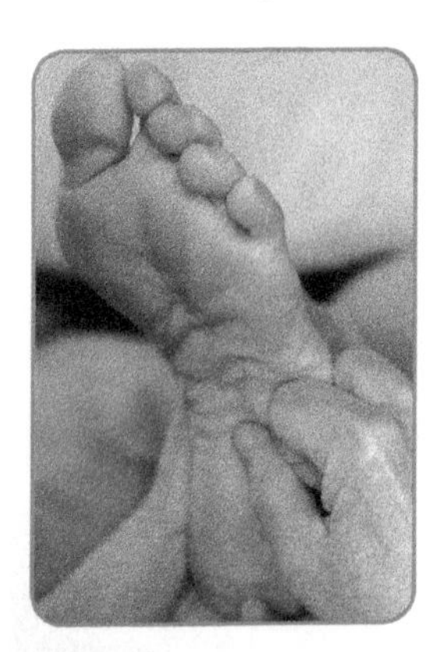

Fig 10.45 - Elbow

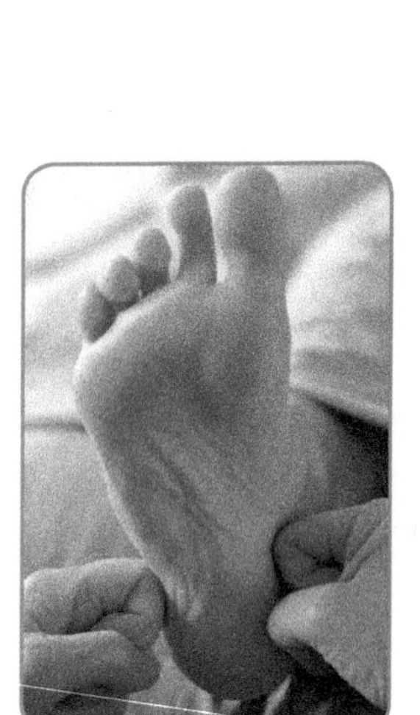

Fig 10.44
Small intestine

29. Hip—Press deeply into the side of the foot with your knuckle to stimulate the hip point. This point may be difficult to reach, so really use your strength here.

a. ***Hip/Sacrum squeeze***—Press points with knuckles. Squeeze together several times.

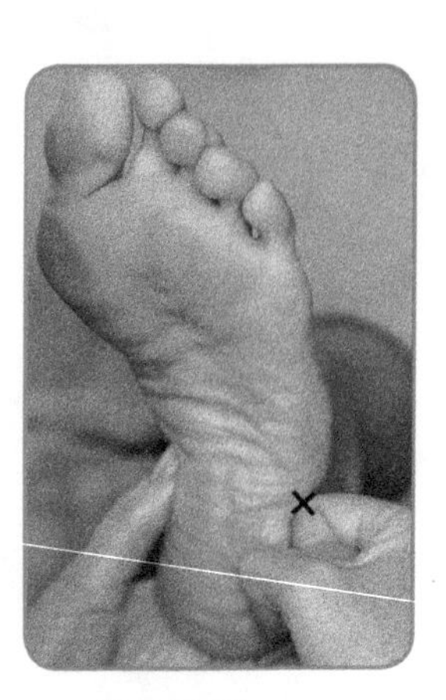

Fig 10.46 - Hip

Fig 10.47
Hip / Sacrum squeeze

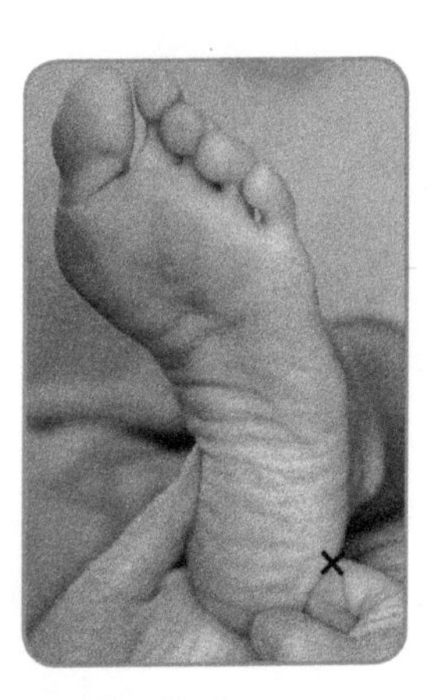

Fig 10.48 - Knee

30. Knee—This is just below the hip point. Again press deeply into the side of the foot. (The knee is the largest joint in the body, and one of the most readily stressed.)

31. Pelvis (Gluteal Muscles/Sciatic Nerve)—Press deeply into heel pad with knuckles or with the heels of your hands. Work entire heel area. This area is so thick, a massage tool or rock may help. Pinch around entire heel to stimulate this area. Notice if there is any cracking—this may be an indication of hemorrhoids or lack of water.

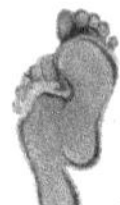

Sciatic nerve pain may radiate down the leg and also be felt deep into the heel.

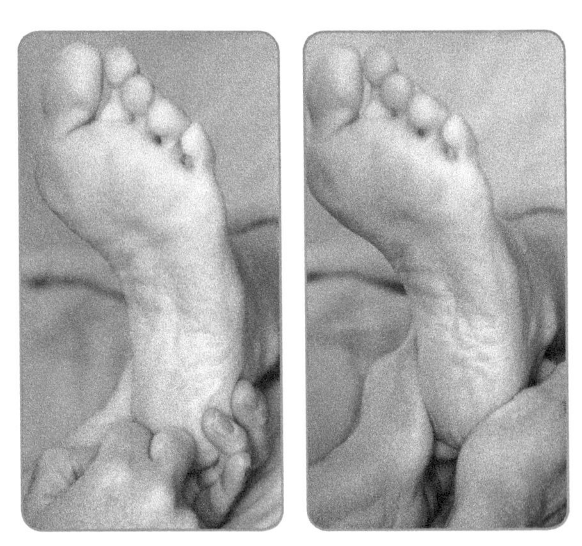

Fig 10.49 - Heel and Gluteals

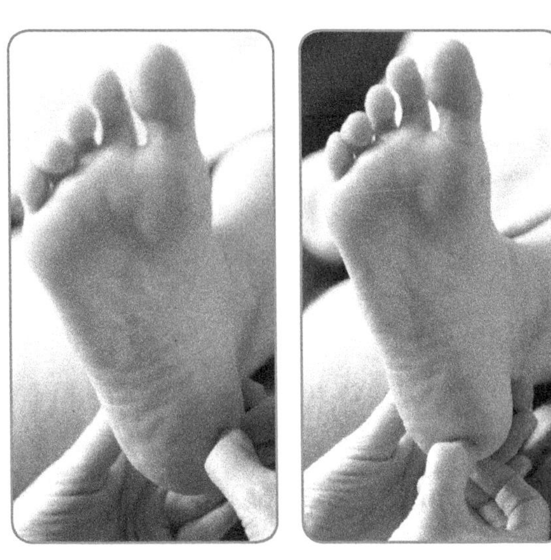

Fig 10.50 - Pinch around the heel

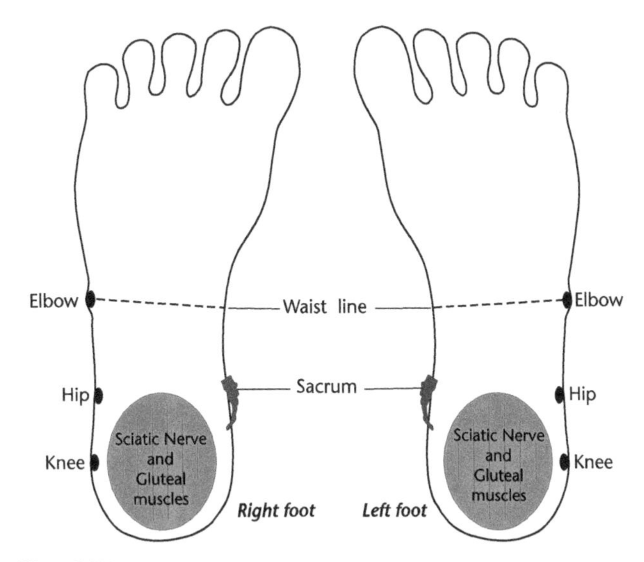

Fig 10.51 - Elbow, hip, knee, sciatic nerve, and gluteal muscles

32. Spine—You may work the spine from the occipital ridge down to the sacrum, or in the reverse, from the sacrum to the occipital ridge. You may also use a spine spread beginning at the waistline, as shown in Figure 10.57.

- For the OCCIPITAL RIDGE, press into the point. Often there is a callous here, indicating tension at the base of the skull. The callous may be massaged with a pumice stone to break up the congestion. You may repeat this whole process for the spine 3 or 4 times.
- At CERVICAL SPINE C7 (defined by the widest bony prominence of the foot), again use circling pressure. Be cautious if there is a bunion.
- Next, massage the larger THORACIC AREA noticing for crystal deposits and tenderness relating to upper back discomfort.
- Massage with circle stroke at the level of the waistline (defined by the cuboid bone) for the LUMBAR SPINE.
- Starting with the SACRUM, use circle stroke with pressure, noticing for softness or swelling indicating possible lower back problems.

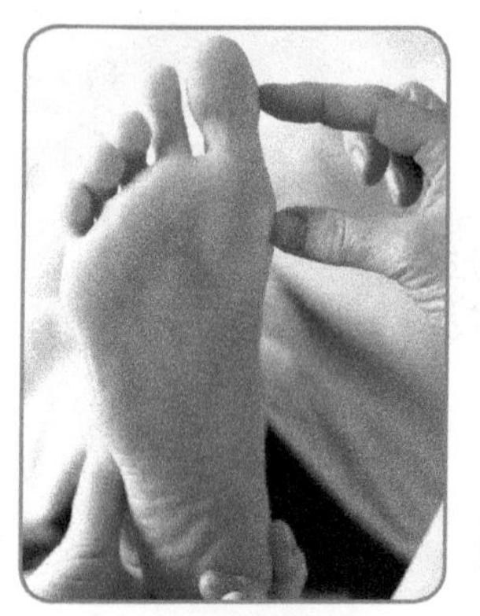

Fig 10.52
Cervical vertebrae

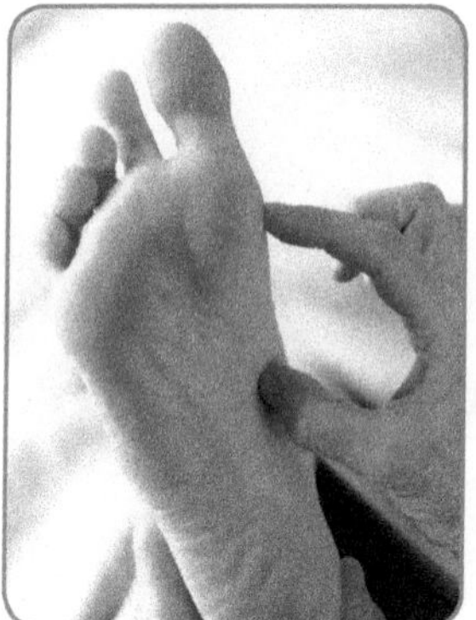

Fig 10.53
Thoracic vertebrae

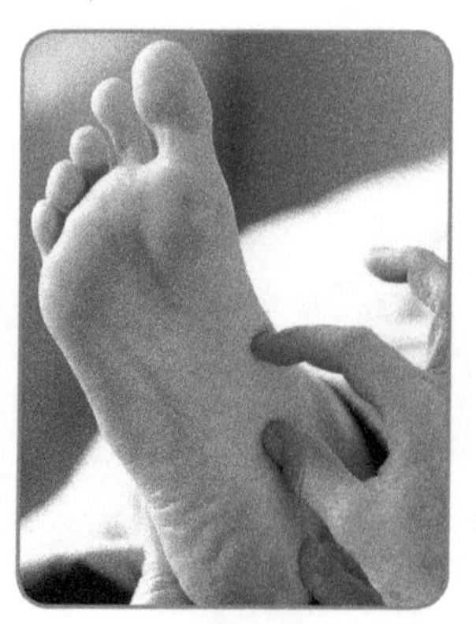

Fig 10.54
Lumbar vertebrae

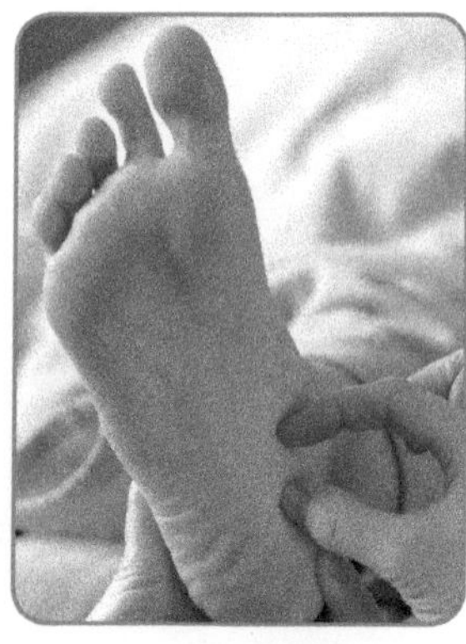

Fig 10.55
Sacrum & coccyx

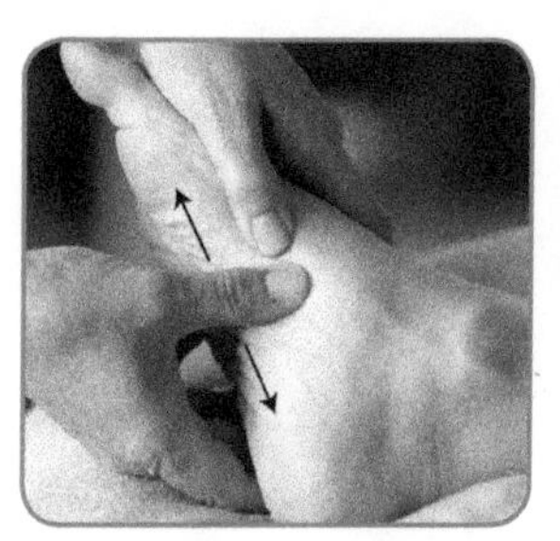

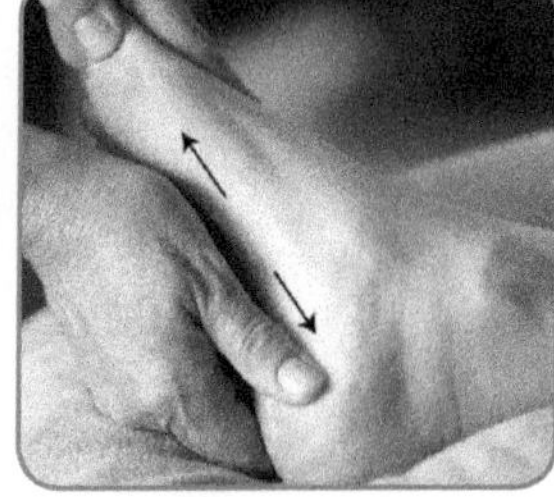

Fig 10.56 - Spine spread

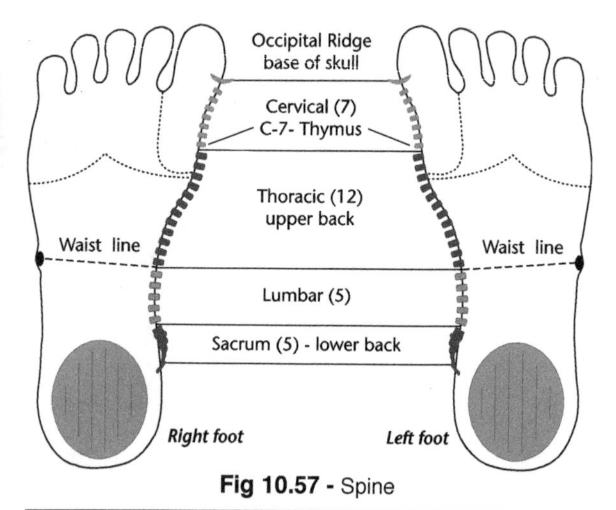

Fig 10.57 - Spine

33. Chest—May work in both directions using long strokes between the bones.

34. Reproductive Points

- Press and circle the point on the inside of the ankle for the UTERUS/ PROSTATE.
- Press and circle the point on the outside of the ankle for the OVARY/ TESTICLE.
- Slide across the top of the ankle from the outside to the inside for the UTERINE TUBE/VAS DEFERENS.

Caution: Never work these points if a woman may be pregnant.

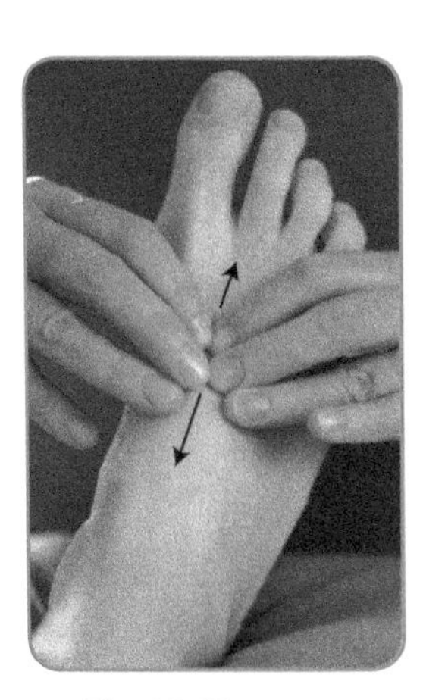

Fig 10.58 - Chest

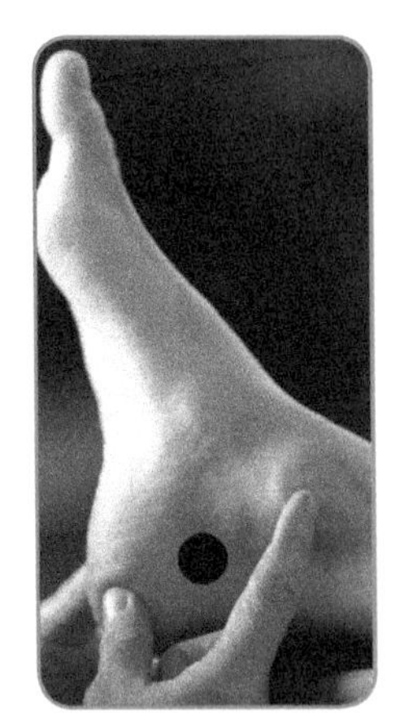

Fig 10.59
Uterus/Prostate

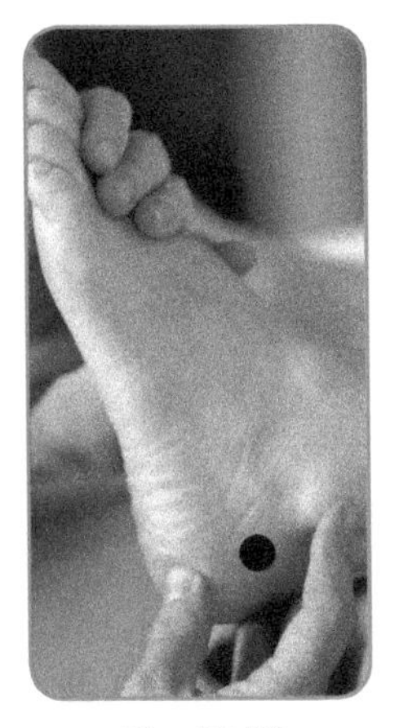

Fig 10.60
Ovary/Testicle

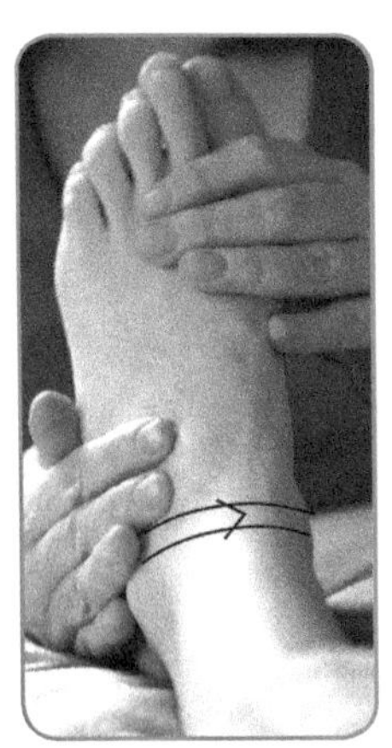

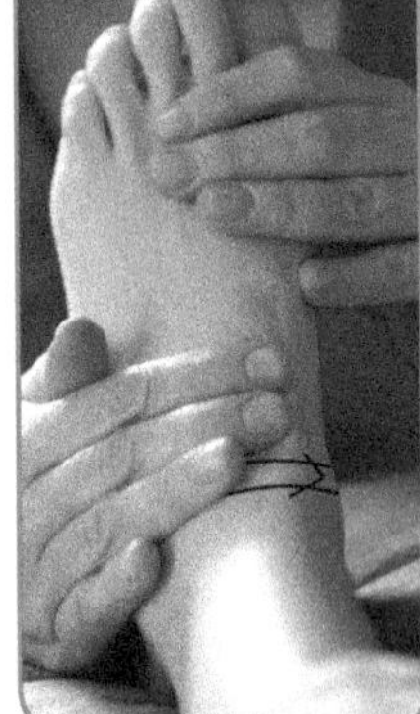

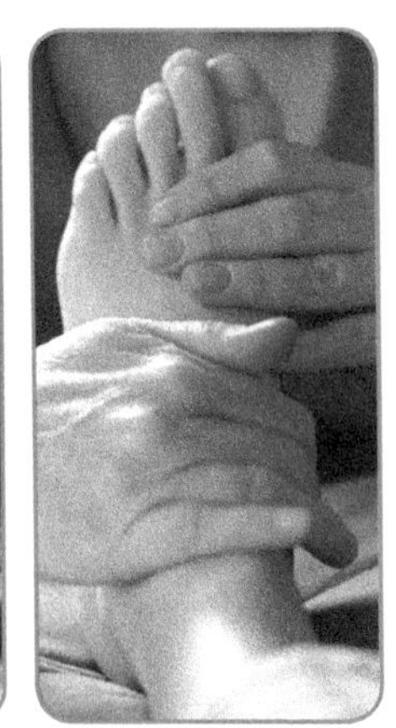

Fig 10.61 - Uterine tubes/Vas deferens

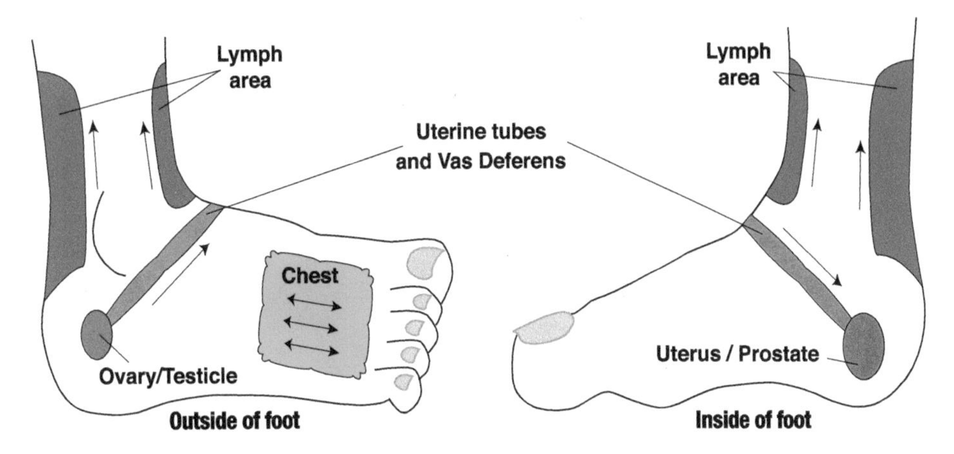

Fig 10.62 - Chest, reproductive points, and lymphatics

35. Lymphatics—Use a light stroke toward the heart on this area. You may squeeze up the back of the ankle. Also, pump the ankle as you work the lymph area on the top. This helps stimulate the lymphatic return.

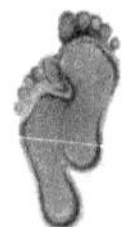

You are moving the lymph fluid in the tissues that you have stirred up with the treatment.

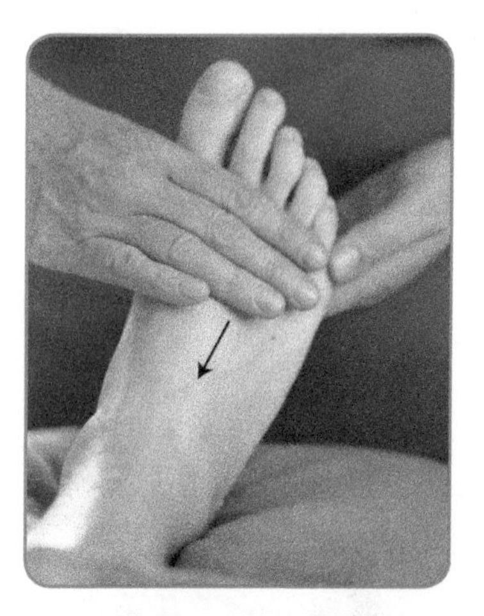

Fig 10.63 - Use a light stroke directed back toward the heart

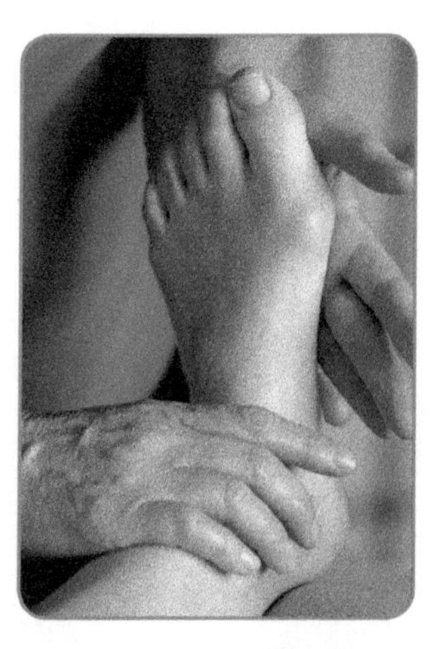

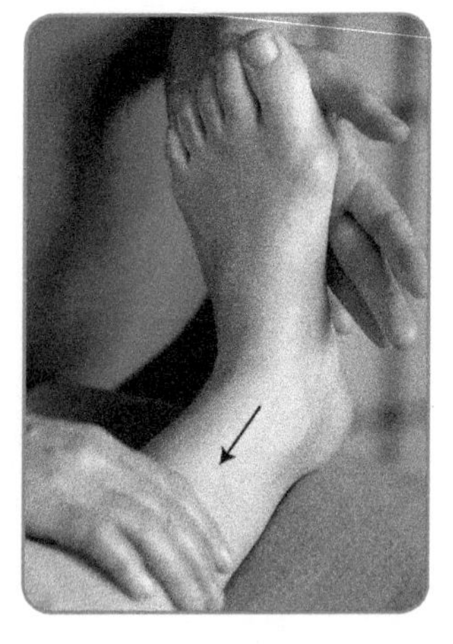

Fig 10.64 - Lymph pumping

36. Kidneys—Locate this point by finding the waist area at the cuboid notch. Gently press with the flat of your thumb. Kidney is one thumb width up from the waistline and one-thumb width in from the spine. Slide down the arch from the kidney to the bladder point, just medial to the sacrum point. Ending with these points may assist in releasing toxins. Client is encouraged to drink water after a treatment.

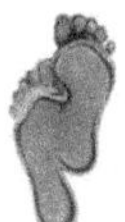

The kidney, ureter and bladder are in the vicinity of the flexor hallicus longus tendon. Be gentle when working this area.

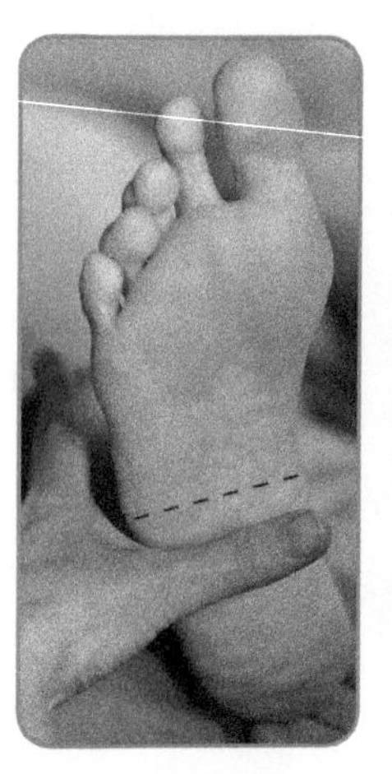

Fig 10.65 Find waistline

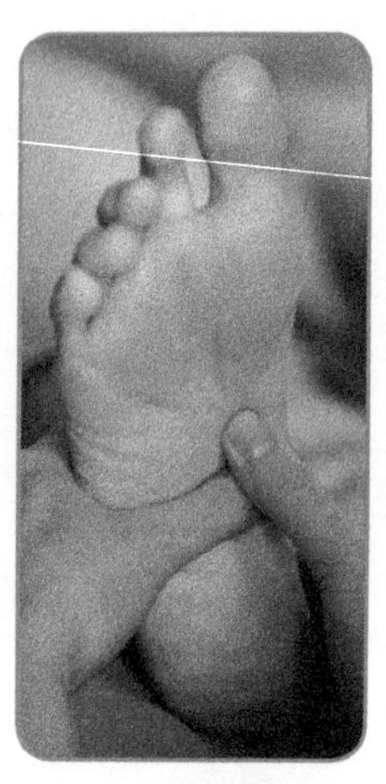

Fig 10.66 Locate kidney just above waistline

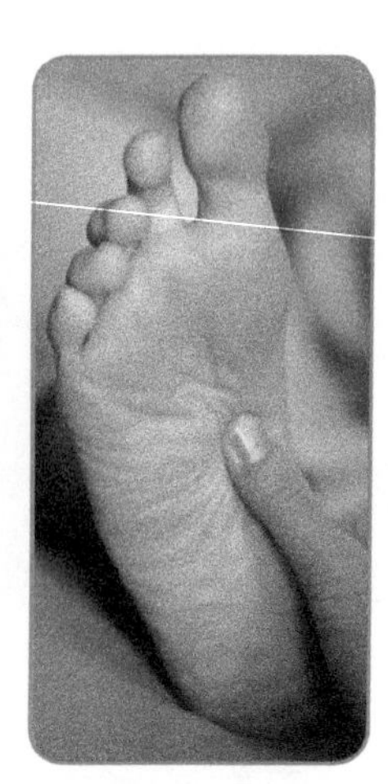

Fig 10.67 - Kidney

37. Adrenals—From the kidney point, press with the tip of the thumb into the adrenal reflex just above the kidney.

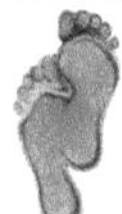

If the adrenal gland is tender, it may be due to stress and caffeine use.

38. Ureter and Bladder—After pressing kidney point, slide down the ureter to just inside the sacrum point and press the bladder. Remember, the bladder is a pelvic organ—you should feel bone. Repeat the series—kidney, adrenal, ureter, bladder—three times on each foot.

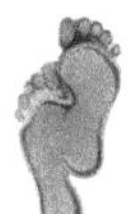

This may have surprising positive results with kidney stones, bladder infections, and fluid retention.

NOTE: Working the kidney, ureter and bladder for the urinary system might stimulate your client's need to urinate, so save it for the end of the session.

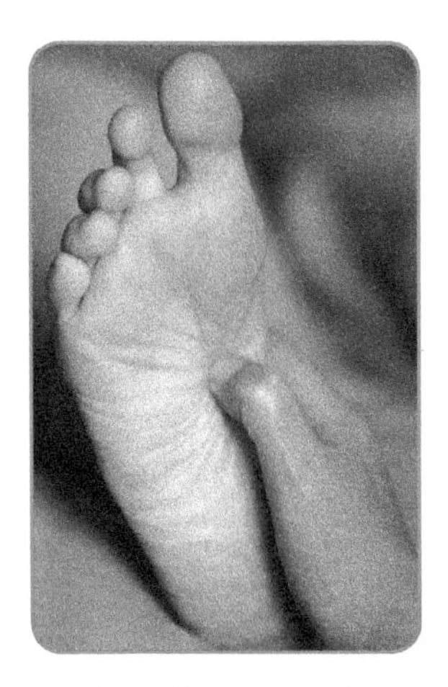

Fig 10.68 - Adrenal

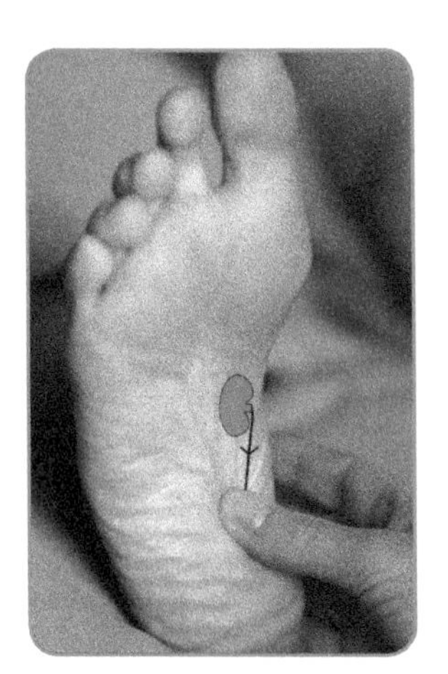

Fig 10.69 - Ureter

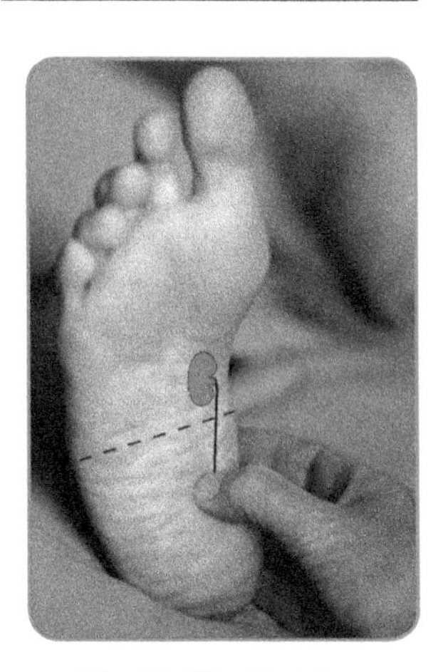

Fig 10.70 - Bladder

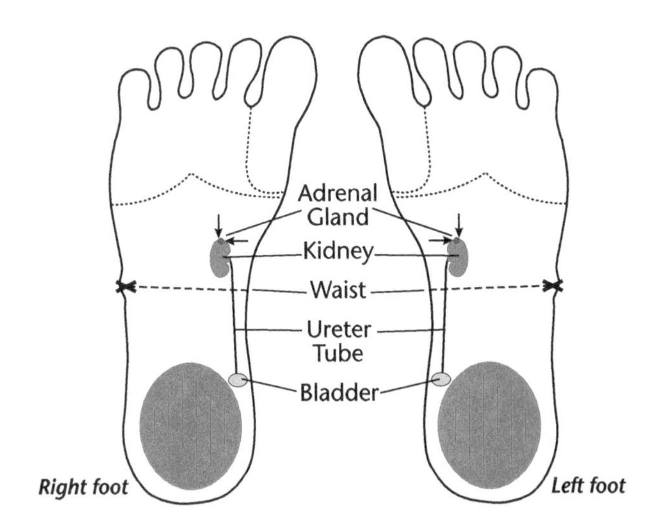

Fig 10.71 - Kidneys, adrenals, ureters, and bladder

39. **Finishing**—Complete the sequence with an all-over squeezing and massage of both feet.

40. **Nerve Strokes**—Use long, light, calming strokes down the legs to the feet.

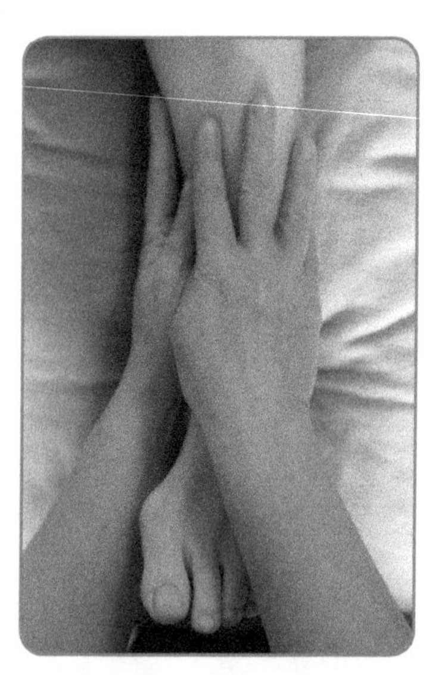

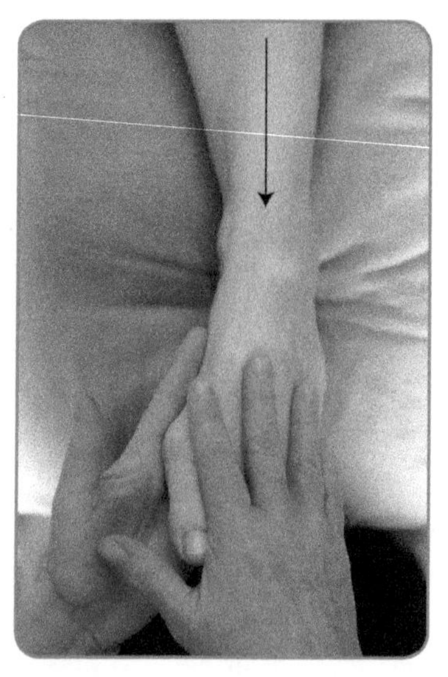

Fig 10.72 - Nerve strokes / Calming down strokes

41. **Solar Plexus**—Gently hold as you did in the beginning of the session to bring your Integrative Reflexology® session to an end.

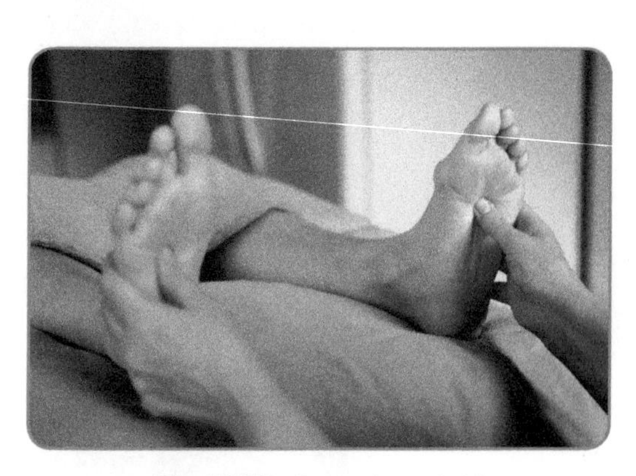

Fig 10.73 - Solar plexus hold

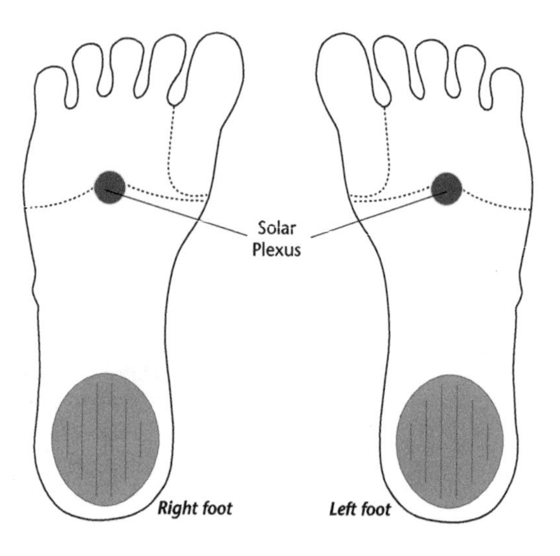

Fig 10.74 - Solar plexus

Remember to always recommend 24 hours of increased water intake following a treatment.

Summary of Integrative Reflexology® Basic 60-Minute Sequence

1. **Leg Release Techniques**
   a. Traction both legs.
   b. Side to side: Rock the hips as you traction the legs.
2. **Solar Plexus**—Center yourself while holding this point on both feet. Set your intention.
3. **Opening Lymph Drainage**—Light and toward the heart.
4. **Toes**—Great toe to little toe—Rotate, massage, and apply gentle traction.

   **** Apply lotion or cream to the whole foot. Try to keep the toes without cream or lotion for now. You will apply lotion/cream there after the sinus work.****
5. **Warm Up the Feet**
   a. Toothpaste squeeze
   b. Wringing
6. **Pineal**—Press the top medial corner of the great toe.
7. **Pituitary**—Press and circle on the pituitary in the center of the great toe.
8. **Sinuses**—Rub/knead and brush.

   ****Apply lotion or cream to the toes if you haven't already****
9. **Throat**—Rub/knead the inner great toe.
10. **Neck**—Rub, knead and work the front, side and back of great toe.
11. **Neck and Shoulder Combo**—Work back and forth between the feet.
12. **Shoulder**—Rub, knead and pinch the entire area, working front, side and back.
13. **Ear, Bronchial, Eye**—Press and circle each point.
14. **Thyroid and Parathyroids**—Hook and press into thyroid. Press parathyroids.
15. **Lungs**—Knead with knuckles and thumbs, diaphragm spread and chest spread.
16. **Solar Plexus**—Work deeper and with client's breath. Press with the exhale and release with the inhale.
17. **Esophagus and Stomach**—Slide down and gently circle the stomach 5-6 times.
18. **Pancreas**—Circle the stomach and then press in on the pancreas reflex.
19. **Liver, Gallbladder, Heart and Spleen**—Press the points on the right foot (liver and gallbladder) and then on the left foot (heart and spleen). Three times on each foot.
20. **Large and Small Intestines**—Follow the flow of the large intestine - work the left foot and then the right foot. Circle and knead the small intestine, left then right foot.
21. **Elbow, Hip and Knee**—Work down the lateral side of the foot.
22. **Pelvis**—Work the entire heel pad with your knuckles or fist.
23. **Spine**—Work the entire spine reflex area.
24. **Chest**—Work the top of the foot and around the ankle to move any lymph fluid up.
25. **Reproductive Area**—Stimulate the uterus/prostate reflex first, then the ovaries/testicles and then slide across from the ovary/testicles to uterus/prostate for the uterine tubes or vas deferens.
26. **Lymph Area**—Drain and pump up the top of the foot and around the ankle.
27. **Kidneys, Adrenals, Ureter and Bladder**—Gently press kidney, roll up to press the adrenal and then slide down to press the bladder. Do this three times on each foot.

   **** Keep this for the end of the 60-minute session. It may stimulate the client's need to use the restroom.****
28. **Nerve Strokes**—Long, light, calming strokes down the legs to the feet.
29. **Solar Plexus**—Gently hold as you did in the beginning of the session to bring your Integrative Reflexology® session to an end.
30. **Closing Intention**

Integrative Reflexology® Variety of Techniques

(Refer to pages 120-136)

Leg Release Techniques

1. **Traction**—See Basic Sequence (Step 1a).
2. **Side-to-Side**—See Basic Sequence (Step 1b).
3. **Shake**—Shake your client's leg like you are shaking hands—hold the outside of their foot under the heel, like it is a hand you are about to shake. Place your other hand on the top of their foot and shake the leg up and down 2-3 times to allow the hip and knee to release (Fig 10.75). Give gentle traction and repeat on the opposite leg.

   NOTE: Do not use this technique with clients who have had injury, surgery or replacement of joints in their legs or hips.
4. **Rattle**—Rattle the entire foot by placing your hands flat on either side of the ankle and sliding your hands back and forth, jiggling the foot (Fig 10.76). This is easier to perform when sitting or kneeling versus standing.
5. **Roll**—Roll the leg by holding the heel in the palm of your hand and rolling the foot in back and forth in your hand. The roll should extend up through the leg, releasing the piriformis muscle in the hip (Fig 10.77).
6. **Circumduction**—Slowly rotate the ankle in a full circle in both directions (Fig 10.78).
7. **Achilles Stretch**—Standing on the side of the table, near your client's feet, use the hand closest to the table to hold the heel in the palm of your hand with your fingers pointing up the leg. Allow your forearm to rest against the ball of the foot and lunge forward as you flex the ankle and stretch the Achilles tendon (Fig 10.79). You can give an additional stretch by using your free hand to compress the quadriceps toward the hip.

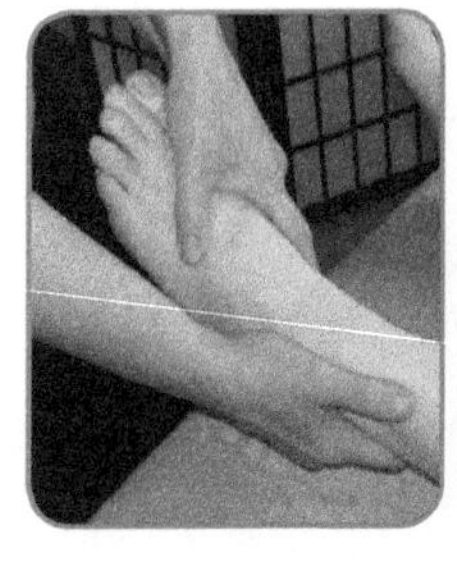
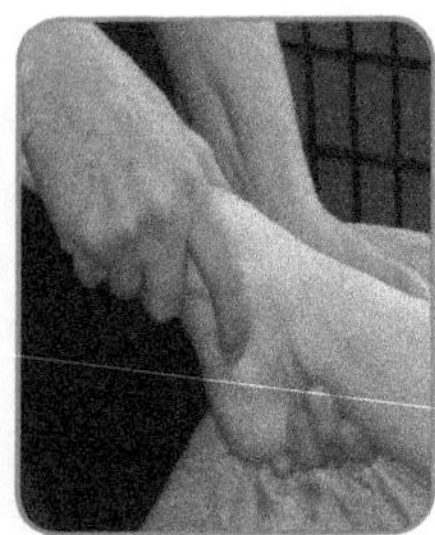

Fig 10.75 - Shake

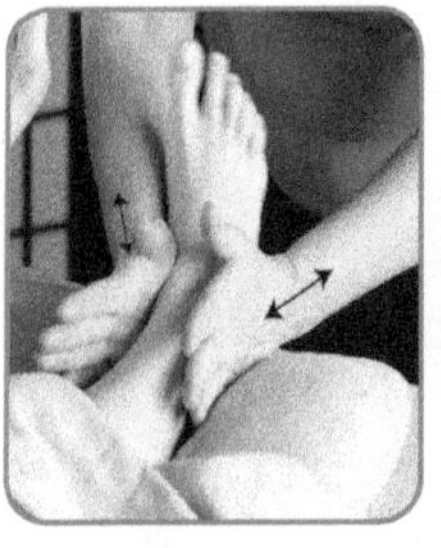
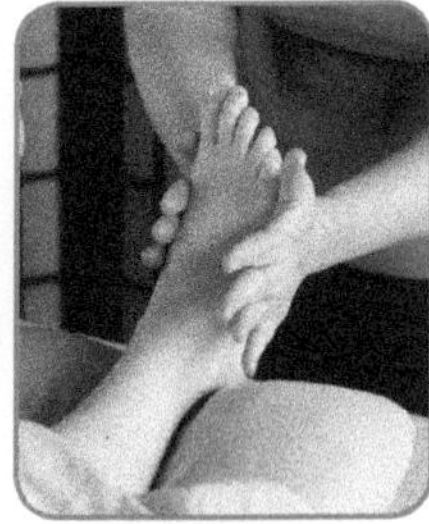

Fig 10.76 - Rattle back and forth

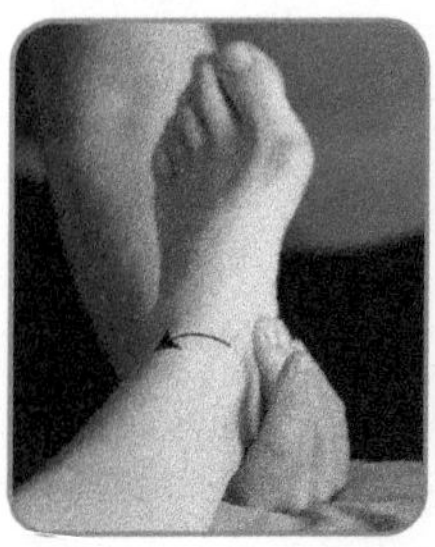
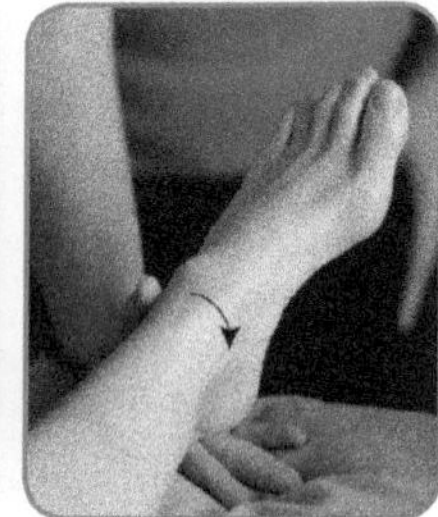

Fig 10.77 - Roll

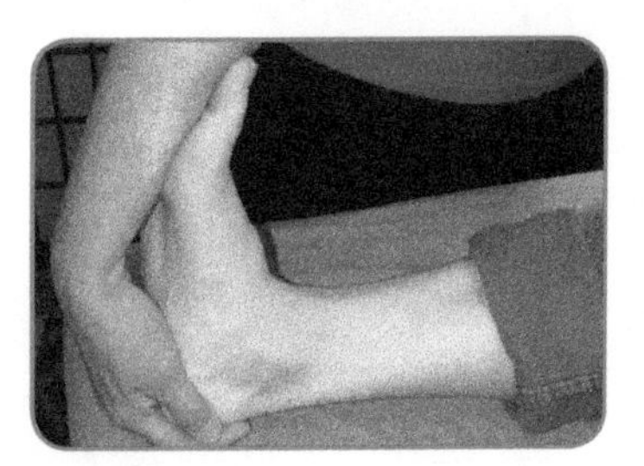
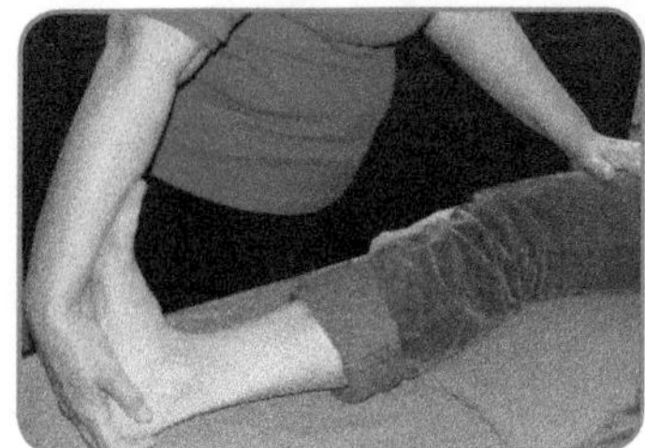

Fig 10.79 - Achilles stretch

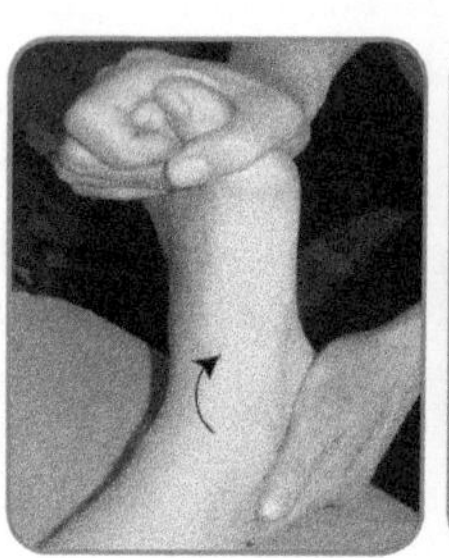
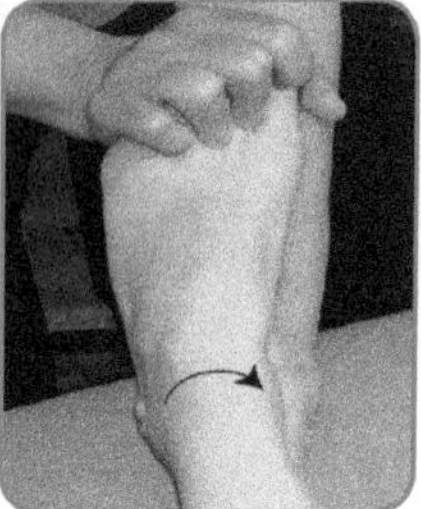

Fig 10.78 - Circumduction

Solar Plexus Techniques

1. **Solar Plexus Hold**—See Basic Sequence (Step 2)
2. **Solar Plexus Press**—See Basic Sequence (Step 19)

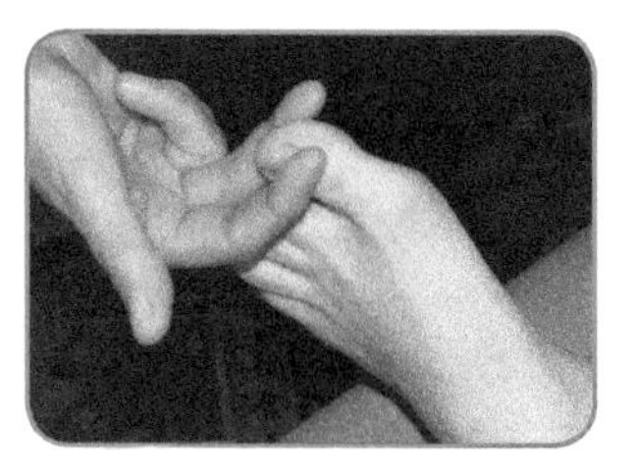

Fig 10.80 - Chinese toe pop

Lymph Techniques

1. **Opening Lymph Drainage**—See Basic Sequence (Step 3)
2. **Lymph Strokes**—See Basic Sequence (Step 35)
3. **Lymphatic Pumping**—See Basic Sequence (Step 35)

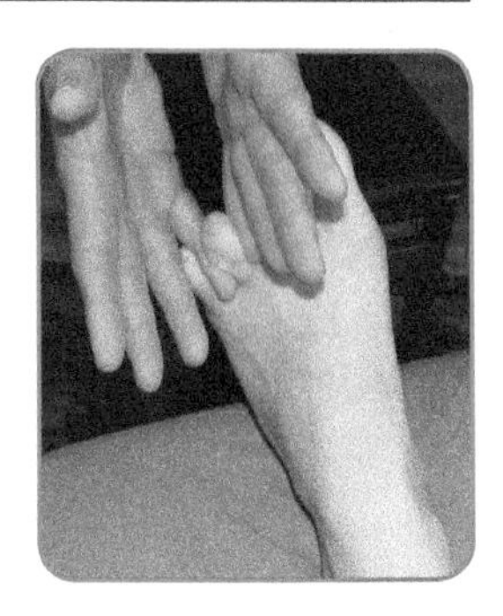

Fig 10.81 - Toe boogie

Toe Techniques

1. **Circumduction**—See Basic Sequence (Step 4)
2. **Chinese Toe Pop**—With your 2nd and 3rd fingers bent clasp the end of the toe between your knuckles. Quickly pull up and off the toe, allowing your fingers to "pop" together (Fig 10.80).
3. **Toe Boogie**—Sandwich one toe between the 4th and 5th fingers of each hand and roll the toe back and forth (Fig 10.81).

Warm Up Techniques

1. **Toothpaste Squeeze**—See Basic Sequence (Step 5a)
2. **Wringing**—See Basic Sequence (Step 5b)
3. **Windshield Wipers**—Use thumbs on the sole of the foot. Make alternating circles up the sole of the foot in a windshield wiper pattern (Fig 10.82).
4. **Yin/Yang Strokes**—Begin with your hands on the medial inner foot, thumbs on the plantar surface. Slide your hands back and forth along the spine reflex area. Then slide your hands over the toes and to the lateral aspect of the foot, sliding back and forth. Then leave one hand on the lateral aspect of the foot while sliding the other hand over the toes and back to the medial aspect of the foot. Slide both hands back and forth and then slide both hands over the toes to the opposite side of the foot (Fig 10.83). Repeat this many times, stimulating opposite aspects of each foot in a yin/yang pattern.

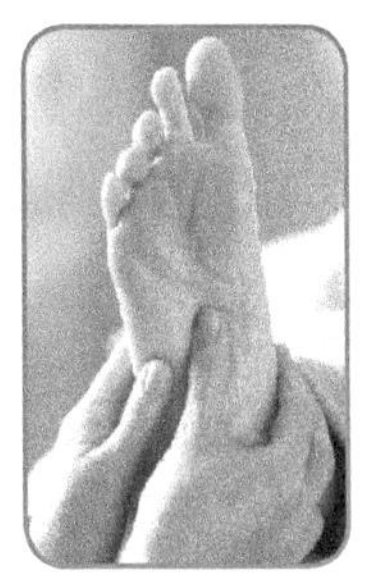
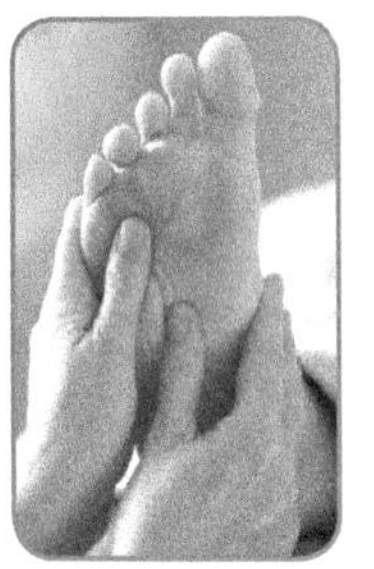
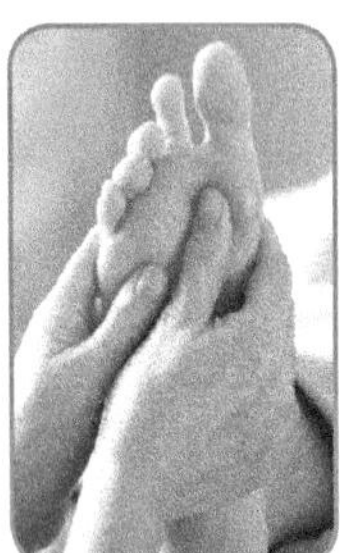

Fig 10.82 - Windshield wipers

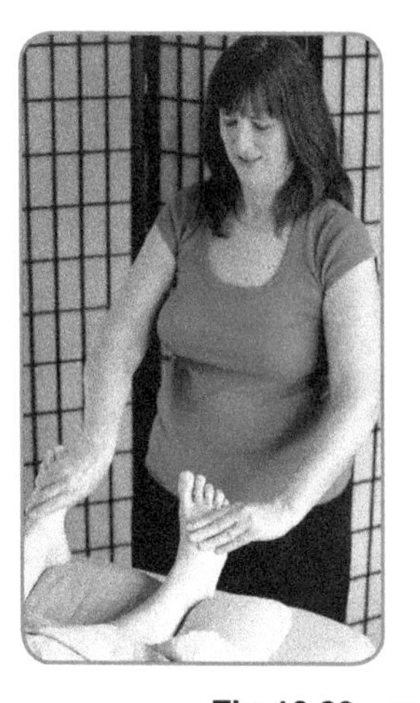
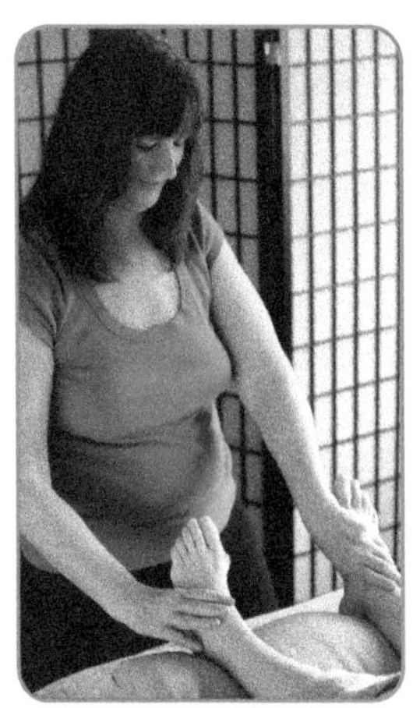

Fig 10.83 - Yin/Yang strokes

Pineal and Pituitary Techniques

1. **Press and Circle/Hold**—See Basic Sequence (Steps 6 & 7)
2. **Pulse Stimulation**—Do point stimulation as a pulsing pressure.

Sinus Techniques

1. **Press and Hold**—See Basic Sequence (Step 8)
2. **Squeezing**—See Basic Sequence (Step 8a)
3. **Scratching**—See Basic Sequence (Step 8b)
4. **Brushing**—See Basic Sequence (Step 8c)
5. **"This Little Piggy"**—See Basic Sequence (Step 8d)

Throat Techniques

1. **Press and Circle**—See Basic Sequence (Step 9)
2. **Slide**—Slide back and forth along the inner space between the great toe and the 2nd toe.

Neck Techniques

1. **Massage Great Toe**—See Basic Sequence (Step 10)
2. **Traction**—See Basic Sequence (Throat/Neck "Foot" Note)
3. **Circumduction**—See Basic Sequence (Figs 10.6 and 10.7)
4. **Neck and Shoulder Combo**—See Basic Sequence (Step 11)

Shoulder Techniques

1. **Pinch and Twist**—See Basic Sequence (Step 12)
2. **Knuckles**—See Basic Sequence (Step 12)

Ear, Bronchial and Eye Techniques

1. **Press and Circle/Hold**—See Basic Sequence (Steps 13-15)
2. **Trumpet**—See Basic Sequence (Fig 10.21)
3. **Three Knuckles**—Press and roll your knuckles into the toe ledge, stimulating all three points simultaneously (Fig 10.84).

Thyroid and Parathyroid Techniques

1. **Thyroid Hook and Press**—See Basic Sequence (Step 16)
2. **Parathyroid Press**—See Basic Sequence (Step 17)
3. **Client Press**—Have the client press their foot into your thumb as you brace and support your thumb against their pressure. The client determines the amount of pressure as you hold your thumb on the thyroid reflex.

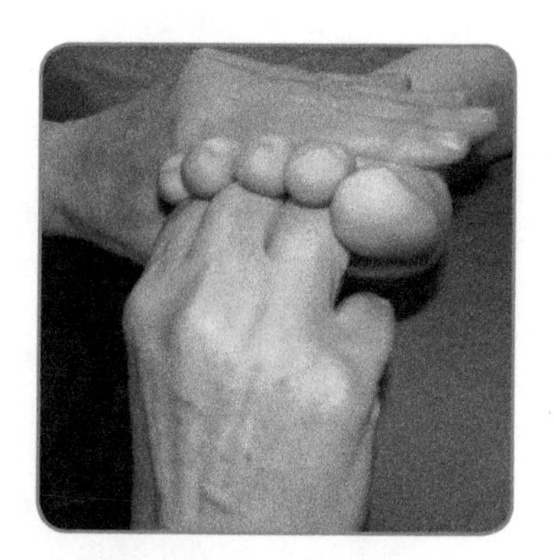

Fig 10.84 - Three knuckles

Lung Techniques

1. **Knuckle Twist**—See Basic Sequence (Step 18)
2. **Pinch and Twist**—See Basic Sequence (Step 18)
3. **Thumb Walking**—See Basic Sequence (Step 18)
4. **Diaphragm Spread**—See Basic Sequence (Step 18a)
5. **Chest Spread**—See Basic Sequence (Step 18b)
6. **Lung Press**—Place one hand on top of the foot to brace the foot. Use the other hand in a fist to press the flat surface of your fist into the lung pad repeatedly (Fig 10.85).
7. **Palming**—Place one flat hand on the chest area and the other flat hand on the lung pad and circle them, stimulating the lung and chest areas between your hands (Fig 10.86).
8. **Pulmonary Pump**—Place one hand on top of the foot to brace the foot. Hold the other hand in a fist and use the first-finger and thumb surface of the fist to pull up the entire plantar surface of the foot, starting at the heel and ending on the lung pad (Fig 10.87).
9. **See-Saw**—Grasp two adjacent metatarsal bones and move them back and forth within the foot, seesawing them with each other. Begin with the metatarsals of the great toe and 2nd toe, then move down the line doing the 2nd and 3rd metatarsals, 3rd and 4th, 4th and 5th. You are grasping the bones in the ball of the foot for this technique, not the toes themselves (Fig 10.88).

Esophagus and Stomach Techniques

1. **Esophagus Slide**—See Basic Sequence (Step 20)
2. **Stomach Circling**—See Basic Sequence (Step 20)
3. **Esophagus and Stomach Combo**—Cross your arms and rest them on the table and grasp the ball of the great toe with your opposite hand (right hand grasps left foot and vice versa) (Fig 10.89). In this position you can work the esophagus and stomach simultaneously on each foot by sliding down the esophagus three times and then gently circling on the stomach six times or more.

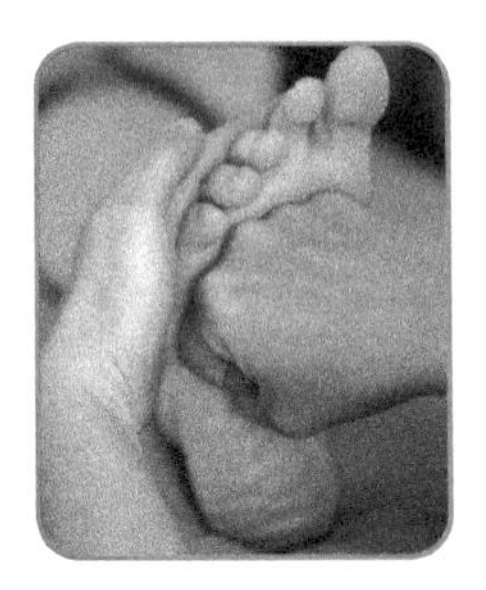
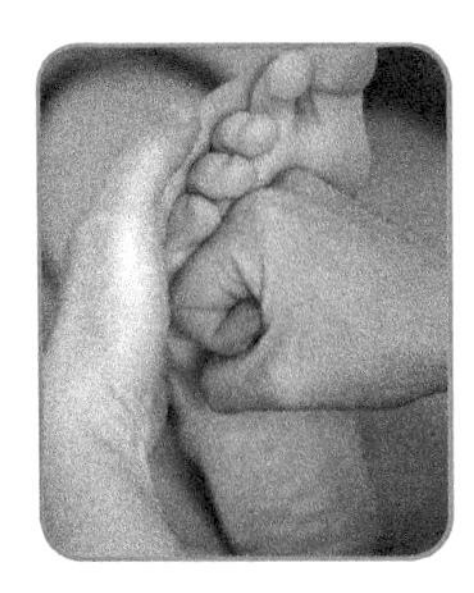

Fig 10.85 - Lung press

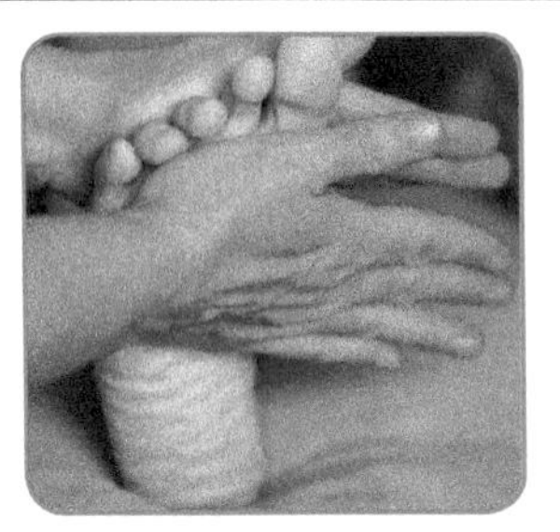

Fig 10.86 - Palming

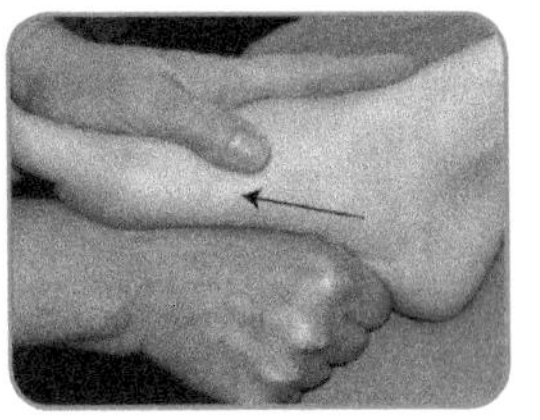
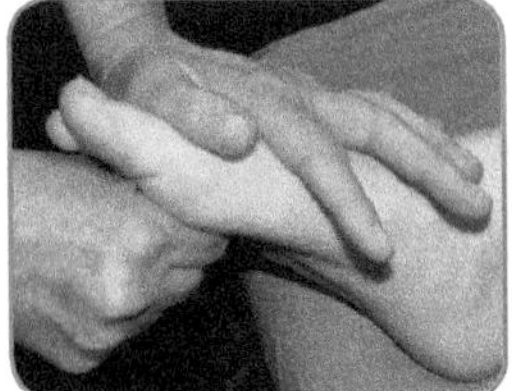

Fig 10.87 - Pulmonary pump

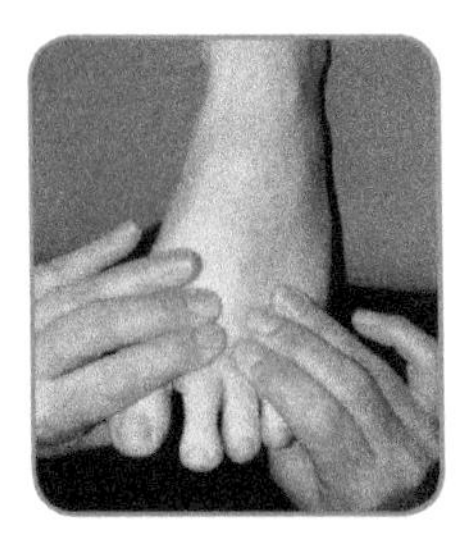

Fig 10.88 - See-saw

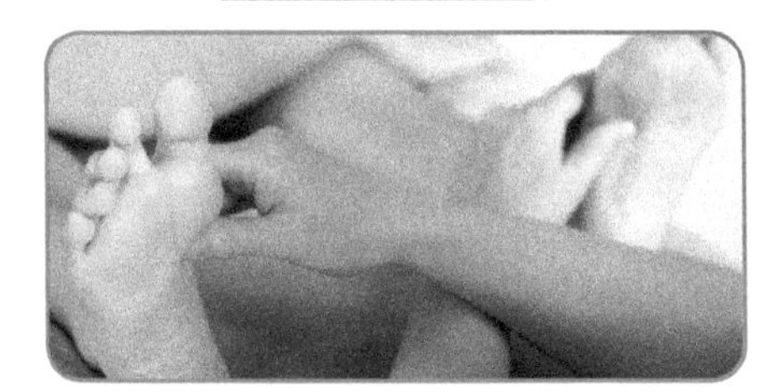

Fig 10.89 - Esophagus and stomach combo

Pancreas Techniques

1. **Press and Hold**—See Basic Sequence (Step 21)
2. **Client Press**—Have the client press their foot into your thumb as you brace and support your thumb against their pressure. The client determines the amount of pressure as you hold your thumb on the pancreas reflex.

Liver, Gallbladder, Heart and Spleen Techniques

1. **Press and Hold**—See Basic Sequence (Steps 22-25)
2. **C-Clamp**—See Basic Sequence (Step 25 NOTE)
3. **Knuckles**—Stimulate each point with one of your knuckles.
4. **Circle-on-Point**—Hold the reflex point with one hand as you grasp all the toes with the other hand. As you rotate the toes in a circular motion, the reflex point receives stimulation (Fig 10.90).
5. **Spread and Press**—Do the diaphragm spread and press on each reflex point at the end of the stroke (you will need to repeat the stroke four times, once for each point).

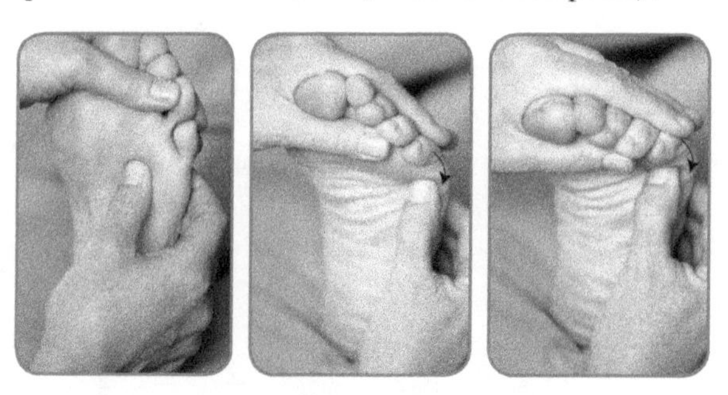

Fig 10.90
Circle-on-point demonstrated here on the heart and spleen points.

Large Intestine and Small Intestine Techniques

1. **Large Intestine Sequence**—See Basic Sequence (Step 26)
2. **Knuckles on Small Intestine**—See Basic Sequence (Step 27)
3. **Thumb-Over-Thumb**—Stimulate the small intestine using a thumb-over-thumb kneading stroke.

Elbow Techniques

1. **Circle and Pinch**—See Basic Sequence (Step 28)

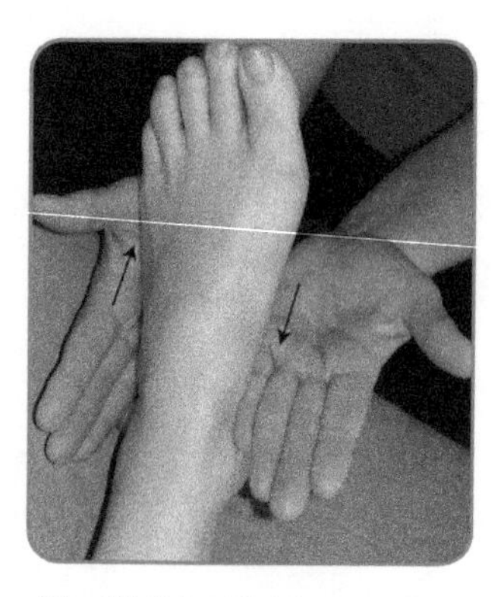

Fig 10.91 - Hip/Sacrum Saw

Hip Techniques

1. **Knuckle**—See Basic Sequence (Step 29)
2. **Hip/Sacrum Squeeze**—See Basic Sequence (Step 29a)
3. **Hip/Sacrum Saw**—Place the edge of each hand on either side of the heel (palms up with the little finger edge against the foot). One hand is on the hip point the other is on the sacrum point. Saw your hands back and forth to stimulate both points simultaneously (Fig 10.91).

Knee Techniques

1. **Press and Hold**—See Basic Sequence (Step 30)

Pelvic Techniques

1. **Pinching**—See Basic Sequence (Step 31)
2. **Knuckles**—See Basic Sequence (Step 31)
3. **Heel on Heel**—See Basic Sequence (Step 31)

Spine Techniques

1. **Thumbs or Knuckles**—See Basic Sequence (Step 32)
2. **Spine Spread**—See Basic Sequence (Fig 10.56)
3. **Spine Twist**—Stand and face the medial edge of the foot. Both hands hold the medial arch of the foot with fingers on top and thumbs on the plantar surface. The hand at the ankle will hold there as an anchor while the distal hand inverts and everts the foot as you slide up and down the spine reflex area multiple times (Fig 10.92).
4. **Spine Saw**—Support the lateral aspect of the foot with your outside hand. Use your inside hand to "saw" up and down the spine reflex area (Fig 10.93).

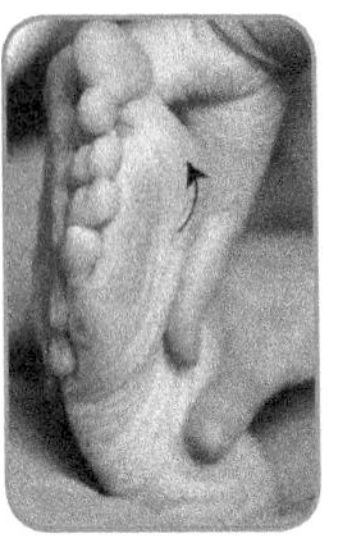
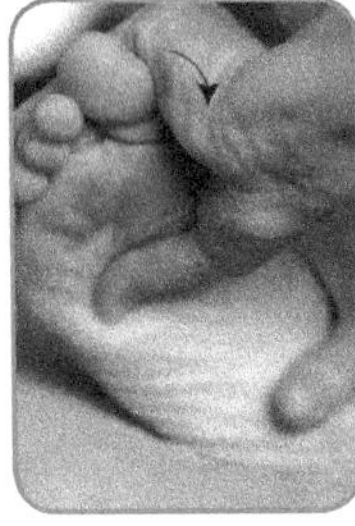

Fig 10.92 - Spine twist

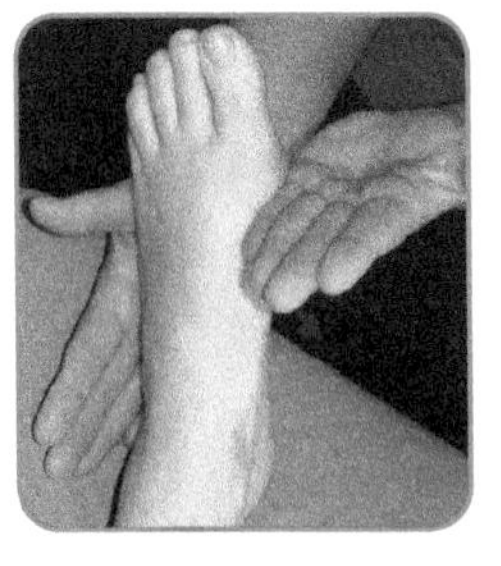

Fig 10.93 - Spine saw

Chest Techniques

1. **Long Strokes**—See Basic Sequence (Step 33)

Reproductive Area Techniques

1. **Uterus/Prostate and Ovary/Testicles Press and Circle/Hold**—See Basic Sequence (Step 34)
2. **Uterine Tube/Vas Deferens Slide**—See Basic Sequence (Step 34)

Kidneys, Adrenals, Ureter and Bladder Techniques

1. **Kidney Press**—See Basic Sequence (Step 36)
2. **Adrenals Press**—See Basic Sequence (Step 37)
3. **Ureter and Bladder Slide and Press**—See Basic Sequence (Step 38)
4. **Client Press**—Have the client press their foot into your thumb as you brace and support your thumb against their pressure. The client determines the amount of pressure as you hold your thumb on the adrenal reflex.

Zone Techniques

1. **Thumb/Knuckle Walking**—Use your thumb or knuckle to "walk" up the vertical zones of the feet from the heel to the toes (Fig 10.94).

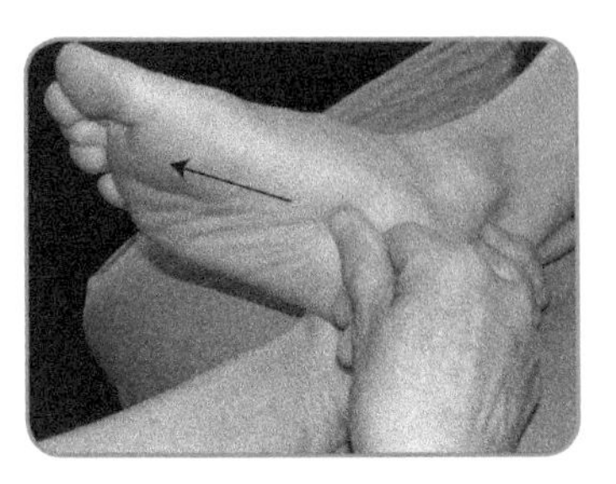

Fig 10.94 - Thumb walking

Percussion Techniques

1. **Toe Drop Soup**—Hold the foot by grasping the great toe, as long as this is comfortable for the client (be cautious if they have a bunion). Gently pound the plantar surface of the foot—first the thoracic pad, then the abdominal arch and lastly the pelvic heel pad. Then slightly raise the foot and allow the great toe to drop out of your grip as you catch the heel of the foot with your other hand.

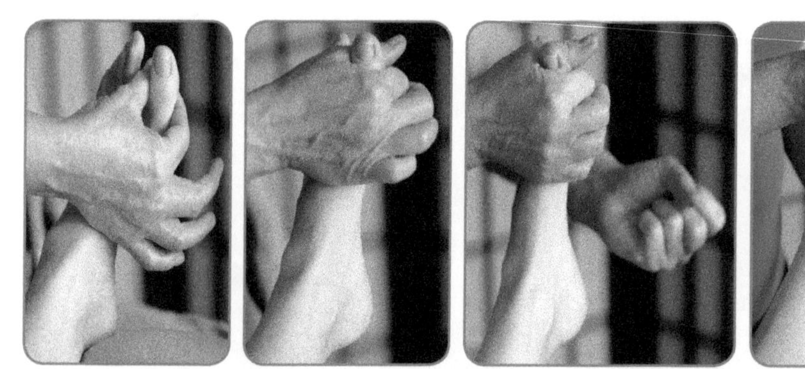
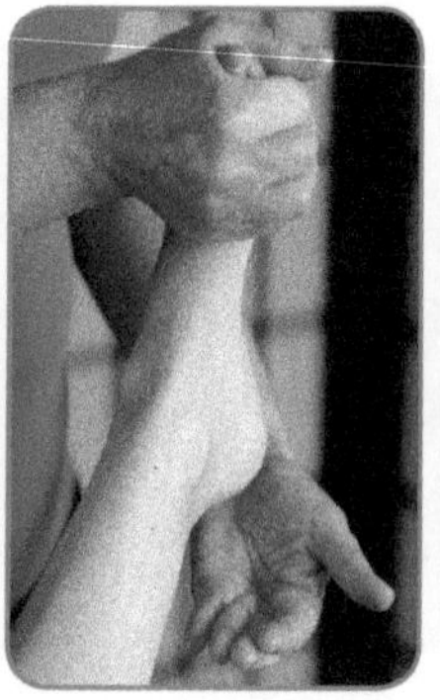
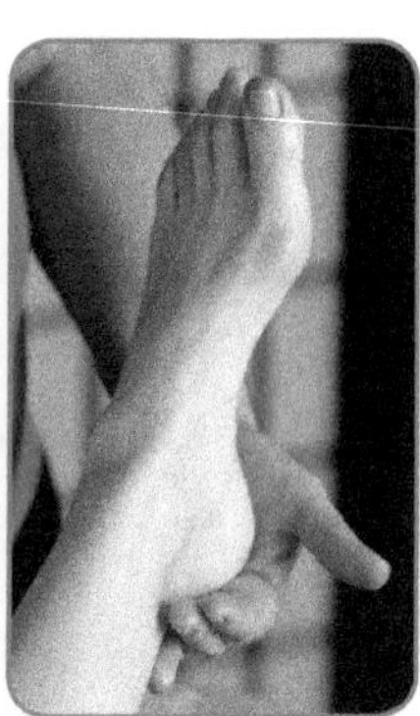

Fig 10.95 - Toe drop soup

2. **Slapping**—Using a flat hand, slap the entire plantar surface of the foot.

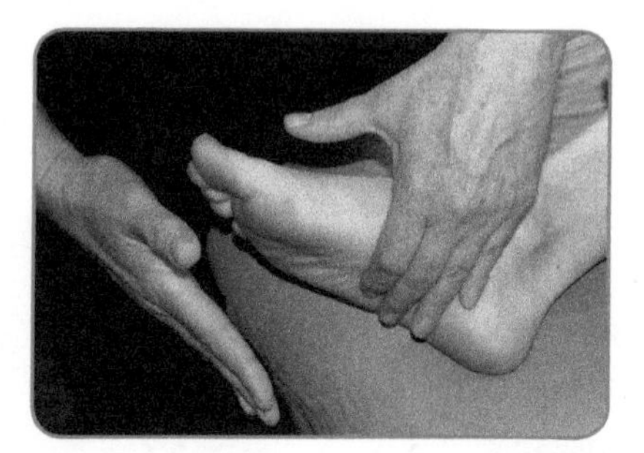
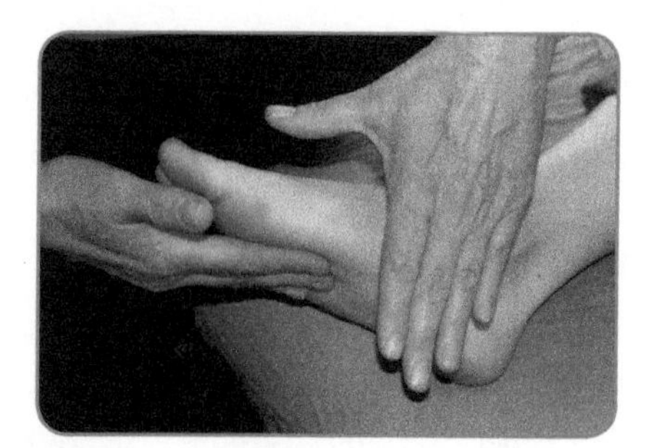

Fig 10.96 - Slapping

3. **Tapping**—Using fingertips, tap the entire plantar surface of the foot.

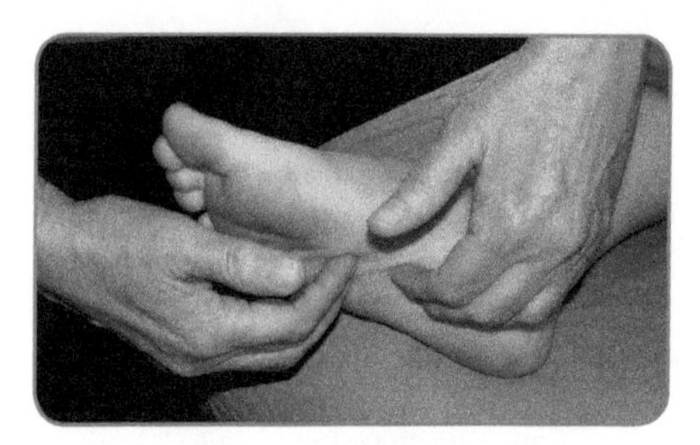

Fig 10.97 - Tapping

Integrative Reflexology® 90-Minute Sequence

1. **Leg release techniques**—Traction, Side to Side, Shake, Rattle, Roll, Ankle Circumduction, Achilles Stretch.
2. **Warm up techniques**—Toothpaste Squeeze, Wringing, Windshield Wipers, Yin/Yang.
3. **Solar plexus**—Hold and breathe with the client for 3-6 breaths. This is where you center yourself and set the intention for the session.
4. **Opening lymph drainage**—Light and toward the heart.
5. **Toes**—Circumduction, Chinese Toe Pops, Toe Boogie.

   **** Apply lotion or cream to the whole foot. Try to keep the toes without cream or lotion for now. You will apply lotion/cream there after the sinus work. ****

6. **Pineal and pituitary**—Press and Circle/Hold, Pulse Stimulation.
7. **Sinuses**—Press and Hold, Squeezing, Scratching, Brushing.
8. **Throat**—Press and Circle, Sliding.
9. **Neck**—Massage Great Toe, Traction, Circumduction.
10. **Neck and shoulder combo**—Work back and forth between the feet.

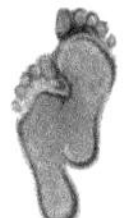

Bodywork on the neck and shoulders may be inserted here to evaluate whether what the therapist is finding in the feet fits with what is in the body. If this is a client stress area, then alternating between the reflexology and the bodywork will give greater relief.

11. **Shoulder**—Knuckles, Pinch and Twist.
12. **Ear, Bronchial, Eye**—Press and Circle/Hold, Trumpet, Three Knuckles.
13. **Thyroid**—Hook and press into thyroid. Press Parathyroids.
14. **Lungs**—Knuckle Twist, Pinch and Twist, Thumb Walking, Diaphragm Spread, Chest Spread, Lung Press, Palming, Pulmonary Pump, See-Saw.

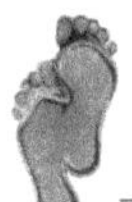

Guide your client to be aware of their breathing. Ask them to breathe in/out slowly and deeply as you work the lungs.

15. **Esophagus and Stomach**—Esophagus Slide, Stomach Circling, Esophagus/Stomach Combo.

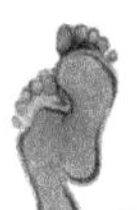

For clients with stomach and digestive challenges, have them rub their stomach as you gently rub the stomach reflex.

16. **Pancreas**—Press and Hold, Client Press.
17. **Liver, Gallbladder, Heart, Spleen**—Press and Hold, C-Clamp, Knuckles, Circle-on-Point, Spread and Press.

18. **Large and Small Intestines**—Large Intestine Sequence, Knuckles on Small Intestine, Thumb-Over-Thumb.

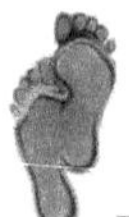

Bodyworkers can guide the client through self-massage of the large intestine, mirroring the same areas in the body as you are working in the feet and in the abdomen.

19. **Elbow**—Circle and Pinch.
20. **Hip**—Knuckle, Hip/Sacrum Squeeze, Hip/Sacrum Saw.
21. **Knee**—Press and Hold.
22. **Pelvis**—Pinching, Knuckles, Heel On Heel.

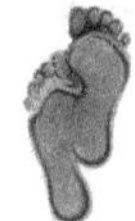

The hips, knees and pelvis are areas that benefit greatly from working the foot reflexes simultaneously with bodywork. For each area, press the reflex point while applying general or deep pressure to the corresponding body part. Try to find the center of pain in both locations and hold those spots until the pain subsides.

23. **Spine**—Thumbs or Knuckles, Spine Spread, Spinal Twist, Spine Saw.

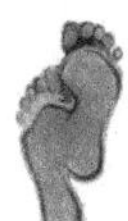

This is an excellent place to have the client prone and palpate the vertebrate. Find the tender areas in the vertebrae and work and hold the corresponding area on the spine reflex. You may try a spinal reflex realignment—work each vertebrate in sync with the spinal foot reflexes.

24. **Chest**—Long Strokes.
25. **Reproductive Area**—Uterus/Prostate and Ovary/Testicle Press and Circle/Hold, Uterine Tube/Vas Deferens Slide.

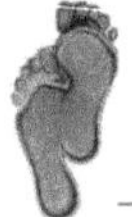

If you are trained in uterus repositioning, this reflexology work supports locating the uterus and assessing it as you realign. The client will be able to feel this as well.

26. **Lymph**—Lymph Strokes, Lymphatic Pumping.
27. **Kidneys, Adrenals, Ureter and Bladder**—Kidney Press, Adrenal Press, Ureter and Bladder Slide and Press, Client Press.

    **** Do the Hand Reflexology Sequence at this point in the session. Then return to the feet to complete the entire session.****

28. **Solar Plexus**—Hold and breathe with the client for 3-6 breaths. You are beginning and ending the session in the same place.
29. **Closing Intention**—Close the session and complete any positive statements or affirmations.

Integrative Reflexology® Spa Sequence

30-40 minute session

Do a foot scrub to begin your spa treatment (See Foot Scrubs on page 113).

1. **Leg release**—Traction, Side to Side, Shake, Rattle, Roll, Ankle Circumduction, Achilles Stretch.

   **** Add the cream with essential oils—only 1 drop of each essential oil and no more than 3 essential oils total. Rub the scented cream in your hands and hold them 8-12" away from the client's face, presenting the scent for the client to inhale three times. This will allow the scent to cross the blood-brain barrier and begin its therapeutic effects on the body. ****

2. **Warm up**—Toothpaste Squeeze, Wringing, Windshield Wipers, Yin/Yang.
3. **Solar plexus**—Hold and breathe with client for 3-6 breaths. This is where you center yourself and set the intention for the session.
4. **Opening lymph drainage**—Light and toward the heart.
5. **Sinuses**—Press and Hold, Squeezing, Scratching, Brushing.
6. **Throat**—Press and Circle, Sliding.
7. **Neck**—Massage Great Toe, Traction, Circumduction.
8. **Shoulder**—Knuckles, Pinch and Twist.
9. **Ear, Bronchial and Eye**—Roll knuckles on the ledge to stimulate all three reflex points.
10. **Lungs**—Knuckle Twist, Pinch and Twist, Thumb Walking, Diaphragm Spread, Chest Spread, Lung Press, Palming, Pulmonary Pump, See-Saw.
11. **Solar plexus press**—Hold and press the solar plexus point on the client's exhale and release with the client's inhale. Do this 3 times. It will help if you follow along with your breath.
12. **Esophagus and Stomach**—Esophagus Slide, Stomach Circling.
13. **Liver, Gallbladder, Heart, Spleen**—Spread and Press 3 times for each point.
14. **Large and Small Intestines**—Large Intestine Sequence, Knuckles on Small Intestine, Thumb-Over-Thumb.
15. **Spine**—Spine Spread, Spine Saw.
16. **Hip**—Hip/Sacrum Saw, Hip/Sacrum Squeeze.
17. **Pelvis**—Pinching, Knuckles, Heel On Heel.
18. **Lymph**—Lymph Strokes, Lymphatic Pumping.
19. **Kidney, Ureter, Bladder**—Press on the kidney reflex point lightly, slide down the ureter, press firmly on the bladder reflex point.
20. **Solar plexus hold**—End the session with this hold and breathe with the client for 3-6 breaths.
21. **Closing Intention**—Close the session and complete any positive statements or affirmations.

Integrative Reflexology® Hand Reflexology Sequence

The hands are the only other area of the body (besides the ears) that contain all the reflex points. The hand reflexology does not give as strong an effect to the organs as working the feet. Hand reflexology offers a wonderful addition to the foot reflexology session and will support the stimulation of both the meridians and the reflex points. The hand reflexology chart is a general reflection of the foot chart and includes the meridian points located on the hands. As you work with the hands, notice the quality of the fingernails and nail beds to determine if there are any imbalances in the particular meridian associated with that finger.

1. **Warm Up Hand**—General squeeze of the hand.
2. **Warm Up Fingers**—Rotate and milk each finger and press the fingertips for the sinuses.
3. **Chinese Pop**—Use this technique to stimulate the meridian points on each finger and press each corner of the nail. Name the meridian as you do the technique.

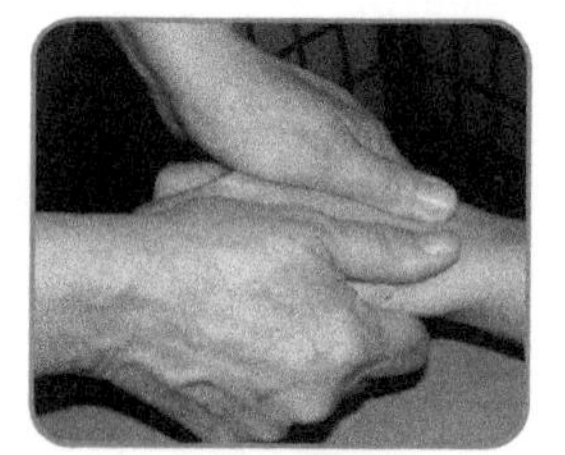

Fig 10.98
Opening strokes

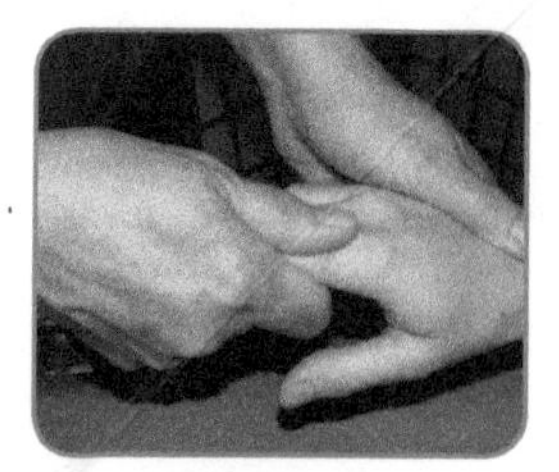

Fig 10.99
Milking

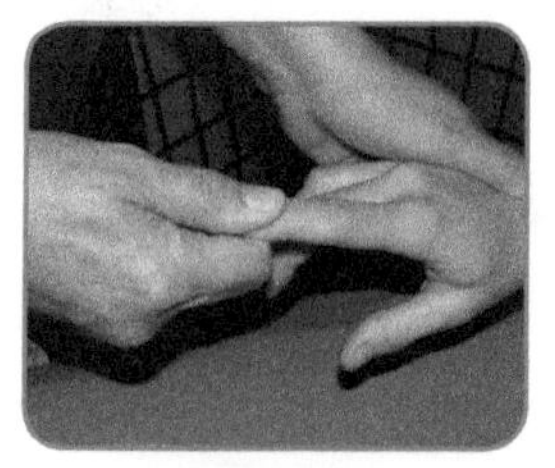

Fig 10.100
Press the sinuses

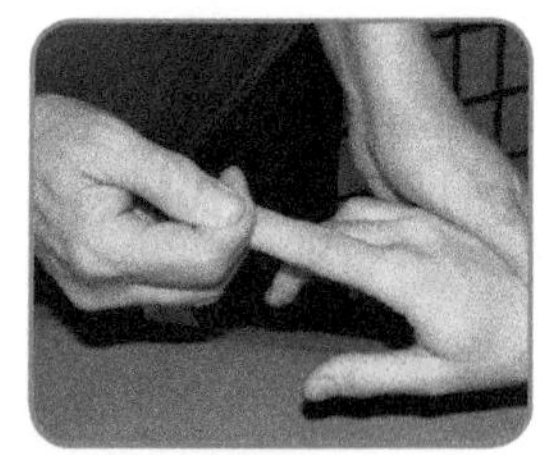

Fig 10.101
Chinese pop

4. **Pineal and Pituitary**—Locate the points on the thumb and apply pressure.
5. **Throat and Neck**—Massage the inside of the thumb for the throat and the entire thumb for the neck.

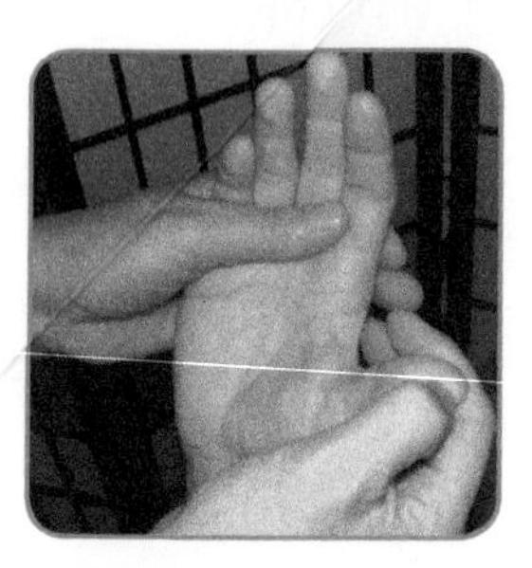

Fig 10.102 - Pineal

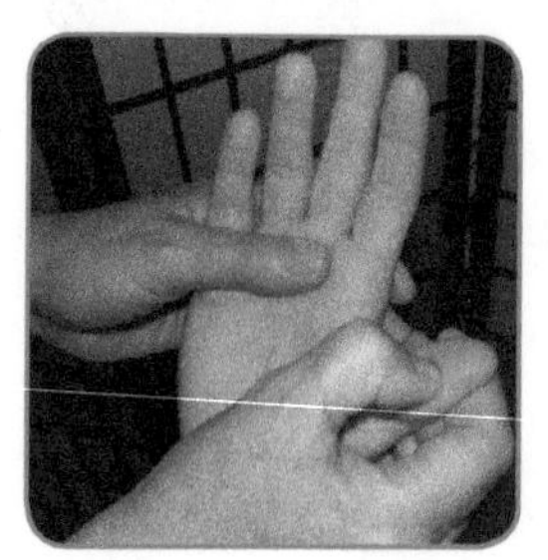

Fig 10.103 - Pituitary

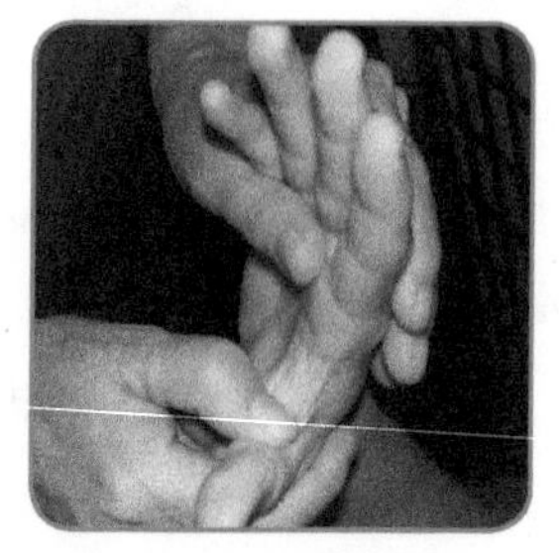

Fig 10.104 - Throat

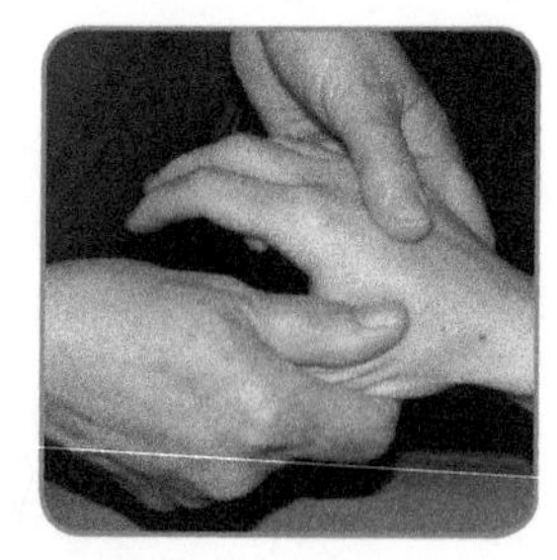

Fig 10.105 - Neck

6. **Neck and Shoulder**—Alternate kneading the thumb and base of the little finger to work both the neck and the shoulder.
7. **Shoulder**—Stimulate the shoulder area just below the little finger.

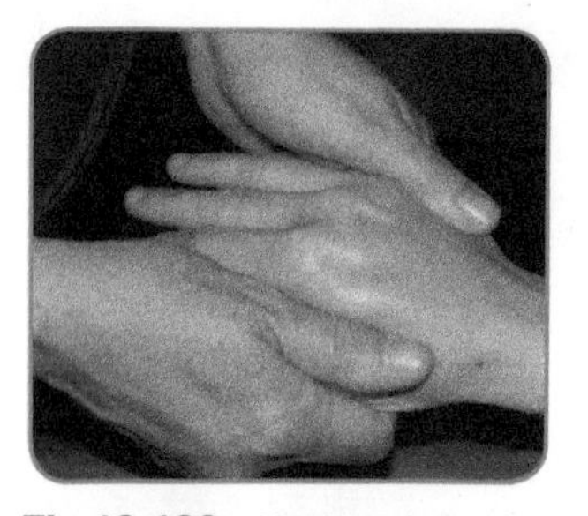

Fig 10.106 - Neck and shoulder

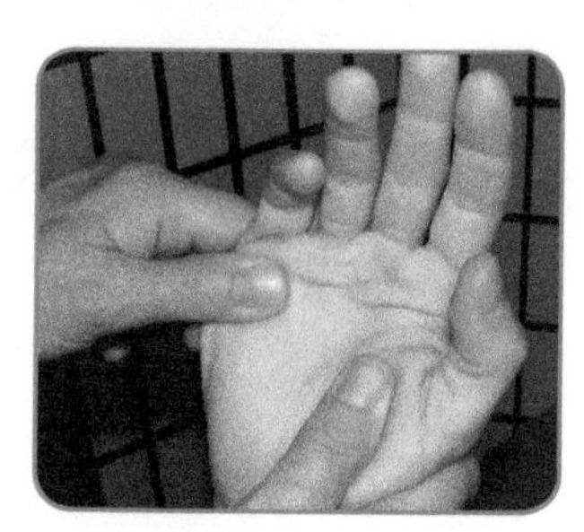

Fig 10.107 - Shoulder

8. **Ear, Bronchial, and Eye**—Push down on the palm side, below the space between the 4th and 5th finger for the ear, 3rd and 4th for the bronchial and the 2nd and 3rd for the eye.
9. **Lungs**—Knuckle twist, thumb over thumb, and thumb presses to stimulate the lungs.
10. **Solar Plexus**—Hold the center area of the palm just under the pad for the calming effect of the solar plexus

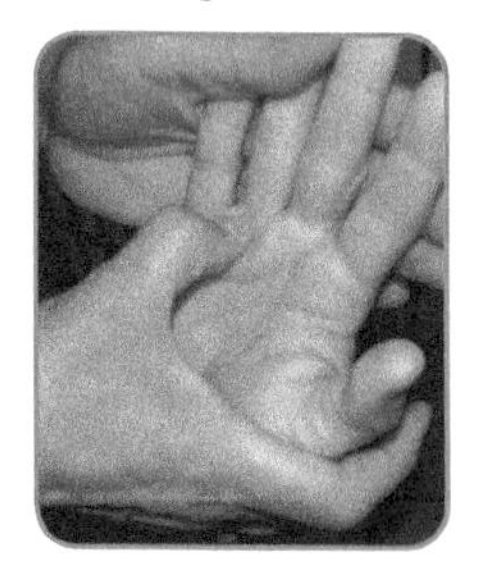

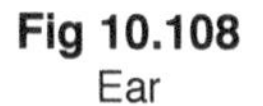

Fig 10.108
Ear

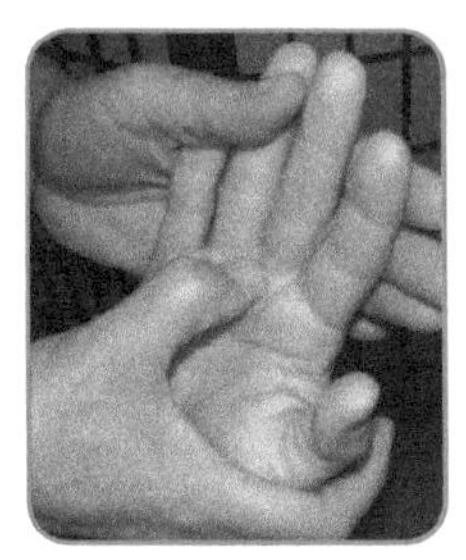

Fig 10.109
Bronchial tube

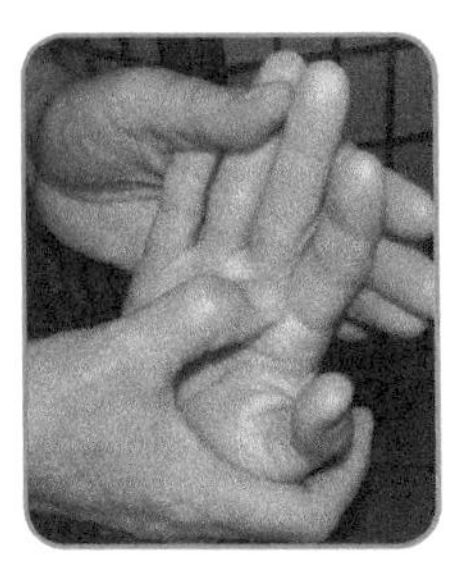

Fig 10.110
Eye

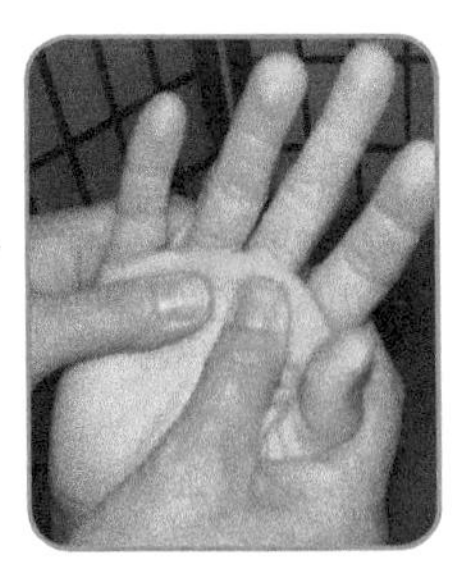

Fig 10.111
Lung

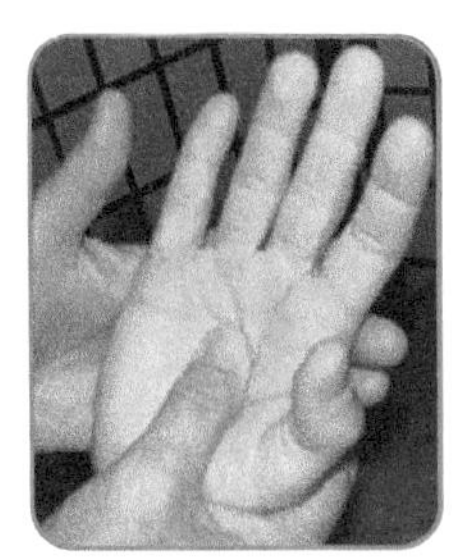

Fig 10.112
Solar plexus

11. **Esophagus and Stomach**—Slide down the web between the thumb and first finger for the esophagus, then circle the stomach.
12. **Liver, Gallbladder**—Press at the joint of the metacarpals at the 5th finger, right hand for the liver and 4th for the gallbladder.

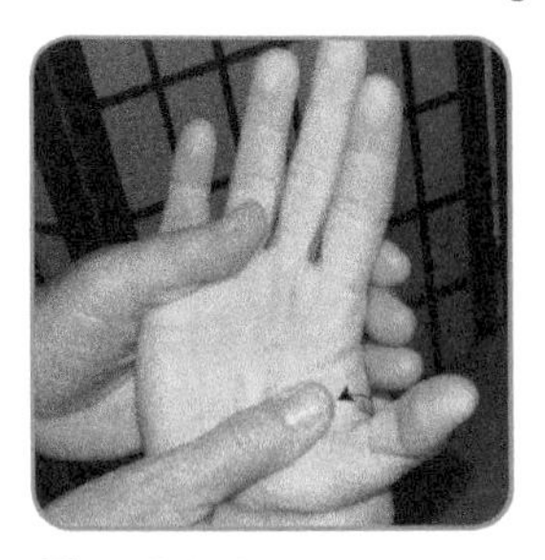

Fig 10.113 - Esophagus

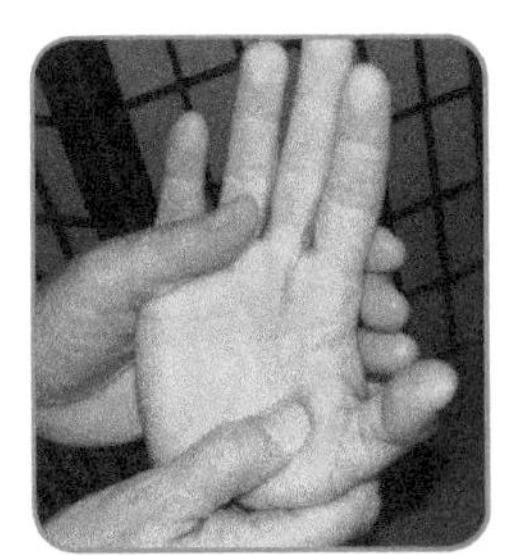

Fig 10.114 - Stomach

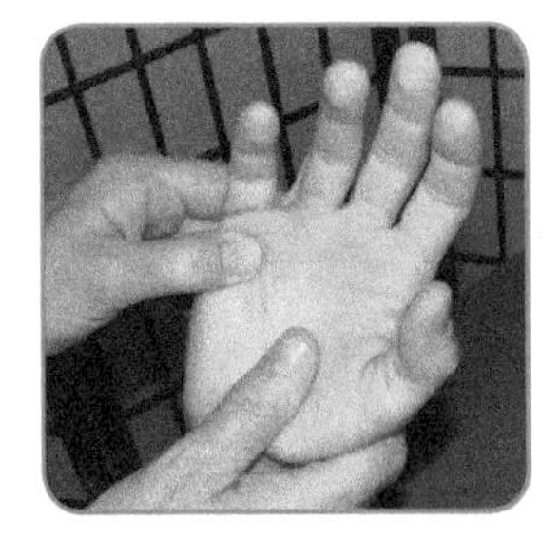

Fig 10.115 - Liver

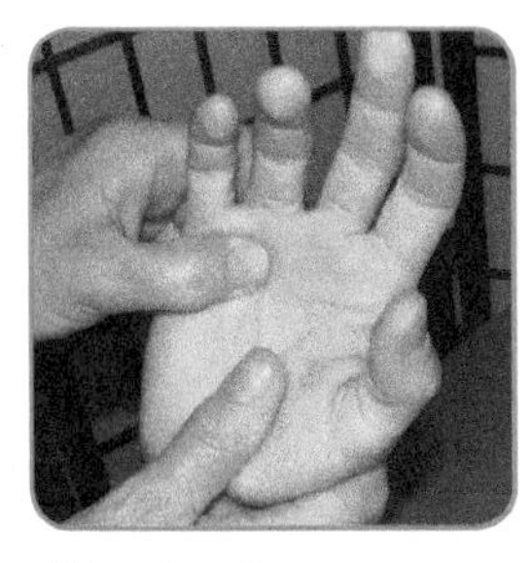

Fig 10.116 - Gallbladder

13. **Heart and Spleen**—Press at the joint of the metacarpals at the 4th finger, left hand for the heart and 5th for the spleen.
14. **Large and Small Intestines**—Use a knuckle twist, clockwise direction in the palm of the hand for the digestive system.

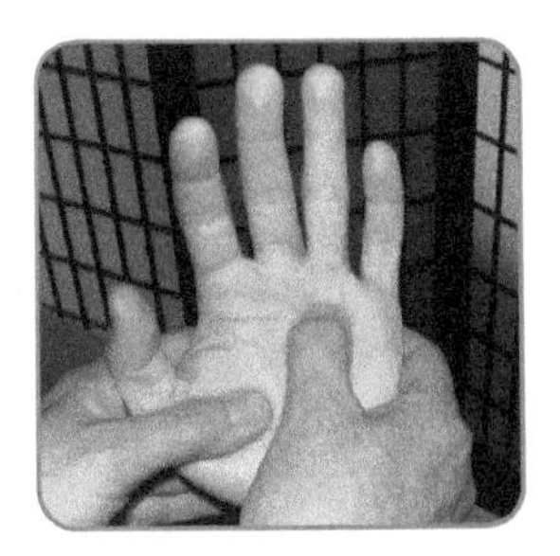

Fig 10.117 - Heart

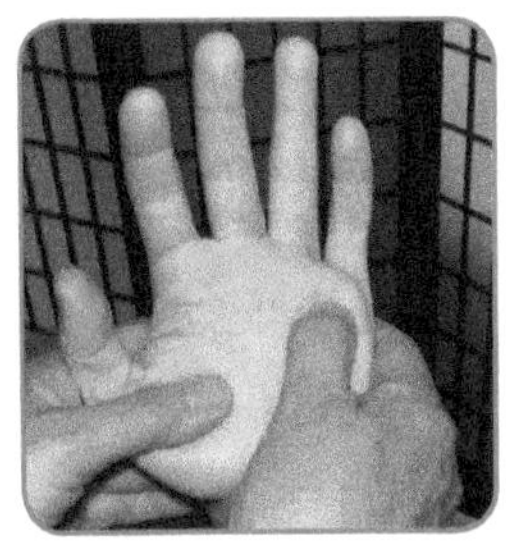

Fig 10.118 - Spleen

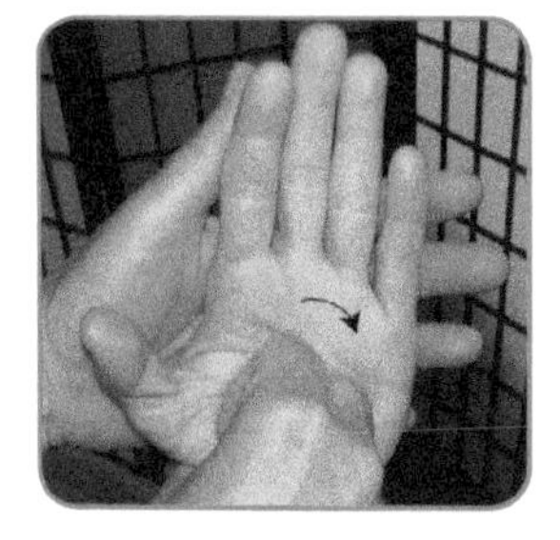

Fig 10.119 - Large intestine

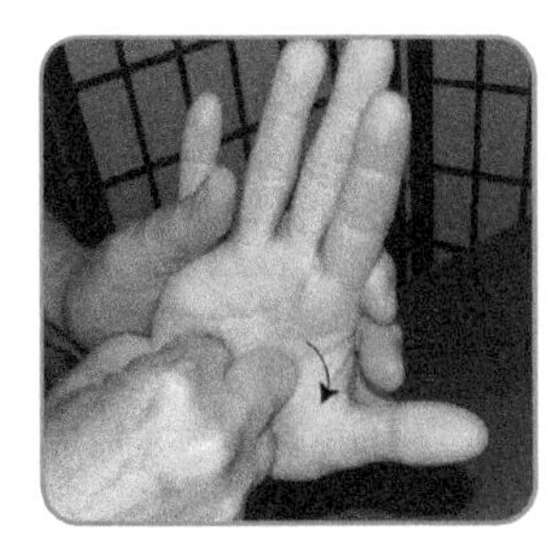

Fig 10.120 - Small intestine

15. **Hoku Point**—Hoku is the point that includes the lung and large intestine meridian. You will find it in the web between the first finger and the thumb. (Avoid this point if client is pregnant). Press and hold.
16. **Spine**—Pinch along the thumb side for the spinal reflex
17. **Shoulder, Elbow, Hip and Knee**—Pinch along the lateral side of the hand for the shoulder, elbow, hip and knee.

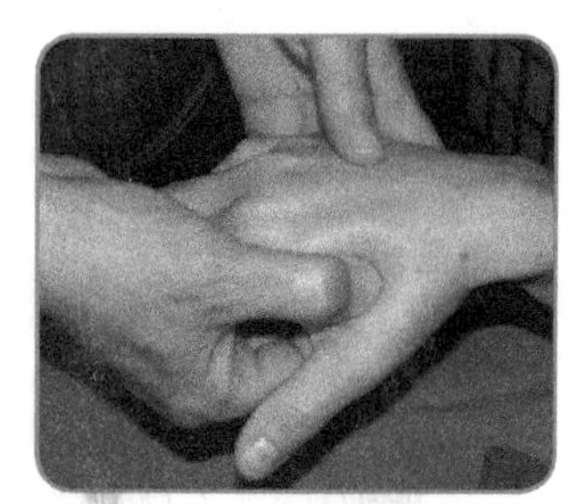

Fig 10.121 - Hoku

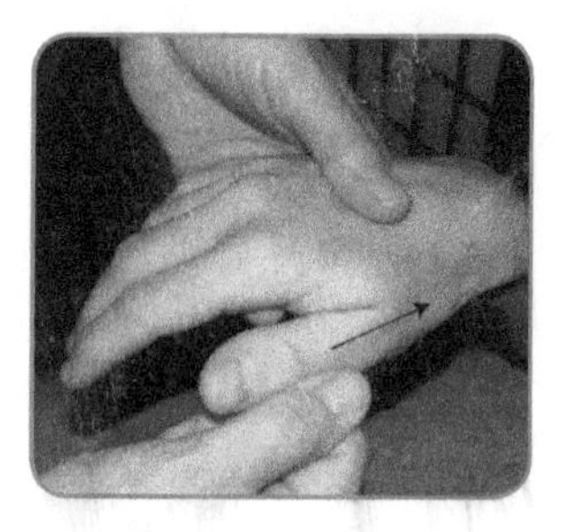

Fig 10.122 - Spine

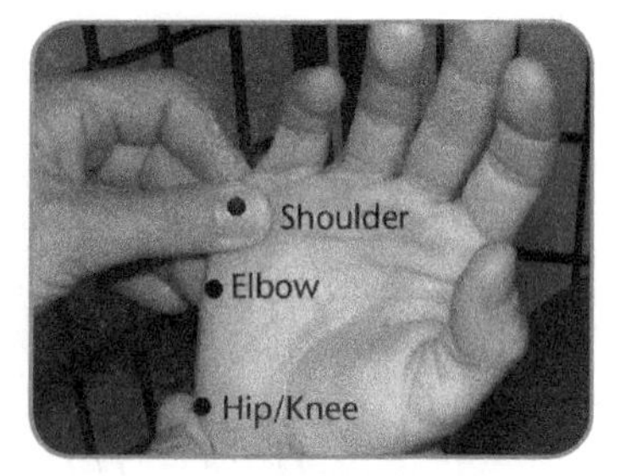

Fig 10.123 - Shoulder, elbow, hip and knee

18. **Reproductive Points**—Use circular thumb movements to work the reflexes on the wrist for the reproductive area. Stimulate the ovary/testicle on the lateral carpal bones, slide across the wrist for the uterine tubes/vas deferens and then press the medial carpals for the uterus/prostate.
19. **Lymph**—Lightly massage the webbing on the top of the hand towards the heart to stimulate the lymph area.

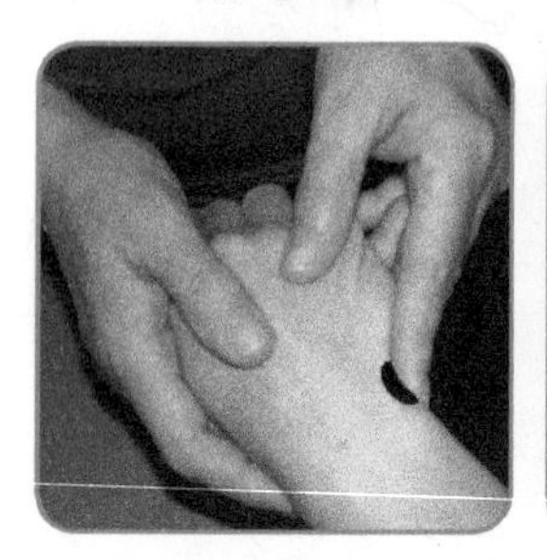

Fig 10.124
Ovary / Testes

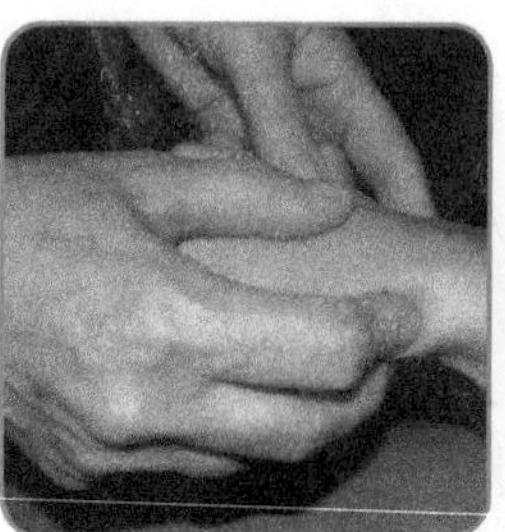

Fig 10.125
Uterus / Prostate

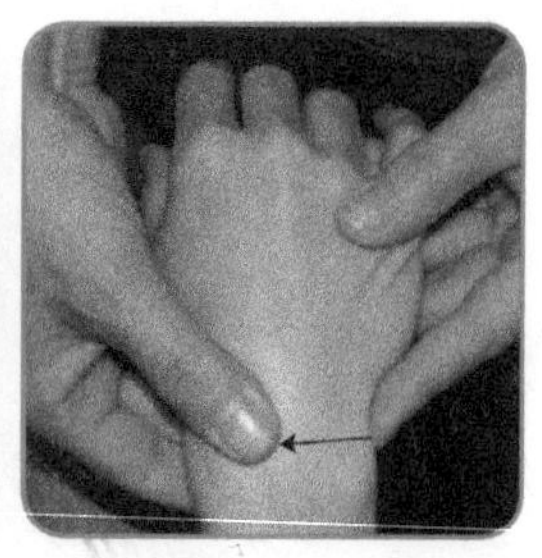

Fig 10.126 - Uterine tubes /Vas deferens

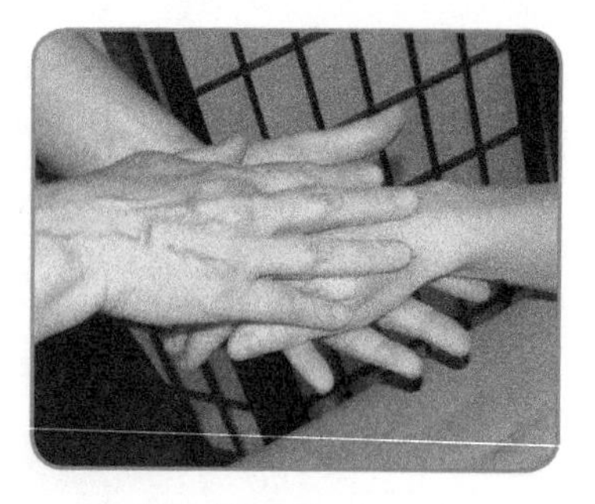

Fig 10.127 - Lymph

20. **Kidney, Ureter, Bladder**—Lightly press the kidney, slide down the ureter and press the bladder.
21. **Massage**—End with a general massage of the entire hand. Add in stretches and any other strokes you already do with hand massage.

Repeat on opposite side.

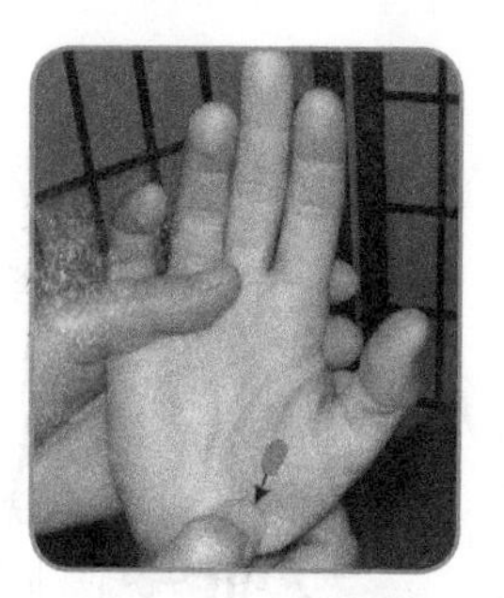

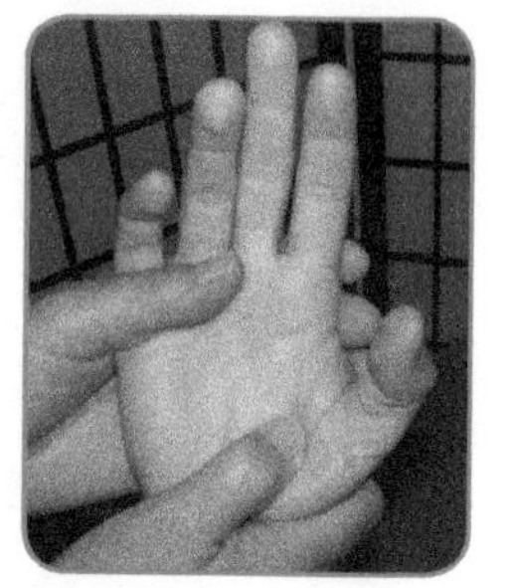

Fig 10.128
Kidney, ureter, bladder

11

Treatmen

Treatment plans are like a road map that you can
The treatment plan will include a combination of re
will best support your client in achieving a great
determine which organs and systems are involved in the imbalances
You will want to include these reflexology areas in your session, along with areas that offer general relaxation and support for the body as a whole.

Your treatment plan will also depend on how long your session is. For a shorter session, you will want to isolate key areas for maximum benefit. For longer sessions, you can include more general techniques and stimulate other areas, in addition to those directly related to your client's expressed condition.

Frequency of treatments will vary with each client based on the severity of their condition, their response to the sessions, and their ability and willingness to administer self-reflexology (which I wholeheartedly encourage). Certain reflexology areas benefit from being stimulated daily, such as the lungs, intestines and spine. You will want to allow a day of rest between stimulation of points such as the liver, gallbladder, heart and spleen. The endocrine glands are the most sensitive, so I recommend at least two days between stimulation of these points. If your client is experiencing strong reactions to the reflexology, it would be best to space out the sessions and allow their system to receive the work at the pace that it needs. It is my opinion that all forms of healing come from within. Your client's body is the ultimate guide to what is most needed at any given time. When you pay attention to their body and its responses you can be a guide for them, to help them notice their body and what it is communicating. Educate yourself about the common reactions to reflexology in Chapter 8 so you can accurately guide your client.

The treatment plans offered below are general suggestions. Use them as a guideline and then notice what you experience doing the work. If your client's condition is outside of your scope of practice as a reflexology practitioner, your client needs to seek medical treatment from his or her own health

...gy is a holistic therapy ... the body's natural healing ... intended to take the place of ... ment when that is necessary.

Conditions

Allergies

Ask your client what triggers their allergic reaction in order to determine where to focus your therapeutic work.

Food Allergies—Stimulate all digestive areas—stomach, pancreas, small intestine, gallbladder, liver and large intestine. Include the areas of the lungs and spleen.

Stimulation of the digestive areas generally results in a quick peristaltic response within 24-hours. Both clients and students have reported this effect. I have had my own experience when students test their skills on me and my digestive system will respond with a bowel movement within hours of the session.

Respiratory Allergies—Stimulate the sinus points and do sinus brushing. Work the throat, bronchials, ears and eyes. Work lung areas. Work the spleen, spine and digestive organs. End with the lymph pumping techniques.

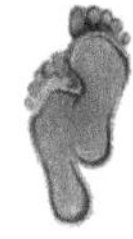

I have used this protocol for my son who has allergy-related asthma. It has provided relief and relaxation for his breathing muscles. Many of my clients and students also report sinuses draining during and post session.

Skin Allergies—Stimulate the digestive areas and the respiratory area. Stimulate the liver with extra focus. Stimulate the lymphatic areas and the spleen. Consider putting castor oil cream on the site of the allergic reaction.

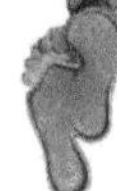

A skin eruption may occur post-session as the body, and particularly the digestive system, goes through a cleansing. I have also experienced this with colon cleansing, colonics and castor oil packs. The state of our skin is reflective of the state of the walls of our intestines. When a client returns with any skin eruptions, I suggest that you notice where the eruptions occur and see if they are on a meridian pathway.

Anemia

Anemia is a state of having low levels of red blood cells. Some of the symptoms are fatigue, pale skin, and reduced pinking of the nail pads when pressed. Most clients will not know if they are anemic, but if your client has already been diagnosed with anemia you can support them by stimulating the following reflexology areas: the kidneys, adrenals, liver, stomach, large and small intestines, spleen points and lung. Also work lymphatic areas and end with gentle cool down strokes (also called nerve strokes).

Anxiety and Panic Attacks

Do gentle holding on the solar plexus point on each foot and have the client focus on slow, easy breathing. Once they are calm, move to working the lungs and suggest that they continue to focus on breathing in a steady rhythm. Gently stimulate the kidneys and adrenals. End with solar plexus followed by nerve strokes.

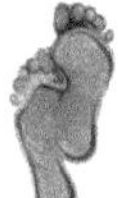

Rescue Remedy is a flower essence that calms the energy field. I have used it on children, myself, and even a small bird during a crisis. I often recommend it to clients as a go-to remedy for stressful situations.

Arthritis

Osteoarthritis—This degenerative disease affects a specific joint. For this condition, you might stimulate the digestive organs (stomach, pancreas, large and small intestines, spleen, liver), the spine area, and the joints affected by the arthritis. Do lymphatic and nerve strokes. Use castor oil, or a cream that has castor oil in it, for your session. Castor oil can also be applied directly to the affected joints. If the arthritis is on the hand or foot, notice which finger or toe is involved, and its corresponding meridian, to gain insights as to where else you might focus your reflexology work.

Rheumatoid Arthritis—This is an autoimmune disease that attacks cartilage and joint linings. The areas to work are the same as osteoarthritis. Since it involves the immune system, give the spleen and liver extra stimulation.

Gout—This is a form of arthritis that causes a buildup of uric acid, which eventually crystallizes around the joints, generally in the foot and ankle. There is a connection to the kidney and bladder. I would gently work them after you have done all the digestive areas.

Asthma

Asthma is a breathing disorder that can be related to allergies, either respiratory or food. It can also be brought on by anxiety and stress. Stimulate the sinus points and do the sinus brushing. Work bronchial points and the lung reflex, especially using the diaphragm spread. Include all lymph drainage areas. Especially focus on adrenals and solar plexus, and include the large and small intestines. End with gentle nerve strokes.

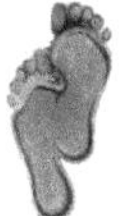

Having had bouts with asthma in my teen and young adult years, I have used the lung stimulation techniques. I also had a plantar wart on the lung area during that time. I treated the wart with Epsom salt foot soaks, scraping the wart and using over-the-counter salicylic acid, followed each time by putting castor oil on the wart. As the plantar wart disappeared, my asthma cleared up. To this day, I no longer suffer from asthma. Soaking and pumicing are other ways to "stimulate" a reflex area

Autoimmune Diseases

With all of the following conditions, stimulate all of these points: spleen, liver, lung areas, large and small intestines and lymph areas. If the client is in an acute stage of any of the autoimmune diseases, reflexology is contraindicated.

AIDS/HIV—Also include stomach and pancreas, as medication can affect digestion.

Cancer—Give general foot massage for pain relief and endorphin release. Stimulation of the intestinal reflexes will help to keep the bowels moving. Often, if pain medication is given, there is a slow down in peristalsis and constipation can occur.

Candida—Include the digestive reflexes and especially take note of tenderness of the pancreas point. Candida often involves too much sugar in the diet. Other areas to stimulate are the reproductive area, since candida can present as a yeast infection, and the kidney and bladder reflexes because bladder infections can also be due to a yeast overgrowth from candida.

Chronic Fatigue—It is important to work the adrenal points to reduce the effects of chronic stress. The deep relaxation effect of reflexology may help balance the stress hormones.

Multiple Sclerosis—Focus on the spine to energize the nervous system.

Fibromyalgia—Pineal and pituitary will help with sleep disorders that are common with this condition. Adrenals should also be gently stimulated for alleviating the stress response. Lymphatic drainage helps to move the chronic tightness in the tissue.

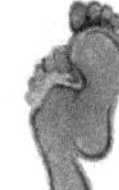

All of my clients diagnosed with fibromyalgia receive both reflexology and lymphatic drainage as treatment protocol. My clients experience a noticeable freedom of movement in their tight muscles after the session and they are able to deeply relax their entire body for 48 hours after the session. I had one client who felt so good she washed the windows of her entire house. Unfortunately, this is exactly the behavior that causes the symptoms to return. And, they did.

Back Problems

If the condition is general and includes the whole spine, stimulate spinal reflexes and traction the great toe. Also work the kidney and bladder areas, since the bladder meridian runs along the erector muscles. Ankle rotation and heel and leg pulling will help with overall stiffness. Work lymphatic areas to keep the fluids moving.

Lower back pain might be from strain, improper alignment, reproductive challenges or digestive challenges. Stimulate lumbar and sacral points, do the spinal twist stretch, ankle rotations and leg and heel pulls. Also, gently rock each leg.

Work the sciatic nerve area (sole of heel), hip and knee points, reproductive areas, large and small intestines, and kidneys. Do lymphatic pumping techniques.

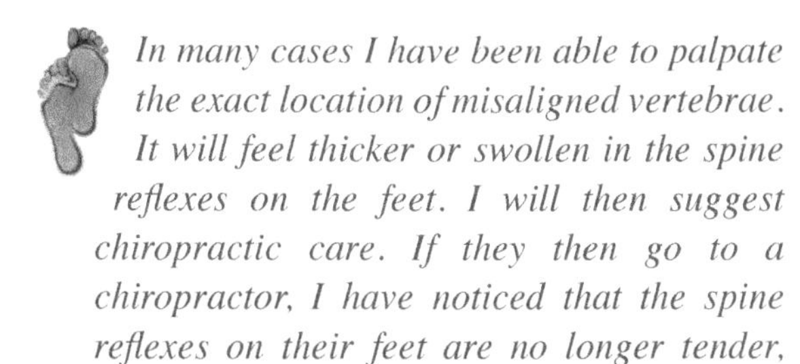

In many cases I have been able to palpate the exact location of misaligned vertebrae. It will feel thicker or swollen in the spine reflexes on the feet. I will then suggest chiropractic care. If they then go to a chiropractor, I have noticed that the spine reflexes on their feet are no longer tender, thick, painful or swollen.

Chronic Constipation

Deeply stimulate the digestive organs with a focus on the large intestine. Consider adding a castor oil pack to your client's abdomen while you are performing the reflexology session. (See Appendix on page 171). If you are a massage therapist, you can teach the client how to do self-massage of the large intestine. Include the Hoku acupressure point on the hand, which stimulates the large intestine. I have been able to associate which hand is more tender to the ascending colon (right hand) or descending colon (left hand). Try checking all three areas—hand, abdomen and foot reflexes to locate the area of the congested organ. It is amazing the information that both the hands and the feet provide.

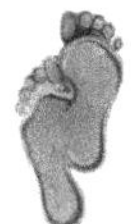

There are numerous stories from students who have received the intestinal reflexology in class and have reported an improvement in the frequency and volume of their bowel movements. It may take several sessions to effect a change.

Common Cold

Stimulate the sinus points and do the sinus brush stroke. Also stimulate the bronchial point, adrenals, spleen, spine, lung, digestive organs and all lymph points. End with the Toe Drop Soup stimulation technique (see percussion techniques on page 144). This helps break up congestion in the entire body. Do lymph-pumping techniques for 3-5 minutes.

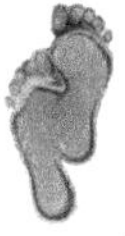

Adding a hot Epsom salt foot soak with a pinch of cayenne pepper to your reflexology session can help heat up the body, open the pores and help the client begin to sweat out the sickness. If you are doing this for self-care, wrap in a wool blanket and drink hot tea with lemon and cayenne pepper in it. This combination of remedies might help move the cold through the body faster, with less residual effects.

Ear Infections

Ear infections are most common in children. My own children had them most often in early childhood while teething. They may also occur in conjunction with colds. For children and adults, I would stimulate the ear reflexes, the sinuses and the lungs and bronchial reflexes. Stimulation of the large and small intestine reflexes will also support pulling the mucous out of the body.

Fertility Support (for both female and male)

Stimulate the endocrine glands—pineal, pituitary, thyroid, pancreas, adrenals, ovaries, and testes at least 3-6 times in each session. Stimulate the liver, spleen, heart and digestive organs. Do ankle rotations to loosen up the reproductive areas. Stimulate the uterus or prostate about 3-6 times each during the session. Work the ovary-uterine tubes (previously "fallopian" tubes) or vas deferens deeply as you move across the top of the ankle from the outer ankle to the inner ankle. Do this 3-6 times.

Fertility Massage is one of my areas of expertise. My clientele includes many who are in the process of conceiving and may be having challenges. I use fertility-focused reflexology on every client.

The uterus repositioning that I perform is validated by the level of tenderness that the client feels on each of her uterus reflexes. First, I palpate the uterus reflex on each foot, then I center the position of the uterus organ. Before centering, the uterus reflex on one side might feel lumpy or puffy, while the reflex on the other side feels hard and flat. After aligning the uterus, both points feel softer and more similar. Clients also report reduction in tenderness and more similar sensation from side-to-side.

Another client had a tubal pregnancy that resulted in surgical removal of her uterine tube (previously "fallopian" tube). She had been a client prior to the event and had a scar on her right ankle, over the reflex for her right ovary-uterine tube. When we spoke after her surgery, I asked if it was the tube on the right that was removed. Indeed it was the very same place. It is quite interesting how often there is a correlation.

Headaches

Ask your client what triggers the headaches. They may be related to food, hormones, allergies, stress, or weather changes (barometric pressure affects sinuses). For all types of headaches, work the Hoku point on the hands (unless the client is pregnant); this point is also called the headache point. Work the lymph drainage areas.

Allergy Headache—Work the sinus points. Stimulate solar plexus points while the client breathes deeply. Work stomach, large and small intestines and spine.

Food Headaches—Stimulate all the digestive organs, especially the large intestine. Stimulate the kidney, ureter and bladder using the press and slide technique.

Hormonal Headache—Stimulate pineal, pituitary, thyroid and adrenal points. If the client is female work the reproductive glands and the ovaries.

Migraine—When the client is in full swing of the migraine, I would only do the solar plexus hold. When the migraine has subsided and the client is able to receive more work, you can increase pressure on the solar plexus, gently work the eye points, and work all the points on the toe ledge—eye, bronchi, and ears. You may also simply hold the points. For nausea, I would do gentle circles on the stomach reflex. End with nerve strokes. You may add cranial-sacral holds or refer them to a cranial sacral therapist.

Weather Changes—Work the sinuses, eyes, ears, and lungs.

Heartburn

Look to see if your client has a long, slender callous along the esophagus reflex area. I have often found this correlation. The esophagus reflex seems to callous more if they are on medication. One student who has such a callous had her esophagus accidentally burned by breathing in a strong, chlorinated cleaning chemical.

Heart and Circulation

Stimulate spine reflexes and include traction of the great toe. Work the heart and solar plexus points.

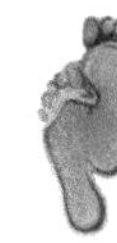

As a massage therapist in Lake Tahoe, I had a client take the time to call me two months post-session to report that he was now in the ICU with an infection of the heart. While he was receiving a session from me, I noticed extreme sensitivity in his heart point. Of course I do not diagnose, but I told the client to keep an eye on that organ. I was as amazed as he was that the correlation was so accurate. I am happy to report that he recovered well. He expressed that, due to our conversation in the session, he was inclined to see a doctor when he experienced pain in the area of his heart. What you notice and share during a reflexology session may inspire your client to be proactive about their health.

High blood pressure

Stimulate spine reflexes. Focus on the adrenals, kidney, heart and solar plexus points. Recommend your client breathe deeply to increase the relaxation effect. End with nerve strokes.

Hypoglycemia

Hypoglycemia is a low blood sugar condition that may be a precursor to type II diabetes. Stimulate the spine reflexes. Work the stomach, pancreas, spleen, adrenals and solar plexus. Include the large and small intestine reflexes. End with lymphatic pumping techniques.

Irritable Bowel Syndrome (IBS)

Stimulate the solar plexus first to calm the system. Then do gentle calming strokes of the entire digestive system—esophagus, stomach, small intestine and large intestine. Do not work deep. Soothing strokes are a better approach. The ileocecal valve should receive some stimulation. It may be tender to the touch. You would hold it and ask the client to do a relaxed breath. End with the lymphatic pumping techniques.

Kidney Problems

For kidney stones, stimulate the kidney-ureter-bladder system 6-9 times to encourage the stone to move. For clients on dialysis, reflexology is contraindicated.

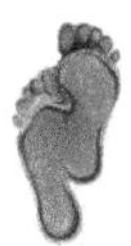

I used this technique on a client who also happened to be pregnant. She passed the kidney stone that night. She said, "labor was still more painful."

During a workshop, one of my students began to pass his stone immediately after the session. He was in pain and left the class to go to the ER for treatment.

In another workshop, I had a student with a very large stone that seemed to enlarge the kidney reflex. It was noticeably thick on the side where the kidney stone was lodged. We chose to avoid that reflex area in this instance because the stone was said to be very large and it would be dangerous to move it.

Liver and Gallbladder Problems

Stimulate the liver, gallbladder, spine, spleen and heart reflexes. Also work the large intestine and small intestine. End with the lymph areas.

Many clients have had their gallbladder removed. If this is the case, you will most likely find that the gallbladder reflex feels hard and thick. Occasionally, I have felt it to be swollen. Be aware that the liver now works harder to process the digestion of food, so the liver reflex may be very tender. I had a student in my class nearly explode at the practitioner when her liver point was stimulated. The liver meridian represents anger and this client was quick to anger. It was an interesting affirmation of the liver being over-stressed. The student who was performing the session was very grateful to understand the cause of the outburst and not take it personally.

Menstrual and Menopausal Symptoms

Stimulate the uterus, ovary, thyroid and parathyroid points, along with the pineal and pituitary points. Include the large and small intestines, as well as the lumbar and sacral areas. End with the lymph areas. Spleen 6 can help relieve menstrual cramps (see Fig 4.18a on page 57).

Urinary Tract Infection (UTI)

Stimulate the kidney, ureter and bladder reflexes. Also stimulate the kidney and bladder meridian points on the feet. Remember solar plexus is K-1 meridian point. The little toe is the bladder meridian. By squeezing the back of the ankle, you will stimulate both the kidney and bladder meridians.

Special Populations

For the following populations you will NOT stimulate the reflexes for the endocrine glands. These include the pineal, pituitary, thymus, thyroid, parathyroids, adrenals, pancreas and ovaries/testes.

Infants

Keep all strokes very gentle and light. You may work the sinuses for any congestion. The lung area may also be worked when needed. The large and small intestines may be massaged with a gentle circular stroke—this will help with colic (gas pains). The spine is also a great place to massage. Babies respond quickly to very gentle massage. (My own adult children still love to have their feet rubbed).

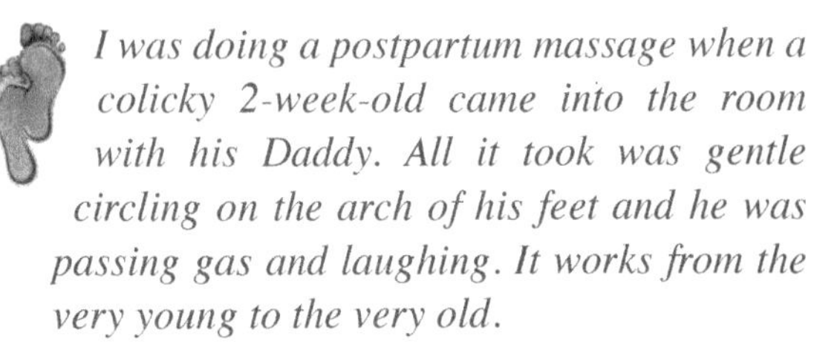

I was doing a postpartum massage when a colicky 2-week-old came into the room with his Daddy. All it took was gentle circling on the arch of his feet and he was passing gas and laughing. It works from the very young to the very old.

Children

Children who grow up with massage as a natural part of their family life enjoy a healthy grounding in safe touch. You may work deeper than with infants, but always keep the pressure at a tolerable level. With both infants and children, avoid the endocrine glands (the pineal, pituitary, thyroid, parathyroids, adrenals and ovaries/testes points). Work any areas that are needed, or just enjoy a wonderful family foot rub.

Pregnant Women

In addition to avoiding the endocrine glands, you will also avoid the uterus, ovaries and the Hoku point on the hand. You may work the sinus points, lung area and digestive organs. Tired and heavy feet respond well to having the spine, hip, knee and sciatic nerve areas massaged. Gentle lymph drainage also works well for swollen feet.

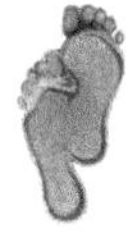

Using reflexology on pregnant women is a safe and effective way to relieve common pregnancy-related discomforts. I have excellent success releasing hip pain with clients by pressing into the sacral reflex and the hip reflex at the same time.

Women In Labor

Stimulate the pineal and pituitary reflexes at this time, as well as the uterus reflex point, Spleen 6 meridian point (four fingers up from the inner ankle) and Hoku on the hand. The large intestine, lung, spine and hips are also excellent to stimulate for labor. You might also apply ice to the Hoku meridian point.

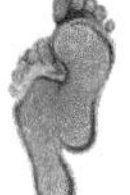

When I was in labor with my daughter Jessica, my PT friend, Diane, worked deeply into the uterus reflex area on the inner ankle. The labor moved quickly after that work—within 3 hours Jessica was born. The next day I felt great, except my ankles were sore!

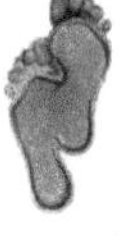

One of my students, a labor and delivery nurse, called me after a workshop and said she used stimulation of the uterus reflex point on a patient and was able to reduce the levels of Pitocin that the woman was receiving. Pitocin is a synthetic drug used to stimulate and intensify contractions during labor. It is usually very painful for the mother and baby, too.

In labor rooms, many massage therapists and even midwives use the uterus reflex point to get labor going or to increase the strength of the contractions. Changes in the uterine contractions have been registered on the fetal monitor that hospitals use for tracking the contractions and heart rates of mother and baby. When the uterus points are firmly stimulated in a circular manner, the contractions increase. When the stimulation of the points is ceased, the monitor strip reflects a marked slow down in the frequency of the contractions.

I have used stimulation of the pineal gland reflex at many births I have attended to increase the natural production of oxytocin. This natural hormone makes it much easier for mother and baby to bear the contractions. In general, foot reflexology releases endorphins (natural pain relief) and is highly indicated to use for laboring women. The uterus point is also indicated in the immediate afterbirth period when they are waiting for the placenta to deliver. Often, the uterus muscle is tired from a long labor and needs the stimulation to get the contractions going to expel the placenta. This might also help to reduce the potential for severe postpartum bleeding.

Postpartum Women

The areas to work about three days after the baby is born are the large intestine, the uterus point (lightly), the chest area (lightly), the spine, hips and lungs. Keep the work calm, gentle and supportive of this powerful transitional period.

Elders

Be sure to take a good health history, and be aware of any contraindications that may prevent you from doing reflexology. I find that this population really loves reflexology. It is easier for them to receive than getting a full body massage. It is best to work lightly and avoid the endocrine glands with the elderly.

Alzheimer's

Touch is crucial during this long, slow, progressive disease. Receiving work on the feet can feel very safe to the anxiety prone Alzheimer's client. The Kidney 1 and solar plexus points will help calm them down. Working on the great toe (brain reflex), lungs and digestive reflexes may help relieve many of their discomforts. The soothing relaxation strokes and nerve strokes down the legs and feet are highly beneficial.

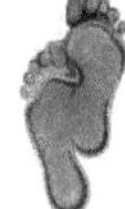

My mother had Alzheimer's. She loved massage and foot reflexology. My parents moved close to me in the last decade of my mother's life so I often gave her bodywork sessions with foot reflexology. Sometimes she would know me and sometimes she would not, but she always loved the touch. When she moved to a facility, I would visit, and,

although she was no longer speaking, she would put her legs up for me to rub her feet. She always remembered that I rubbed her feet, and she loved it. It was both beautiful and bittersweet for me. I think it is important that touch remain in the life of the elderly. It definitely kept my mom and me in touch!

End of Life Care

This is such a wonderful time to share reflexology. Reflexology gives an endorphin release that assists in dealing with pain. Working the large and small intestines and kidney reflex points help those organs continue to release. Working the lungs and solar plexus will stimulate a relaxation response. The gentle and simple therapy of reflexology is easily shared with family members. In some cases, I feel that it helps families ease the transition through death.

The terminally ill can experience the following benefits from reflexology:

1. Improved function of the organs of excretion (kidneys, intestines, skin, lungs)
2. Increased control of the bladder and bowels
3. Alleviation of pain
4. The social engagement of touch and human contact

Reflexology and End-of-Life Care

My Experience with Jon-Paul

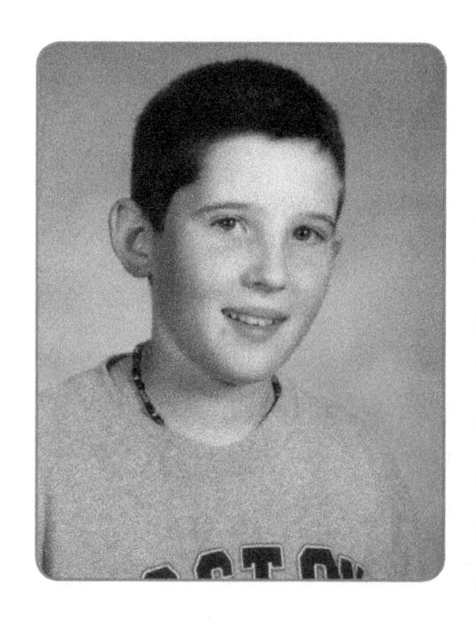

In 2004, I learned that my printer's 13-year-old son, Jon-Paul, was receiving chemotherapy to treat bone cancer. He was facing surgery in the future and I offered my services, especially reflexology, to help. His mom was immediately receptive to the idea of my coming to work with him. Jon-Paul was not quite as enthusiastic as his mother, but he decided to give it a try. At that time, my intentions were to support his appetite and help him build strength for the surgery ahead. Jon-Paul seemed to like the reflexology. He rested after the first session and I worked on his mom, Diana, as well. It seemed to provide some rest and peace to both of them. I enjoyed connecting with Jon-Paul during that first session.

The next time I worked on Jon-Paul was in the hospital and my intention was to move the chemotherapy out of his system so that he could go home. I began with calming and relaxing strokes to relieve the stress of his hospital stay. I stimulated Kidney 1 to deepen the calming effect. Next, I followed the nerve pathways in his legs with long, light, downward strokes. When I felt that Jon-Paul was in a receptive, relaxed state, I began working on his large intestine to help remove the toxic chemotherapy from his system. I followed this with the kidney/ureter/bladder points, sliding down the system several times on each foot. I noticed swelling in his bladder reflex and suggested that he might need to pee. At first he said "no," but minutes later he changed his mind. Both the nurse and Jon-Paul were surprised that I could tell from a point in his feet that he needed to pee. The news was amazing and proved reflexology's usefulness. I think Jon-Paul became a believer, too! I continued to work on Jon-Paul throughout his journey with cancer.

Another time when I worked with Jon-Paul, the skin on his feet was sloughing off from his latest round of chemotherapy. I think he was a little embarrassed by the amount of skin coming off his feet. We had to use a lot of paper towels to catch it all. Once I was able to clear his feet, it seemed that he received deep relaxation from the session.

I don't know all about the various types of chemotherapy nor their different effects on the body, but when I went home I could feel it in my body. I felt a nauseating, queasy feeling and I was a little run down and tired. I took a nap after that session and wondered if it was possible to absorb the chemicals of chemotherapy through your hands. Having interacted with his skin coming off into my hands, I believe it is possible.

My last session with Jon-Paul was the most profound. I had hoped that he would pull through his battle with cancer and come out with a healthy body to live a long and joyous life. Even though it seemed that he would not live much longer, I still went to that last session with the hope of recovery. When I arrived, the emotions of his family and friends were intense. I had to calm my own emotions so that I could be present for Jon-Paul. My intentions were to provide relief. I soon found that I also wanted to move the excess fluids that were causing him a lot of discomfort. I worked gently on his feet as he moved in and out of hallucinations. At times, he apologized for the dark things he might say. I told Jon-Paul that I really could not hear what he was saying. I was completely focused on his body and its messages to me. For the session, I first worked the Kidney 1 meridian point to calm his system. Then, I began gentle relaxation strokes to help quiet his nervous system. At one point, he asked that we be alone in the room for the session. I did diaphragm spreads and lung and chest stimulation to alleviate his breathing difficulty. A friend of his, who was also a nurse, commented at some point that he needed less oxygen when I was working on him.

During the session, he began to lay flatter in the chair. The energy in the room felt calmer. I also sensed that Jon-Paul needed to release the fluids in his kidneys, and within minutes after doing the kidney/ bladder strokes he asked for a urinal. He peed about two cups, which was the most he had released in 24 hours. Jon-Paul asked me to work up by his right shoulder. I could feel or sense the congestion in his lungs. I did lymphatic strokes to move the fluid out of his lungs and ease his breathing. I followed this with meridian strokes down to each of his fingers, especially the lung meridian. I repeated this on the other side and Jon-Paul started coughing up mucous. I then returned to the feet to continue the lung and chest strokes. I suggested that he not force too much coughing because it might cause irritation. I ended with the same calming point that I started with – Kidney 1/solar plexus. I prayed for healing and relief. His breathing was much easier.

The deep and pure spiritual energy in his family and home was palpable. I was profoundly touched by my experience with this young man and his loving family.

During this last session Jon-Paul mentioned that he was craving peaches. I offered to return that day with some that I had just purchased in South Carolina. I am again grateful that I was able to return a few hours after the session and see Jon-Paul up and playing on the computer, very alert and being with his family and friends. His mom, Diana, expressed her gratefulness with one of the best hugs I have ever received. I am grateful to have experienced the power of healing and to have learned to surrender to spirit during my journey with Jon-Paul. Jon-Paul passed away on July 23, 2004, two days after my final session with him.

I woke up about a month later, in the early morning hours and wrote Jon-Paul's story. I felt Jon-Paul's presence urging me to tell about this experience and about the importance of alternative health care. Alternative practices need to be valued, studied and utilized.

12

Ethics and Marketing

Laws

The profession of reflexology is always evolving and expanding, and there are a few organizations that play instrumental roles in this ancient healing modality gaining acceptance as a profession. The most widely known of these organizations is the Reflexology Association of America (RAA). A reflexology practitioner can join the RAA at different membership levels based on the amount of training hours that have been achieved. As a member of the RAA, a practitioner is able to claim accreditation as a reflexology professional. The American Reflexology Certification Board (ARCB) offers certification for reflexology practitioners who pass their written exam and practical exam. A practitioner must achieve 300 hours of reflexology training in order to qualify to take the ARCB exam. Both the RAA and the ARCB exist to offer a standardized and accredited system of certification in order to legitimize the professional field of reflexology as well as ensure the safety of the public.

If you are a licensed massage therapist, reflexology is considered within your scope of practice. My entry into the field of reflexology was through my massage school training. I have used reflexology as a stand-alone session as well as within the massages that I perform. Integrative Reflexology® Certification was created with the intention for massage therapists to incorporate reflexology into their bodywork services. Integrative Reflexology® was never intended to compete with the 300-hour training that non-massage therapists may need in order to safely and effectively practice reflexology. If you have little to no training in anatomy or physiology, it is highly advisable that you seek further training before you begin to practice reflexology with paying clients.

For many states, there are no laws governing the practice of reflexology. Currently, there are three states where you will need to be licensed in order to practice reflexology. Those states are North Dakota, New Hampshire and Washington state. Tennessee has a requirement to be registered to practice reflexology, but not licensed. In some states, such as Nebraska and Florida, you will need to be a licensed massage therapist to do any hands-on work. For over 32 states, the practice of reflexology is exempt from the requirements of a massage license, and in some of those states it is considered to be strictly energy work, not bodywork. This wide range of variability with regard to licensure requirements continues to create confusion when practitioners cross into other states to practice. It is wise to research each state where you plan to practice reflexology in order to clearly understand their requirements before you set up a practice and begin to advertise your services. If you are intending to practice reflexology in one of the states listed above that requires licensure or registration, you can find information about that process at the following websites:

- **ND**—North Dakota Reflexology Board (www.reflexology-nd.com/)
- **TN**—Reflexology Registry (www.tn.gov/health)
- **NH**—Bureau of Licensing and Certification under the Department of Health and Human Services (www.dhhs.nh.gov)
- **WA:** Department of Health (www.doh.wa.gov)

You can further research the laws for reflexology on the RAA website (reflexology-usa.org). You can research information on massage therapy and bodywork laws through the American Massage Therapy Association (www.amtamassage.org) or the website of Associated Bodywork and Massage Professionals (www.abmp.com).

Professional Conduct

As a practitioner of Integrative Reflexology®, you are a member of the health care profession, which requires you to consider certain ethical responsibilities. As the practitioner, you will need to establish ethical boundaries with your clients in order to ensure safety for yourself and your client, and also to prevent potential conflict or miscommunication.

Today, we are all familiar with HIPAA, the Health Insurance Portability and Accountability Act, which ensures confidentiality for patients. In alignment with these principles, all client information that you obtain is to remain private between you and your client, unless your client consents for it to be shared. Confidentiality creates a foundation of safety and respect within a therapist-client relationship. Maintaining confidentiality means that, outside of your sessions, you do not discuss who your clients are or what they share with you during a session. It is possible to share with other practitioners about specific conditions or experiences you have during a session without naming your client, thus maintaining their confidentiality. Confidentiality is a basic tenet of professional ethics in the healing arts.

You must also be considerate of the way in which you communicate with your client before, during and after the session. We have already discussed how to frame things in a positive, healthful way, rather than focusing on what might be "wrong." Clients are vulnerable and impressionable when receiving therapeutic work. They are coming to you because you are a trained professional. You need to be willing to listen to what they say in words and in body language as much as you are willing to communicate and educate. You are the expert in reflexology, but your client is the expert on their body. It is important that you honor and respect the feedback they offer, even if you are sensing something different. You might share with your client if you notice something during the session and then ask if that is consistent with their experience of their body. We absolutely do not diagnose. That is out of the scope of our practice. If you notice something, do not name it as a specific pathology. If you feel that it is something that your client needs to seek a medical opinion about, share with them what you notice, in objective terms, and recommend that they ask their physician about it.

The treatment plans offered within this book are suggestions for how to support your client achieving a balanced, healthy state of being. The treatment plans offered here, or the treatment plans that you create with your client, are not a prescription. Any recommendations you offer to your client need to be conveyed in the manner of a suggestion, not as a guaranteed treatment. Knowing when a condition is out of the scope of your practice and being willing and able to refer your client to the appropriate health care professional will ensure that you maintain your role as a responsible member of the healing arts community.

A reflexology session does not require the client to undress in any capacity other than removing socks and shoes. Even though the work is generally experienced as safe touch, every client is different. It is important that you honor this intention throughout your relationship with your clients.

All of the above ethical guidelines will ensure that you behave in a responsible, professional manner. This behavior will create trust and safety between you and your clients, which will serve you, your business, and the profession of reflexology as a whole.

Marketing

Before you can begin to market yourself and your practice, you will need to determine how you intend to use reflexology. Are you a massage therapist who is now going to incorporate reflexology into your menu of services? Are you a Reiki practitioner, or do you perform other forms of energy work, and now you also offer reflexology? Perhaps you are venturing into reflexology with the intention of making it your primary career. Or maybe you have training in other hands-on health care modalities such as nursing, physical therapy, midwifery or occupational therapy, and reflexology is another skill you bring to the table. There are infinite ways that you can incorporate reflexology into your life and your career. In order to market your new skill, you will need to understand how you want it to fit with the skills you already have.

If you are adding reflexology to your menu of services for massage and bodywork, you already have an established clientele to whom you can begin to offer your services. If you are wanting to practice reflexology but do not want to venture into establishing an individual private practice, there are other areas where you can offer your reflexology skills. Below are some examples:

- **Spas**—They often have reflexology on the menu. It has become very popular with the public.
- **Foot spas**—These have been growing in popularity.
- **Medical podiatry and medical pedicures** — In Richmond, VA, Integrative Reflexology® is used in conjunction with a medi-foot spa.
- **Other health care practitioners**—Some of the professions that might appreciate the services of a reflexology practitioner are chiropractors, acupuncturists, medical doctors, midwives, naturopaths, osteopaths, neurologists, podiatrists and other massage therapists.

Fees

An average price for a one-hour reflexology session can range from $50-75. It is wise to price your session according to the prices in your area. The amount you charge will vary depending on the length of your sessions and if you charge for add-ons, such as foot scrubs and essential oils.

Create Marketing Material

Before you can really get out there and market yourself, you will want to create business cards and perhaps, brochures, flyers or discount cards to distribute at various places around town. You are not only educating potential clients to who you are and what you offer, but you are educating them to what Integrative Reflexology® is and why they would want to experience a session. Each practitioner of Integrative Reflexology® will offer a unique approach to the therapeutic reflexology session. You will want to communicate to your potential clients what you, specifically, offer in your sessions. You might consider including the following information:

1. **Benefits of an Integrative Reflexology® Session:**
    - Creates a state of deep relaxation.
    - Improves digestion.
    - Can reduce constipation.
    - Supports sinus drainage.
    - Clears mucus from the lungs.
    - Can induce labor contractions for full-term babies.
    - Relieves premenstrual symptoms.
    - Reduces muscular tension throughout the body, including the neck, shoulders, hips, gluteals and spine.
    - Reduces swelling in the feet and lower limbs, which results in greater range of motion.
    - Cleanses fluids through increased kidney function and urination.
    - Elicits an overall sense of well-being.

2. **What is Integrative Reflexology®?**

    Integrative Reflexology® is a form of foot and hand reflexology that uses whole-hand strokes to stimulate reflex areas to achieve therapeutic effects throughout the body. Integrative Reflexology® is based on the four theories of Structural Alignment, Zones, Meridians and Psychoneuroimmunology.

3. **Through foot and hand reflexology, your Certified Integrative Reflexology® practitioner will:**
    - Work with the structural alignment of the feet and improve function in the body, by freeing the fascia that is holding tension.
    - Work with the Chinese meridians in order to achieve greater balance in the system.
    - Improve function within each cavity of the body through the reflexology zones.
    - Activate the calming effect in your body while improving your mood through stimulation of the nerves on the bottom of your feet.

4. **What to expect in a session**

Your session might include:

- A therapeutic foot soak with essential oils.
- A foot scrub with either salt or sugar and essential oils.
- The use of a hydrating foot cream.
- Hand reflexology, to further enhance the relaxation and therapeutic effects.
- Foot and toe stretches.
- Sessions generally are performed on a massage table or in a reclining relaxation chair.
- Massage as needed.

Promote, Promote, Promote

If you want to build up clientele for a private practice, or even if you want to spread the word about your services within another local business, it is important that you get yourself out in the community so people know where you are and what you are offering. Some ways that you might do that are:

1. **Community events**—Any local fair or fund raiser can be a great way to market yourself. If you bring a reflexology chair and offer free 10-minute sessions, or even charge $1 per minute, you can educate people about reflexology in general, while giving them the opportunity to experience your services. You might even give them a discount pass for their first session. Events to consider are the Walk for Alzheimer's, Crop Walk, Susan G. Komen runs, any walking or running event, local fairs, music and dance festivals, professional appreciation days (teachers, nurses, e.g.) and farmers markets. I have personally participated in a Ronald McDonald House event called "Girls Just Want to Have Fun." During that event, there was always a long line at my reflexology station.

2. **Create a Foot Reflexology Party**—Make this a fun Sunday afternoon event with food and games for happy feet. Offer foot scrubs and foot soaks while you give away foot rollers or other reflexology prizes. You can teach the participants about certain reflexology areas that they can work for their family and friends to keep everyone healthy and in touch.

3. **Volunteer**—Consider volunteering with groups such as the Ronald McDonald House, hospice, Wounded Warriors, Support for Caregivers, cancer support groups and so many more.

4. **Offer free lectures to the public**—You can do this at your local library, church, women's center, YMCA or alternative health centers. Even a local health food store may be open to a lecture on reflexology and optimal foot health.

When it comes to your business, marketing is your big opportunity to be creative. You might join a local networking group that meets monthly and provides you with a community of contacts who might refer clients to you while you can refer clients to them. Wherever you are already connected in the community is a great place to start sharing about your new business.

Appendix

Castor Oil

Properties, Benefits and Uses

What is castor oil?

Castor oil is a fatty liquid extracted from the seeds of the castor bean plant (Ricinus communis), which is native to India and Brazil. Castor oil is a triglyceride of fatty acids composed primarily of ricinoleic acid, which is a monounsaturated fatty acid that is responsible for most of castor oil's beneficial properties, including its anti-inflammatory properties. Castor oil also contains oleic and linoleic acids.

What is castor oil used for?

Castor oil is used mainly for its industrial and medical applications. It is a raw material for manufacturing fibers, lubricants, synthetic resins, varnishes and various chemicals. This plant-based oil is also used in manufacturing commercial skin care and conditioning products like shampoo and lipstick. When it comes to its medical uses, castor oil is a laxative, which is famous for providing temporary relief to constipation. It is also considered an alternative treatment to many kinds of health conditions.

Nature and Characteristics

Castor oil is a rich, amber substance that is produced by the tropical castor bean plant. This thick liquid is rich in fatty acids, thereby making it a natural emollient perfect for moisturizing. Pure castor oil also contains anti-inflammatory, anti-bacterial and antioxidant properties, which make it good for cleansing, healing, and removing scars.

Castor oil can be used to treat many everyday conditions, such as:

- **Digestive challenges**—Castor oil is a very effective laxative. It provides temporary relief for diarrhea and constipation. Castor oil removes waste matter from the small and large intestines by loosening the bowel. The moisture it provides helps in the smoother passage of waste matter through the excretory system.
- **Ringworm**—Undecylenic acid, which is one of the active compounds of castor oil, helps fight ringworm, a fungal infection.
- **Skin Challenges**—The ricinoleic acid in castor oil provides anti-inflammatory benefits for the skin. It penetrates the skin and removes all of the dirt clogging the pores. Castor oil is also a natural emollient, so it cleans the skin while also stimulating the production of collagen and elastin that hydrates and moisturizes the skin. Castor oil also reduces scarring and serves as a treatment for minor cuts, burns, abrasions and sunburn. It can help prevent skin disorders such as acne and eczema. It can be used to reduce wrinkles by repairing and rejuvenating the skin to make it look flawless and smoother. When applied regularly, castor oil also helps diminish dark circles under your eyes.
- **Labor Induction**—Castor oil has been used to induce labor in pregnant women.

NOTE: Seek consultation with your doctor or midwife before ingesting the oil as it may cause potential side effects in the mother and baby.

- **Sciatic Nerve Pain**—When applied topically, castor oil relieves sciatica, a painful condition characterized by lower back pains and soreness in your lower limbs.
- **Hair Growth**—Castor oil helps increase hair growth and makes hair healthier, softer, shinier and fuller. The moisture penetrates the scalp and gives a protective coating to the hair from roots to tips. Meanwhile, the anti-bacterial qualities of castor oil will thoroughly cleanse the scalp, thereby preventing dandruff and other scalp infections. Having clean and hydrated hair will not only prevent hair from falling out, it will also stimulate more hair to grow. Usually, castor oil therapy for the hair comes in the form of applying castor oil to the scalp. You will want to cover your head and sleep with the castor oil on, then wash it out in the morning. Pure castor oil can also

be applied to the eyelashes and eyebrows for thickening effects. You simply dab a very small amount on the area every night before sleeping.

- **Arthritis**—Castor oil acts as a natural remedy for arthritis. Its anti-inflammatory properties bring relief to arthritic joints and sore, tired muscles.
- **Lymph Conditions**—Another medical benefit of castor oil is in lymph treatment. Castor oil stimulates the activity of the lymph system, which is responsible for eliminating the body's metabolic wastes.
- **Tumors**—The use of a castor oil pack (a piece of flannel soaked in castor oil) with heat, placed over a tumor can help reduce the size of the tumor.
- **Neurological Problems**—Castor oil is believed to deliver medical benefits to certain neurological problems, such as Parkinson's disease, multiple sclerosis and cerebral palsy.
- **Natural Remedy**—Castor oil treats yeast infections, migraines, menstrual disorder, and athlete's foot.

Considering the many health benefits of castor oil, it is no wonder why it is one of the most beneficial oils available today. Castor oil is truly a valuable, organic remedy that can help improve your body's overall wellness.

Side Effects of Castor Oil

Castor oil, when used in moderation and in small doses, is perfectly safe. Applying too much of it on the skin or hair can lead to excessively oily skin and sticky hair. More precaution is required when the users are pregnant, lactating or menstruating, and especially when the castor oil is going to be ingested. Ingesting too much castor oil can lead to side effects such as vomiting, diarrhea and even poisoning. For pregnant, lactating and menstruating women, it is best to consult a doctor or midwife before using this organic remedy. As with any natural remedy, moderation is the best approach (www.castoroilhome.com).

Applications

Taken Internally—The recommended dosage for purging the system is 1 tablespoon for adults and 1 teaspoon for children. This application is most associated with a memory of grandma and the large spoonful of the sticky, thick oil. It is not always pleasant, but can be very therapeutic in its cleansing of whatever ails you.

Topically—Castor oil can be applied topically to any area that has a skin condition or anything internal that is ailing you. Castor oils seeps into the skin as deep as six inches, so it can bring relief to sore muscles and joints as well as reduce inflammation and bruising when applied topically. Castor oil can also be used as a massage oil for lymphatic stimulation or cleansing the colon. In this way, the massage therapist should always follow the lymphatic pathways or the path of the intestines if using it for a colon cleanse.

Castor Oil Packs—Castor oil packs can be used to relieve muscle strain, menstrual cramps, pain caused by arthritis or rheumatism and digestive challenges, and to increase blood circulation. Heat applied to the pack will help relieve the body pain (www.castoroilhome.com).

Supplies needed:

- Cold-pressed castor oil.
- A 100% cotton or flannel cloth prewashed and folded so it is at least four layers thick and still covers the treatment area.
- Hot water bottle half filled with hot water, or a heating pad.
- Hand towel.

Directions

1. Apply castor oil liberally over the abdomen (or other treatment area).
2. Place folded cloth over the abdomen.
3. Cover the cloth with a hand towel.
4. Place the prepared hot water bottle or heating pad over the hand towel.

For best results, leave the castor oil pack on for a minimum of 20-45 minutes, preferably for 1½–2 hours. It is a good idea to do this at bedtime since castor oil packs are very relaxing and sleep inducing. Once the pack is removed, there is usually very little residue left on the body. You can wash the excess oil off with a solution of baking soda and water. Used cloths can be stored in a sealed plastic bag at room temperature or in the refrigerator for future use. Each person should have his/her own cloth to use for a castor oil pack. The recommended frequency of application of a castor oil pack is three or four nights on, then three nights off.

NOTE: Castor oil packs should be avoided during ovulation due to the release of toxins that occurs in the body from the cleansing effects of castor oil. If pregnancy occurs and there is a history of miscarriage, stop using the packs. Otherwise, one can continue to use castor oil packs without heat application on the abdomen.

If castor oil packs are used while menstruating, there may be an increase in bleeding. This should occur in a comfortable, cleansing way. Edgar Cayce spoke of menstrual cramps being caused by poor eliminations, which can be improved by the use of castor oil packs.

This information was compiled by Kim Schultz and Claire Marie Miller.

References:

The Oil That Heals, by Dr. William McGarey, A.R.E. Press Virginia Beach, VA.

Edgar Cayce: The Sleeping Prophet, by Jess Stearn, Bantam Books, 1968.

Bibliography

Structural Alignment

http://www.health.harvard.edu/blog/try-tai-chi-to-improve-balance-avoid-falls-201208235198

https://www.anatomytrains.com/fascia/

"Fascia: Fascia and Tensegrity." *Anatomy Trains*. Anatomy Trains. Web. Jan. 2016.

Howell, Daniel, PhD. *The Barefoot Book, 50 Great Reasons to Kick off your Shoes*, Hunter House, Alameda, CA, 2010.

Myers, Thomas W., *Anatomy Trains: Myofascial Meridians for Manual and Movement Therapists*. Harcourt Publishers Limited, London, UK, 2001.

Rolf, Ida P. *Rolfing: Reestablishing the Natural Alignment and Structural Integration of the Human Body for Vitality and Well-Being*, Healing Arts Press, Rochester, VT, 1977.

Watson, Stephanie. "Try Tai Chi to Improve Balance, Avoid Falls." *Harvard Health Blog*. Harvard Health Publications, 23 Aug. 2012. Web.

Zones

Ingham, Eunice. *Stories the Feet Have Told*. Ingham Publishing Inc., St. Petersburg, FL, 1951.

Issel, Christine. *Reflexology: Art, Science, History*. New Frontier Publishing, Sacramento, CA, February 1990.

Marquardt, Hanne. *Reflex Zone Therapy of the Feet*. Healing Arts Press, Rochester, VT, 1983.

Meridians

Dougans, Inge. *The Art of Reflexology: A Step-By-Step Guide*. Element Books, Rockport, MA, 1992.

Psychoneuroimmunology

http://emedicine.medscape.com/article/1875813-overview

Buczynski, Ruth, PhD. with Porges, Stephen, PhD. "Polyvagal Theory: Why This Changes Everything" *Webinar from The National Institute for the Clinical Application of Behavioral Medicine*. 2012.

Hay, Louise L., *You Can Heal Your Life*, Hay House, Inc., Carlsbad, CA, 1984.

Pert, Candace B. "The Wisdom of the Receptors: Neuropeptides, the Emotions, and Bodymind". *Advances*, Institute for the Advancement of Health, Vol. 8, No. 8: Summer 1986.

Seaward, Brian Luke. *Managing Stress: Principles and Strategies for Health and Well-Being. Sixth Edition*. Jones and Bartlett Publishers, Sudbury, MA, 2009.

Tewfik, Ted L., MD. "Vagus Nerve Anatomy." *Medscape*. Aug. 17, 2015. Web. Feb. 2016.

University of Virginia Health System. " Missing link found between brain, immune system; major disease implications." *ScienceDaily*, 1 June 2015. <www.sciencedaily.com/releases/2015/06/150601122445.htm>

Recommended Reading for Reflexology

The Art of Reflexology: A Step-by-Step Guide by Inge Dougans.

This is Dougans' second book and my favorite. The first book presented a nice introduction to her work and her third book is called *The Complete Illustrated Guide to Reflexology*. I like *The Art of Reflexology* best because it clearly explains the meridians and their importance in reflexology. Dougans includes illustrations of meridians and muscles.

Body Reflexology: Healing at your Fingertips by Mildred Carter.

In her book, Carter, a pioneer in reflexology and a student of Dr. William Fitzgerald, incorporates techniques of whole body reflexology. She pioneered the use of tools within a reflexology session. Her tools can be explored and purchased through Stirling Enterprises at Mildred Carter's Reflexology website (www.mcreflexology.com). I find her body reflex charts clearer than her foot charts, which can be confusing.

The Complete Guide to Foot Reflexology by Kevin and Barbara Kunz.

This is an excellent book. It is well worth your time and study. Their work brings both variety and an open mind to the study of reflexology. They have written several other good books as well.

Reflex Zone Therapy of the Feet, a Textbook for Therapists by Hanne Marquardt.

This book is a good resource for the new reflexologist and provides plenty of information on observations, techniques, and treatments. Great text, but the charts are confusing.

Stories the Feet Have Told Thru Reflexology by Eunice D. Ingham.

Eunice Ingham wrote her first book, *Stories the Feet Can Tell Thru Reflexology* in 1938. Both books are a must. They are now in print as one edition and they provide important historical and foundational information gleaned from Ingham's pioneering work in reflexology. The stories are great and the photo of Eunice shows us what a powerful woman she was. We owe her a debt of gratitude for the information she has shared with the world. Her work is being carried on by the International Reflexology Institute in St. Petersburg, Florida.

Structural Alignment

Rolfing: Reestablishing the Natural Alignment and Structural Integration of the Human Body for Vitality and Well Being by Ida P. Rolf, Ph.D.

This book is a classic look at Rolf's work. The chapter on feet is a "must-read" in terms of gaining understanding on how foot imbalances play into structural alignment.

The Barefoot Book: 50 Great Reasons to Kick Off Your Shoes by Daniel Howell, PhD.

Dr. Daniel Howell is an anatomy professor at Liberty College in Lynchburg, VA. His book is a well-documented essay on why humans were designed to be barefoot. Dr. Howell explains how we have been brainwashed by our culture to believe that going barefoot is unsafe, when in reality it may be safer. This book is full of fun facts that will inspire you to explore the world in your bare feet.

Anatomy Trains by Tom Myers.

Tom Myers is a Rolfer who trained under Ida Rolf herself. His book offers a thorough roadmap to how fascia functions in our bodies. This book has created new awareness in the structural alignment community. It offers fundamental knowledge and awareness of fascia and its journey through the body.

Meridian Theory (Asian Medicine and Theory)

Staying Healthy with the Seasons by Elson M. Haas, M.D.

This was the first book I studied after my training in acupressure at the Boulder School of Massage Therapy. It has an easy-to-understand manner, and it explains the five seasons and their place in maintaining balance and good health. The information is timeless, and each time I re-read it, I learn something new. I have worn out several copies. It is a *must* for your library and a great book to recommend to your clients. Don't lend it to them however, you may never get it back.

The Five Elements of Self-Healing: Using Chinese Medicine for Maximum Immunity, Wellness, and Health by Jason Elias, L.Ac. and Katherine Ketcham.

This book offers a fascinating look at the power of Chinese Medicine. There is a test in the book that helps you tune into your own physical weaknesses and suggests ways to strengthen and balance your body.

Traditional Acupuncture: The Law of the Five Elements by Dianne M. Connelly, Ph.D.

This is a short but informative book. It has helped me deepen my understanding of the five elements and five seasons, and their interconnectedness with body systems and meridians.

Between Heaven and Earth: A Guide to Chinese Medicine by Harriet Beinfield, L.Ac. and Efrem Korngold, L.Ac., O.M.D.

This book is not for the beginner. It delves deeply and with complexity into Chinese Medicine, the elements, seasons and meridians.

Psychoneuroimmunology

Molecules of Emotion: The Science Behind Mind-Body Medicine by Candace Pert.

In the late 1970s, research at the National Institute of Health was done primarily by male scientists. It was at that time that a new and brash young woman named Candace Pert was doing research on opiate receptors that would change our language and perception of the neurological chemicals that affect our brain and body. This book is her story. Anyone with an interest in the chemistry of emotions and health should read this book. It is truly inspiring.

The Biology of Belief: Unleashing the Power of Consciousness, Matter and Miracles by Bruce Lipton, Ph.D.

Dr. Lipton is a cellular biologist from the University of Wisconsin in Madison. His work describes the intelligence of our cells and how our genes and DNA do not dictate our biology. His book explains how thoughts play into the actions of our cells and our biology. Dr. Lipton states that we can rise above our genetics to live a healthy life, not doomed by the diseases of our grandparents.

You Can Heal Your Life by Louise Hay.

Louise Hay created an empire based on positivity. She experienced personal healing that inspired her to want to help others. Louise experienced the power of releasing negative emotions due to past trauma, in order to heal her cancer. Using positive affirmations, and targeting the language to specific conditions in the body, she created a movement in the self-help community that shows that healing comes from within. This book is an excellent addition to everyone's home library. The companion book, *Heal Your Body*, is a great go-to resource for positive affirmations to use with a wide variety of conditions.

Castor Oil

The Oil that Heals: A Physician's Successes with Castor Oil Treatments by Dr. William McGarey

This book shares the value of and anecdotal evidence for the healing properties of castor oil as used by Dr. McGarey on countless patients.

Edgar Cayce: The Sleeping Prophet by Jess Stearn.

This book is an historical account of the fascinating life of Edgar Cayce, one of the most studied psychic's ever known. Over 15,000 readings were recorded when Edgar went into a trance and offered readings to clients on health, past lives and other information. His work is still researched today at Edgar Cayce's Association for Research and Enlightenment (A.R.E.) in Virginia Beach, VA.

Website Resources

www.clairemariemiller.com: For all of Claire's products and seminars in Integrative Reflexology®, Nurturing the Mother® Pregnancy and Postpartum Massage, Nurturing the Mother® Fertility Massage and more.

www.foot-reflexologist.com and **www.reflexology-research.com:** Both sites are by Barbara and Kevin Kunz.

www.botanicallyrooted.com: Formerly lovingscents.com, created by Cynthia Loving (now retired), this is an excellent source for high quality essential oils. Cynthia Loving is the co-creator of Sweet Feet© products used in Integrative Reflexology®.

www.ctslabsinc.com: Website and store for high quality castor oil.

www.peoplespharmacy.com: An excellent resource for natural remedies and holistic health.

www.unshod.org: They offer the website, "Parents For Barefoot Children," a source for information on all things barefoot.

Integrative Reflexology® Products

Integrative Reflexology® DVD—The Integrative Reflexology® DVD is for both the beginner and the seasoned student of reflexology. Claire walks you through the foundations of bones, landmarks and points. Then you get to follow along with a complete reflexology session. Information on the DVD includes:

- Bones of the feet
- Landmarks on the foot
- A complete reflexology session protocol
- Stimulating the points on the feet in sequential order
- Additional foot reflexology stimulation techniques
- Foot Soak
- Hand Reflexology

BONUS material—DO-IN Chinese self-massage techniques. This DVD is an excellent companion to the Integrative Reflexology® Book. Video run time: 55 min.

Hot Rockin' Reflexology and Sweet Feet© Aromatherapy DVD—72 minutes with a lecture and demonstration of this incredible sequence combining hot rocks and aromatherapy in a reflexology session.

Sweet Feet© cream (8 oz and 4 oz)—This cream was created by Cynthia Loving and Claire Marie Miller specifically for use with Integrative Reflexology®. It is made with a combination of Shea butter and castor oil and has a shelf life of one year.

Sweet Feet© Kit—This kit includes the customized Sweet Feet© foot cream that was created by Cynthia Loving and Claire Marie Miller and contains only Shea butter and castor oil. It also includes eight essential oils—lavender, peppermint, rosemary, ravensara, lemongrass, cypress, geranium, and rosewood. The laminated Sweet Feet© card gives the practitioner the recommended use for each essential oil as well as suggested recipes. The kit also includes a 4"x 5" foot reflexology card.

Foot Chart—8.5"x 11" Easy to read, laminated Integrative Reflexology® foot chart.

Hand Chart—8.5"x 11" Easy to read, laminated hand reflexology chart, includes locations for meridian points on the hands.

4"x 5" Foot Card—This is the same chart as the 8.5"x 11" foot chart, in an easy-to-carry size.

4"x 5" Hand Card—This is the same chart as the 8.5"x 11" hand chart, in an easy-to-carry size.

Foot Roller—This is an excellent tool for plantar fasciitis, neuropathy and swollen feet and ankles.

Castor Oil and Flannel Pack—A 100% cotton flannel cloth for a reusable castor oil pack with an 8 oz bottle of castor oil and an instruction sheet.

Cloth Reflexology Poster—(24" x 40") Printed on cloth. Easy to carry and post on the wall.

About the Author

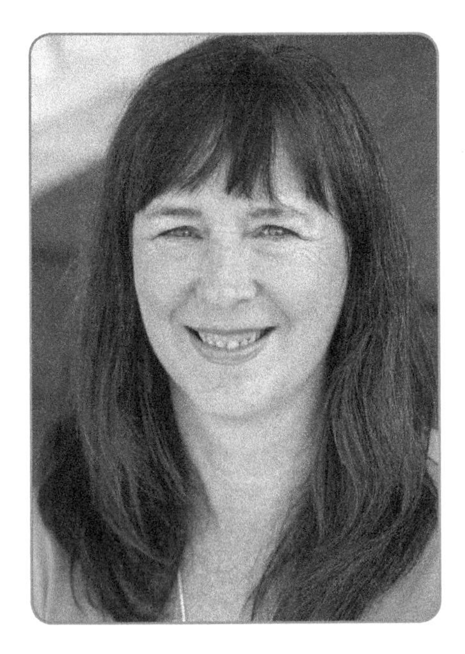

Claire Marie Miller is a Licensed Massage Therapist in the state of North Carolina. She is Nationally Board Certified and has been a member of the American Massage Therapy Association since 1982. Her background in health started at the age of 17 when she began her training in radiology technology, receiving the technologic award for her class. Her career path eventually led her to holistic health care and the premier Boulder School of Massage Therapy, where she graduated in 1979 with honors. Her love for reflexology began with her training in massage school. She has spent over 30 years developing this unique, massage-based, whole hand approach to reflexology. Her integrated method offers a deepening journey into the body through the feet. In 2010, Claire was inducted into the Massage Hall of Fame for her innovation in the massage therapy field. She has been a presenter at the AMTA National Convention and at the Reflexology Association of America's national conference.

Claire has maintained a private massage therapy practice since 1980. In addition to her certification workshops in Integrative Reflexology®, Claire has developed continuing education and certification workshops in Nurturing the Mother® Pregnancy and Postpartum Massage as well as Nurturing the Mother® Fertility Massage. She teaches a variety of other courses related to her innovative work in massage and reflexology.

Visit the website to inquire about workshops and certifications: www.clairemariemiller.com

Index

Italicized, bold page references indicate single or multiple graphic, photographic or illustrated figures on that page.

CPSIA information can be obtained
at www.ICGtesting.com
Printed in the USA
BVHW021619230120
570263BV00001B/1